Psychotropic Drugs

A Guide for the Practitioner

PSYCHOTROPIC DRUGS

A Guide for the Practitioner

H. M. VAN PRAAG

Psychiatric University Clinic
University of Utrecht
The Netherlands

Brunner/Mazel, Publishers • New York

Library of Congress Cataloging in Publication Data

Praag, Herman Meir van.
Psychotropic drugs.

Bibliography: p.
Includes index.
1. Psychopharmacology. I. Title. [DNLM:
1. Mental disorders—Drug therapy. 2. Psychotropic drugs.
QV77 P895pa]
RC483.P723 616.8'918 77-21009
ISBN 0-87630-157-X

Exclusive sales rights for
United States of America and Canada *Brunner/Mazel, New York*
United Kingdom and the Commonwealth (except Canada) *Macmillan, London*
All other countries *Van Gorcum, Assen*

Translated from the Dutch by Th. van Winsen

Published by
BRUNNER/MAZEL, INC.
19 Union Square, New York, New York 10003

MANUFACTURED IN THE UNITED STATES OF AMERICA

To the memory of my parents

To my wife and children

In our branch of science (i.e. psychopharmacology), it would seem we are as attracted to substance as we are to symbol; we are as interested in behavior as we are aware of the subtleties of subjective experience. There is here no conflict between understanding the way things are, and the way people are, between the pursuit of science and the giving of service.

Where else does one find a field as rich and powerful as ours?

J. Elkes,
Discoveries in Biological Psychiatry
Lippincott Company, 1970.

Preface

This book is intended for physicians—general practitioners and specialists—who are prescribing psychotropic drugs, and for future physicians who will. Although this is a practice-oriented book, I have avoided presenting the subject matter in the manner of a cookery-book: for depressions give 3 × 50 mg imipramine daily, for psychoses give 3 × 100 mg chlorpromazine daily, etc.

Ideally, the decision to prescribe a particular psychotropic drug should be based on three series of data:

1) the nature of the behaviour disorders, or the syndromal diagnosis;
2) the nature of the disorders of cerebral function underlying the behaviour disorders;
3) the mechanism of action of the drug, that is to say the functional changes which occur in the brain in response to its administration.

It looks as if we are still far away from this ideal situation. For the time being, the only more or less reliable beacon to guide our course is the nature of the psychopathological manifestations, and this criterion accordingly demands our full attention. Careful syndromal diagnosis in a sine qua non for a responsible use of psychotropic drugs. Chapters II, VI and XII were written on the basis of this conviction.

The other two criteria cannot yet be applied; our knowledge is insufficient for this. On the other hand, there is no question of a status quo. On the contrary, I believe that the situation is changing. A striking example can be found in studies of the biological determinants of disorders of mood regulation. However fragmentary this research may still be, yet some understanding is dawning. On the mechanism of action of certain groups of psychotropic drugs, particularly antidepressants and neuroleptics, hypotheses have been evolved which are beyond the speculative phase and, what is most important, can be clinically tested. In actual practice, insights of the type I am referring to are not yet of any use. But I believe they will be, and this is why I briefly discuss them in chapters XI and XVI. The reader of these chapters needs some elementary knowledge of the mode of transportation of stimuli in central monoaminergic neurons. Chapter IV has been included to provide such knowledge.

Each of the three principal groups of psychotropic drugs—neuroleptics, antidepressants and ataractics—has many representatives. However, these are so closely similar in action profile that they can be discussed under the same heading (in chapters VII, VIII, XIII and XIX). The individual compounds are discussed in separate chapters (X, XV and XX), which discuss their dosage as well as deviations from the general action profile, if any. The lists presented in these "specific" chapters are not comprehensive. They comprise compounds in conventional use and more or less adequately studied. Also included are some compounds which are not commercially available in the United States. It seemed useful to me to inform the American physician on a number of drugs commonly used in Europe.

Some psychotropic drugs are available under scores of trade names. In this respect, too, I made a choice which, whenever possible, was guided by the popularity of the compound in question. My choice expresses no preference. For a comprehensive survey of the trade names I refer to the Index Psychopharmacorum of Pöldinger and Schmidlin (1972).

In the conventional classification of psychotropic drugs, lithium is placed in the principal group of the psycholeptics, because it is used in the treatment of the manic syndrome. Nevertheless, I discuss this compound in part III, which deals with the treatment not of psychoses but of affective disorders. I had two reasons for doing this. The first was the consideration that mania, even if it assumes psychotic forms, can be interpreted as a manifestation of disturbed mood regulation. The second was the fact that lithium owes its unique significance not to its antimanic effect but to its prophylactic effect in unipolar and bipolar depressions.

The psychotropic drugs evolved in the past 25 years are of importance not only therapeutically but also scientifically. They have vigorously catalysed three types of research.

1) *Research into biological determinants of (disturbed) human behaviour.*

Psychotropic drugs produce changes in the brain and in behaviour. In this way they provide a natural point of crystallization of hypotheses on relations between brain function and behaviour regulation. The present heyday of biological psychiatry would have been unthinkable without the psychotropic drugs.

2) *Psychopathological research.*

In the thirties of this century the great German psychiatrist Kurt Schneider believed that human behaviour disorders had been fully charted. The psychotropic drugs have shown that he was wrong and have led to a productive re-orientation on problems of psychopathological description and differentiation.

3) *Psychometric research.*

The effects of psychotropic drugs on disturbed behaviour had to be registered in a standardized way. Moreover, the effects of individual compounds had to be compared. This necessitated a measuring of human behaviour, and consequently behaviour-rating scales appeared in the psychiatric clinic in the wake of the psychotropic drugs. Although far from ideal as measuring instruments, these scales can be regarded as a revolutionary development. For with the introduction of the rating scale several myths were destroyed: the myth that the individual human behaviour program is unique; the myth that human behaviour cannot be measured; the myth that verifying, hypothesis-testing research is impracticable in psychiatry.

It is no exaggeration to state that the psychotropic drugs gave impetus to the trend of "scientification" now discernible in certain sectors of psychiatry. For this reason I have been unable to present this practical book on psychotropic drugs without adding chapter V, which discusses precisely this scientific aspect.

BIBLIOGRAPHY

PÖLDINGER, W. and P. SCHMIDLIN (1972). *Index Psychopharmacorum.* Bern and Stuttgart: Hans Huber Verlag.

Contents

PART TWO
PHARMACOTHERAPY OF PSYCHOSES

PART THREE
PHARMACOTHERAPY OF DISORDERS OF MOOD REGULATION

PART FOUR
PHARMACOTHERAPY OF NEUROTIC CHANGES AND OTHER PERSONALITY DISORDERS

PART ONE

Scientific Aspects of the Practical Application of Psychotropic Drugs

Acquisition of basic knowledge is now threatened by strong social, economic and political pressures. These forces discourage financial support of basic research and question its importance. They drive scientists to undertake excessively complex problems in a gamble for quick payoffs. They make scientists into entrepreneurs and administrators. It is just such times that test the temper of men. Whether he is a basic scientist, a clinical investigator or a practitioner of medicine, the investigator must adhere to the fundamental discipline of science by asking discrete and well defined questions. It is out of these small and numerous contributions of knowledge that we build the grand edifices of nature.

Arthur Kornberg,
New Engl. J. Med., 27 May 1976.

I

Classification of Psychotropic Drugs

Psychotropic drugs are compounds which, via a selective influence on the central nervous system, cause more or less characteristic changes in mental activity and experiencing. In the past, too, the psychiatrist prescribed drugs in suitable cases, e.g. opium, scopolamine, bromides and later also barbiturates; but it was not until after the introduction of chlorpromazine (Largactil, Thorazine) in 1952, and of reserpine (Serpasil) in 1954, that pharmacotherapy took a wider scope in psychiatry—to such an extent, in fact, that we can no longer do without a system of classification. A system based on the mechanism of action of psychotropic drugs cannot be achieved for lack of adequate knowledge. For the time being, only a relatively gross classification is possible on the basis of the disease symptoms which these compounds control or provoke. On this basis the French psychiatrists Delay and Deniker (1961) proposed a classification which, apart from some minor modifications, has been almost universally accepted. They started from the following tripartition (Table 1):

1. Psycholeptics, i.e. compounds which depress certain psychological functions.
2. Psychoanaleptics, i.e. compounds which activate certain psychological functions.
3. Psychodysleptics, i.e. compounds which provoke certain psychopathological manifestations.

Two further groups, not included in the system of Delay and Deniker, comprise the compounds used in addictive diseases and sexual aberrations. These groups are still small, but tend to grow larger.

The nomemclature used by Delay falls back directly on the psycholepsy concept of the 19th-century French psychiatrist Janet. By this term the latter indicated a reduction of what he described as "tension psychologique," i.e. psychological tension. Psycholeptics, therefore, are compounds which reduce this tension, psychoanaleptics stimulate it, and the term psychodysleptics denotes a deformation of this function.

Within the category of psycholeptics, four groups can be distinguished: sedatives/hypnotics, neuroleptics, lithium compounds and ataractics. Compounds of the first group allay excitement, but only at the price of a degree of dullness; they include the barbiturates, bromides and opiates. As sedatives, most of these compounds are obsolete. In somewhat larger doses the barbiturates in particular are still being used as hypnotic agents.

Neuroleptics, otherwise known as neuroplegics or antipsychotic drugs, are strikingly strong sedatives with only a limited hypnotic effect even in larger doses. In addition they exert a so-called antipsychotic influence. This action component is ill-defined. In some cases the psychotic symptoms disappear completely. In other cases these compounds "only" reduce the emotional tonus, thus causing a degree of affective flattening which becomes manifest as indifference. The psychotic disorders do not disappear but are more bearable. The complex of antipsychotic effects is unique, and it is from this that the neuroleptics derive their identity. Another characteristic feature of these compounds is a more or less pronounced influence on the extrapyramidal system and on the mechanisms of central vegetative regulation. It is to this "neurological syndrome" (Delay) that they owe their name.

In the group of the psycholeptics, lithium compounds occupy a special position. Like neuroleptics, they are strong inhibitors of psychotic restiveness with only a limited hypnotic effect. But their indications are limited to maniacal agitation. They have no antipsychotic effect and virtually no effect on the extrapyramidal system. Lithium is unique also because of its prophylactic effect in unipolar and bipolar depressions.

Ataractics (from the Greek ataraxia: peace of mind) can be characterized as more or less strong sedatives, indicated in: restiveness, anxiety and tension states of non-psychotic origin. Unlike the classical sedatives they cause no or little drowsiness, and their influence on anxiety and tension is therefore a more selective one. Moreover, they lack the antipsychotic potency so characteristic of the neuroleptics, and they provoke no "neurological syndrome."

The fashionable term tranquillizer (from the Latin tranquillus: quiet, calm, serene) is to be defined as a compound which sedates without untoward effect on the level of consciousness and the degree of alertness. The term therefore applies equally to neuroleptics and ataractics. In the Anglo-American literature the neuroleptics are sometimes called major tranquillizers, and the ataractics minor tranquillizers.

Psychoanaleptics can be divided into stimulants and antidepressants. Both groups of compounds have a central stimulating effect, but the action of the stimulants is largely confined to the energy regulation. The antidepressants, however, exert an additional profound influence on affective life in certain types of depression.

The psychopathological symptoms provoked by psychodysleptics show a certain similarity to those commonly observed in certain psychoses. These compounds, therefore, give rise to a state of disintegration. The term "model psychoses" has been used in this context. The group comprises natural as well as synthetic compounds. Some of them disturb consciousness and lead to a state resembling intoxication (e.g. hashish and opiates); others cause disintegration but leave consciousness undisturbed or sometimes even unusually clear (e.g. LSD and psilocybine), which means that the experience does not fade away as the state of intoxication abates. Compounds of the latter type have been therapeutically applied, but their significance is controversial.

So much for the classification of psychotropic drugs according to effect or, to put it more precisely, according to their site of action in the range of psychopathological manifestations. Table 1 shows that the above discussed groups can be further differentiated. This, however, yields only gradual, not essential differences in effect. The subdivision is based on heterogeneous criteria, namely: chemical structure, pharmacological effects and biochemical sites of action. The classification of psychotropic drugs in its totality can therefore be justifiably called multidimensional, and it is multidimensional for want of a better one.

Table 1. Classification of psychotropic drugs.

I. PSYCHOLEPTICS

A. Sedatives/hypnotics
1. Barbiturates
2. Bromides
3. Mono-ureids
4. Aldehydes and halogenated alcohols
5. Opiates
6. Other sedatives

B. Neuroleptics
1. Phenothiazines
   a. aminoalkyl derivatives
   b. piperidine derivatives
   c. piperazine derivatives
2. Thioxanthenes
3. Butyrophenones
4. Diphenylbutylpiperidines
5. Dibenzazepines
6. Indoles
7. Rauwolfia alkaloids
8. Benzoquinolizines

C. Lithium compounds

D. Ataractics
1. Benzodiazepines
2. Substituted dioles
3. Diphenylmethanes
4. Tricyclic and tetracyclic compounds
5. Beta-blockers

II. PSYCHOANALEPTICS

A. Stimulants
1. Amphetamine derivatives
2. Compounds with piperidine group

B. Antidepressants
1. Tricyclic antidepressants
   a. dimethyl compounds
   b. monomethyl compounds
2. Tetracyclic antidepressants
3. MAO inhibitors
   a. hydrazine compounds
   b. non-hydrazine compounds

III. PSYCHODYSLEPTICS

A. Compounds which reduce the level of consciousness

B. Compounds which virtually do not reduce (sometimes increase) the level of consciousness

IV. OTHER PSYCHOTROPIC DRUGS

A. Compounds used in addictive diseases

B. Compounds used in sexual aberrations

BIBLIOGRAPHY

AYD, F. J. AND B. BLACKWELL (Eds.) (1970). *Discoveries in Biological Psychiatry*. Philadelphia: Lippincott.

BAN, TH. A. (1969). *Psychopharmacology*. Baltimore: Williams and Wilkins.

BENKERT, O. AND H. HIPPIUS (1974). *Psychiatrische Pharmakotherapie*. Berlin-Heidelberg-New York: Springer Verlag.

DELAY, J. AND P. DENIKER (1961). *Méthodes Chimiothérapiques en Psychiatrie*. Paris: Masson et Cie.

DELAY, J. (1965). Psychotropic drugs and experimental psychiatry. *J. Neuropsychiat.* 1, 104.

HOLLISTER, L. (1973). *Clinical Use of Psychotherapeutic Drugs*. Springfield, Ill.: Charles C Thomas.

JANET, P. (1908). *Les Obsessions et la Psychasthénie*. Paris.

KLEIN, D. F. AND J. DAVIS (1969). *Diagnosis and Drug Treatment of Psychiatric Disorders*. Baltimore: Williams and Wilkins.

KLEIN, D. F. AND R. GITTELMAN-KLEIN (Eds.) (1976). *Progress in Psychiatric Drug Treatment*. Vol. 2. New York: Brunner/Mazel.

LEVITT, R. A. (1975). *Psychopharmacology*. New York: John Wiley.

SILVERSTONE, T. AND P. TURNER (1974). *Drug Treatment in Psychiatry*. London: Routledge and Kegan Paul.

SIMPSON, L. L. (Ed.) (1975). *Drug Treatment of Mental Disorders*. New York: Raven Press.

WHEATLEY, D. (1973). *Psychopharmacology in Family Practise*. London: William Heinemann Medical Books.

II

Classification of Psychiatric Syndromes

1. Classification: basis of diagnosis

Psychiatrists cannot claim a rich tradition of classification. They have long regarded classification with contempt, as an unproductive activity (and a dangerous one to boot) which leads to a "labeling" of patients, thus disregarding their "essential" features. Of course this point of view is untenable. Classification of phenomena in which one is interested precedes their scientific study. Classification is the foundation on which diagnosis rests; and without adequate diagnosis, therapy as well as research inevitably must remain patchwork.

Few psychiatrists will overtly oppose this statement today. The system of classification available to them, however, is not a solid one. In this respect psychiatry appears to lag far behind other medical disciplines. Following are a few factors which make psychiatric classification so imperfect and opaque.

2. Two-dimensional diagnosis

Psychiatric classification could be based on three pillars: symptomatology, aetiology and course. In actual practice, however, all three are rarely used systematically. For example, the term "endogenous depression" gives some indications about the aetiology and the symptomatology of the psychopathological state but supplies no information on its course. Another example: the term "unipolar depression" refers to a particular symptomatology and a certain course, but supplies no information on its aetiology.

Two-dimensional diagnosis would be justifiable only if the definition of two criteria would virtually establish the character of the third criterion. This is not the case. Taking the example of unipolar depression, we are confronted with a phasic vital depressive syndrome without (hypo)manic periods (Chapter XII). These data, however, do not by any means establish its aetiology. The conditions for repeated depressive phases could be created not only by some hereditary disposition, but equally well by a given personality structure and/or a particular situation of life.

Another example: a diagnosis such as "psychogenic schizophrenia" gives no information on the course. Yet this is by no means certain, given a particular aetiology and a particular syndrome. The disease can take several different courses: a single disease period with complete recovery to the premorbid level; a recurrent course with complete recovery after each phase; or a recurrent course with gradual deterioration of the personality.

Finally, a concept such as pre-oedipal neurosis with recurrent decompensations provides an example of a diagnosis which indicates aetiology and course but gives no information on the symptomatology, although this can vary widely.

3. One-dimensional diagnosis

While a two-dimensional diagnosis is inadequate, a one-dimensional diagnosis is totally unacceptable. An example of a one-dimensional diagnosis is the term "vital depression" (Chapter XII). It indicates a syndrome (described in Anglo-American literature as endogenous depression), but is aetiologically quite "vacuous," although in this respect the vital depression is non-specific. It can develop largely as a result of hereditary factors, but equally well in response to intrapsychic tension, pressure exerted by the environment, acquired somatic diseases, or a combination of these factors. In some cases, no cause at all is demonstrable (idiopathic type). The aetiology of a vital depression, therefore, should certainly be indicated. The same applies to its course, which is likewise variable. There may be a single depressive phase in the course of a lifetime; or a recurrent course with complete recovery after each phase; or a recurrent course with incomplete recovery after each phase and transitions to chronic depressivity. In the case of a recurrent course, finally, there may be exclusively phases of depression (unipolar depression) or a combination of depressive and manic or hypomanic phases (bipolar depression).

My second example is the personal depression—a term I use to refer to the *syndrome* which is described as neurotic or reactive depression in Anglo-American literature (Chapter XII). The term personal depression does not account for aetiology and course. Psychological factors play an important aetiological role in many of these cases, but environmental factors are also involved to a varying extent. The significance of heredity is often refuted in advance and rarely evaluated. But this has no justification, for there are strong indications that this factor indeed plays a role. The natural history of this syndrome has hardly been studied systematically, but is undoubtedly variable. A neurotic breakdown can occur once in a lifetime; but it can also recur frequently, and may in the long run tend towards chronicity. By this I merely mean to say that the "diagnosis" personal depression is an incomplete one and should be supplemented with data on aetiology and course.

The term compulsive neurosis (to give a final example) describes a syndrome but gives no information on aetiology and course. Compulsive symptoms can occur as the disastrous terminal point of an abnormal psychological development; but they are also observed in association with (vital) depression, certain types of schizophrenia and morphological brain lesions. The course can be malignant—with intractable, progressively increasing ritual and erosion of the personality structure—or relatively benign and responsive to psychotherapy or antidepressant medication.

4. One-word "diagnoses"

Apart from one-dimensional or two-dimensional diagnoses, there is another custom which causes confusion in psychiatric practice. It is the custom of giving one-word "diagnoses" which, as should be evident from the above, are multi-interpretable by definition. Take the term schizophrenia. It evokes the suggestion of a nosological entity in the sense of Kraepelin, as if its use establishes with fair accuracy the aetiology, symptomatology and prognosis of a syndrome. Nothing could be less true. About what schizophrenia is, or is not, the greatest conceivable confusion prevails (Chapter VI).

Another disadvantage of one-word "diagnoses" is that they can be used in several different ways, in some cases with reference to an aetiology (usually conceived in psychodynamic terms), in other cases to indicate a syndrome. Typical examples are such "diagnoses" as neurosis, and hysteria. These are ambiguous terms and for this very reason should be avoided.

5. Pathogenesis: a future fourth dimension in psychiatric diagnosis

Medicine recognizes a fourth principle of classification beside the triad "aetiology, symptomatology and course"—that of pathogenesis. This is classification on the basis of the somatic substrate which generates the disease symptoms. In principle, this criterion is valid in psychiatry also. I define *pathogenesis* as the complex of cerebral functional disorders which enables psychopathological symptoms to occur. I define *aetiology* as the complex of (somatic, psychological and social) factors responsible for the development of these functional disorders. I shall revert to this subject in chapter V.

Recently there have been indications that the criterion "pathogenesis" is applicable in psychiatry not only in principle but also in actual fact. For the time being this pertains in particular to the depressions and, so far as the cerebral dysfunctions are concerned, to disorders of the central monoamine metabolism. This subject will be discussed in chapter XVI. For the psychoses, a comparable evolution seems likely to occur in future. The pertinent data will be discussed in chapter XI. There are no sound reasons for assuming that this evolution will be confined to depressions and psychoses. I am convinced that biological data and arguments will come to play a role also in the diagnosis (and treatment) of neurotic disorders and psychopathies. These are precisely the disorders which, according to many psychiatric and non-psychiatric behavioural scientists, should not be touched by the biologically-oriented psychiatrist.

6. Conclusions

Three criteria have so far been available for the classification of psychiatric syndromes: symptomatology, aetiology and course. Many diagnoses are being established without accounting for each of these three criteria. One-dimensional or two-dimensional diagnoses, however, would be justifiable only if with the definition of one or two criteria the nature of the remaining one or two were established with a high degree of certainty. But this is not the case. This is why one-dimensional and two-dimensional "diagnoses" make psychiatric diagnostics more opaque than would be necessary. Consistent three-dimensional diagnosis is the only way out of the labyrinth in which psychiatric diagnosis now finds itself.

Medicine recognizes as a fourth principle of classification: pathogenesis, i.e. the material substrate which generates the disease symptoms. It seems likely that this criterion will be introduced in psychiatric diagnosis as well.

BIBLIOGRAPHY

Jaspers, C. (1959). *Allgemeine Psychopathologie*. Berlin: Springer.

Katz, M. M., J. O. Cole, and W. E. Barton (Eds.) (1968). *The Role and Methodology of Classification in Psychiatry and Psychopathology*. Washington: U.S. Department of Health, Education and Welfare Publ.

Kendell, R. E. (1975). *The Role of Diagnosis in Psychiatry*. Oxford: Blackwell.

Praag, H. M. van, and B. Leijnse (1965). Neubewertung des Syndroms. Skizze einer funktionellen Pathologie. *Psychiat. Neurol. Neurochir.* 68: 50-66.

Wing, J. K., J. E. Cooper, and N. Sartorius (1974). *The Measurement and Classification of Psychiatric Symptoms*. London: Cambridge University Press.

III

Clinical Evaluation of Psychotropic Drugs

1. Problems in the clinical study of psychotropic drugs

The development of a new therapeutic agent takes place in three phases. To begin with, it is established that a given chemical substance produces a potentially useful biological effect in the living organism. Next, animal experiments are carried out in order to obtain information on the toxicity of the agent. Thirdly, the agent reaches the clinic for evaluation of its effects and side effects. The first and second phases will be left undiscussed here. The third phase—that of clinical pharmacological research—will be concisely discussed.

Clinical pharmacological research is a young branch of science, in the evolution of which England has pioneered. As early as 1931, the Medical Research Council of England appointed a committee (the Therapeutic Trials Committee), which was to concern itself with the study of the therapeutic properties of new drugs. Yet clinicians were long hesitant to give this new branch of research its due. New drugs, many thought, could be sufficiently evaluated on the basis of uncontrolled experience gained by individual physicians prescribing them to individual patients. In the past two decades, however, a rapid change has occurred. A scientifically sound approach to pharmacological trials proved to be a necessity rather than a luxury. Clinical pharmacology was soon recognized as a fully fledged subspeciality with its own position, between pharmacology and clinical medicine. In several countries, physicians are now being trained especially in research of this type.

The field of clinical pharmacology is especially difficult because the effect of a therapy depends not only on the drug under investigation, but also on a variety of non-pharmacological factors.

2. Pharmacological influences on the action of a drug

Factors of influence on the action of a drug, of course, include first of all the changes which the drug causes in the organism (the *pharmacodynamic* properties of the drug). A second group of action determinants comprises the factors which determine what happens with a drug in the organism: how quickly it is absorbed in the intestine; how it is distributed over the various compartments of the organism; how and how quickly it is degraded. These and other *pharmacokinetic* factors determine whether a sufficient concentration of the drug reaches its sites of action. The pharmacokinetics of a given drug are not constant within a given species. In different healthy individuals of the human species, for example, its degradation rate can differ widely. Differences of this kind are largely determined genetically, and the study of this aspect is known as *pharmacogenetics*. These differences are an (not *the*) explanation of the fact that psychotropic medication sometimes produces surprises. Drug A has a favourable effect in one patient, whereas another patient with similar symptoms shows an unsatisfactory response. Or else: a given patient shows no improvement in response to drug A whereas drug B, chemically closely related to and pharmacodynamically indistinguishable from drug A, produces the desired effect. These surprises may be related to differences in the way in which the organism handles the drug.

3. Non-pharmacological influences on the action of a drug

Psychological influences

The action profile of a drug, however, is influenced also by factors which have nothing to do with the drug itself but with the individual's somatic and psychological condition and with the environment in which he lives. This applies to all drugs, but particularly to psychotropic drugs. Let us consider the principal non-pharmacological factors in some detail.

To begin with, there is the complex of psychological factors which comprises: a) the patient's condition at the time of the medication, and b) his premorbid personality structure.

a) Many drugs produce a discernible effect only if certain well-defined symptoms are present. A characteristic example is found in the tricyclic antidepressants. It is in particular the vital depressions (chapter XII) that often show striking improvement in response to these compounds. Patients with other types of depression and healthy individuals, however, experience not much more than a sedative effect. Careless selection of patients, therefore, can lead to underevaluation of a drug.

b) The personality of the test subject is of importance also. In 1934 Lindemann and Malamud wrote: "Each drug undoubtedly has certain characteristics but these are quite closely related to the conditions of the patients which are present when these specific effects are produced. The changes produced by a given drug will not only be elaborated on in the light of the pre-existing psychic state but totally new types of reaction may result from such an interrelationship." They were far ahead of their time, for it was not until 1955 that von Felsinger demonstrated experimentally that the effect of phenobarbital, morphine, heroin and amphetamine is partly dependent on certain personality traits (not further discussed here); and they were among the pioneers in this field. The same applies to the newer psychotropic drugs. Frostad et al. (1966) divided neurotic patients, on the basis of their scores with a given test, into an "action-oriented" and a "non-action-oriented" group. With the Taylor Manifest Anxiety Scale, moreover, they rated the degree of anxiety. All these patients received the ataractic diazepam (Valium). Its therapeutic effects were most pronounced (and its side effects also) in the non-action-oriented group with high anxiety scores. The effects (and side effects) were least marked in the action-oriented group with low anxiety scores. A systematic study of the relation between premorbid personality structure and drug effect can be found in the work of Eysenck (1963). The literature on animal experiments also comprises striking examples. For instance: the central depressing effect of physostigmine in rats proved to depend partly on the initial degree of irritability. Irritable animals were inhibited more markedly than the less irritable individuals (Leavitt 1974).

Placebo effect

The influence of the personality structure can go much further than a degree of interference with the specific effect of a drug. A pharmacodynamically inert substance which passes as a therapeutic agent—a so-called placebo—can, in fact, behave like a therapeutic agent in certain cases, even including side effects. This is known as placebo effect. In such cases it is psychological rather than pharmacological factors that initiate the therapeutic process. A legitimate agent can have placebo effects as well as its specific effects. I referred to "certain cases" above. Not all persons are apparently placebo-sensitive. Numerous investigators have tried to define the predisposing factors in psychological terms. Predictions concerning sensitivity to placebo effect, however, have thus far not been very reliable. Moreover, the placebo effect is not linked to illness but is observed as well in healthy individuals. Normal test subjects were found to perform better at work when, during rest periods, they were given air to breathe with the announcement that it was oxygen than when they were given oxygen which was described as air (De Jongh 1954).

The occurrence of a placebo effect is dependent not only on personality characteristics but also on various environmental influences. The physician's attitude and his relation to the patient, the attitude of the nurses, the mentality of fellow-patients are all factors which can either potentiate or attenuate the placebo component in the effects of a drug. A detailed discussion of the aetiology of the placebo effect may be found in Shapiro (1964).

Of course the placebo effect is not a novelty. It has been known as long as physicians have existed. Only in our times, however, is the phenomenon being experimentally studied and efforts being made systematically to separate the specific effect of a new drug from its non-specific placebo effect.

Somatic factors

The patient's physical condition also influences the results of a medication. Age and sex are of importance in this respect. Although phenobarbital usually behaves like a sedative, it often produces a paradoxical effect in children and elderly patients; instead of sedating, it provokes or aggravates restiveness.

The significance of sex is confirmed, for example, by the observations of Goldberg et al. (1966), who found that male schizophrenics were more sensitive to a placebo effect than females, but that females showed a better response to phenothiazines than the males.

We should finally mention a factor which is often overlooked in this context: the fact that various biological processes, including metabolic processes, are subject to certain rhythmic variations. One example: rats given pentobarbital at 6 a.m. slept an average of 91 minutes; when the drug was given three hours later, however, the sleeping time did not exceed 53 minutes (Scheving et al. 1968). The significance of biological rhythms in human psychopharmacology has so far hardly been studied.

Environmental factors

Of special importance for the effect of a drug is the manner in which it is prescribed and administered (with skepsis or in a climate of confidence and expectation), and where it is administered (at home, in an environment which for the psychiatric patient is often fraught with tensions, or in the attentive, protective climate of a hospital; in a chronic ward or in one with a high turnover of patients. Not infrequently, moreover, the convalescing patient exerts an important therapeutic influence on his environment.

There is another way in which the physician plays a role with regard to the effect of a drug. Not only does he prescribe it but he also evaluates the therapeutic result. This evaluation is not a strictly objective process. It has been found that the physician's judgement is determined not only by the actual condition of the patient but also by his own confidence in or skepsis of the medication, by the knowledge that the effect was obtained with a drug or with a placebo, and by the degree of his commitment to the research being done. In spite of all good intentions, a physician's judgement is never entirely unbiased, particularly in a research situation.

4. The design of clinical studies of psychotropic drugs

Elimination of non-pharmacological factors

The clinical (psycho)-pharmacologist makes efforts to ensure that the influence of the non-pharmacological factors discussed above is eliminated or controlled so far as possible. I am of course referring to an experimental situation, i.e. a situation which focuses not on curing the patient but on obtaining optimally objective information on the specific effect of a given drug. Under normal (i.e. non-experimental) conditions, the physician is more than happy to use the non-pharmacological factors. As Beckman once wrote: "I would say: Do not deny to the gods the thanks due for making man the impressionable animal he is. Unless the doctor is willing to admit that his role as a dispenser of placebos, whether of drug or other nature, is upon occasion an important part of the doctor-patient relationship, he had better quit dealing with people and go into veterinary medicine." With all due respect for the medical conscience, he is of course right.

The pillars on which clinical research into the therapeutic value of drugs rests, are: the control group and the double-blind arrangement.

Control observations

These are indispensable because the investigator has to demonstrate with plausibility that the changes (if any) which followed administration of a drug would not have occurred without this administration. To use an image derived from another empirical science: the effect registered should always be compared with a blank observation.

The control group is treated in the same way and under the same conditions as the test group, the only difference being that the compound administered contains no pharmacodynamically active substance. Placebo and drug should, of course, be of identical shape, colour and taste.

The composition of the control group and the manner in which this composition is achieved are of great importance. There should be no selection, or as little as possible. Yet the patients in the control group should be symptomatologically similar to those in the test group. In actual practice this problem often solves itself in that a group of patients considered to be suffering from the same illness is divided into two groups at random, i.e. on the basis of chance, whereupon one group is treated with the test drug and the other with the placebo. An optimal situation prevails if each member of the control group corresponds with a member of the test group not only in terms of pathology but also in terms of age, sex, social status, etc. (matched controls). Such perfect matching, however, often cannot be achieved.

The requirement that test group and control group should be symptomatologically well-defined and congruent poses grave problems, particularly in clinical psychiatry. Yet, in view of the rapid developments in pharmacotherapy, this requirement cannot be disregarded. In any case, these problems have proved to be less inaccessible than they may seem to be. By virtue of new methods of registration such as (self)-rating scales and standardized interviews, and more sophisticated statistical analysis of the data thus obtained, substantial progress has been made in the past few years in the standardization of psychiatric diagnosis (chapter V).

It is not always necessary to form a separate control group. It is also possible to have the patient serve as his own control, treating him with the drug and with the placebo during alternate periods. In this way the difficulty of forming homogeneous groups can be avoided; that is why there exists a certain preference for this method. It is occasionally overlooked, however, that this method is valid only if the syndromes studied show no great spontaneous fluctuations in intensity, and if the test drug can be expected to produce its effect fairly quickly. A major disadvantage of this arrangement is that the drug may have an after-effect during the placebo period, thus influencing the findings.

In some cases a third group is formed beside placebo and test group; this is done if other drugs are already available for the purpose for which the test drug has been recommended. The third group receives the drug with the already established effect. In this way it is also possible to gain an impression of the relative value of the new drug. If an adequate standard substance is available, then the formation of a placebo group is sometimes omitted. Of course such a simplified test arrangement yields less information. It can only provide an answer to the question whether the new drug is superior or inferior to the standard drug, while the question whether the test drug really has a specific effect remains unanswered.

Double-blind arrangement

Evidently the patient himself must not know whether he is receiving the drug or the placebo. Whenever this requirement is fulfilled, the arrangement can be called "blind." It becomes "double-blind" if not only the patient but also the observers (physician, nurses) are ignorant of the nature of the agent administered. It is only after completion of the experiment that the code is broken. It is the purpose of the double-blind arrangement to keep the evaluation of the therapeutic result free from subjective impurities. Of course the double-blind arrangement does not eliminate such errors, but it distributes them evenly over test group and control group and thus reduces the risk that these errors may influence the test results.

An experiment is called *controlled* if a test drug is compared with a control substance (placebo or drug with a known effect) under double-blind conditions.

Pros and cons of the controlled experiment

The uncontrolled experiment, in which no control group is formed and the investigator is aware of the nature of the agents administered, still has its attractions. This is not surprising. The proper designing and analysing of a controlled drug experiment require methodological and statistical knowledge, and always involve a great deal of work. Indeed, an experienced investigator is certainly able to obtain general information on the efficacy of a given drug from uncontrolled observations. This method is, therefore, undoubtedly suitable in pilot studies. But one should not go further, although some do. The uncontrolled approach has its true advocates, who maintain that the controlled experiment is too rigid and that psychotropic medication should be adjusted to the needs of the individual patient if optimal results are to be obtained. Of course this is true, but it is irrelevant in this context. The psychopharmacological experiment does not primarily focus on determination of optima, but is carried out in order to establish whether a compound has any specific activity at all, or functions exclusively as a placebo. The question of optimal dosage becomes meaningful only after the efficacy of the compound has been established with certainty.

Moreover, the double-blind arrangement is by no means incompatible with a flexible dosage scheme. Personally, I like to make use of the following set-up if the action of substance A is to be compared with that of substance B. Identical capsules are prepared which contain different amounts of substance A or substance B. The patients in both groups receive a capsule on a fixed number of occasions every day, and every day a psychiatrist who does not participate in evaluation determines the amount required by each patient. In my opinion this is an elegant method, but it is also an "expensive" one because a psychiatrist has to be added to the research team as the one who determines the dosages.

It has also been called a disadvantage of the controlled experiment that the system is not infrequently less foolproof than it may seem to be. This is supposedly due to side effects of the drug tested. In fact, such side effects do occur, but it is to be borne in mind that serious mistakes can be made because a placebo, too, can produce "side effects" (the so-called negative placebo effect). However, if the code has to be broken prematurely for any reason, then of course the experiment has to be considered a failure.

Other arguments against the controlled experiment are: the fact that it is often of limited duration, for organizational reasons; the use of inadequate dosages; insufficient homogeneity of the groups. All these arguments, however, concern technical imperfections which, in principle, can be avoided.

Finally, ethical arguments have been advanced. It is maintained, for example, that it is not justifiable to deprive a group of patients of the expected advantages of a new therapy. The obvious flaw in this argument is that it presumes the validity of a new therapy although it is precisely this validity that has to be demonstrated—and this can be done only via a control group. If this is omitted, then one runs the risk of sacrificing the future interests of many patients to the *presumed* interests of a few patients involved today. To turn the tables, this could be described with some justification as unethical.

To put it briefly: the controlled experiment is by no means infallible, but the simple truth is that it yields more reliable results than the uncontrolled method. One would throw out the baby with the bath water if one preferred the uncontrolled experiment to the controlled experiment on the basis of the abovementioned arguments. There are no other, more convincing arguments against the controlled experiment.

BIBLIOGRAPHY

Beckman, H. (1961). *Pharmacology*. Philadelphia and London: Saunders.

Byar, D. P., R. M. Simon, W. T. Friedewald, J. J. Schlesselman, D. L. de Mets, J. H. Ellenberg, M. H. Gail and J. H. Ware. (1976). Randomized clinical trials. *New Engl. J. Med.* 295, 74.

Chassan, J. J. (1976). *Research Design in Clinical Psychology and Psychiatry*. New York: Appleton-Century-Crofts.

Controlled Clinical Trials. A conference organised by C.I.O.M.S., Blackwell Scientific Publ., Oxford. (1960)

Eysenck, H. (1963). *Experiments with Drugs*. New York: Macmillan.

Felsinger, J. M. von, (1955). Drug-induced mood changes in man; 2. personality and reactions to drugs. *J. Am. Med. Ass.* 157, 1113.

Fisher, R. A. (1952). *The Design of Experiments*. Edinburgh: Oliver and Boyd.

Frostad, A., G. Forrest and C. Bakker (1966). Influence of personality type on drug response. *Am. J. Psychiat.* 122, 1153.

Goldberg, S., N. Schooler, E. Davidson and M. Kayce (1966). Sex and race differences in response to drug treatment among schizophrenics. *Psychopharmacologia* 9, 31.

Hamilton M. (1974). *Lectures on the Methodology of Clinical Research*. London: Churchill/Livingstone.

Harris, E. L. and J. D. Fitzgerald (eds.) (1970). *The Principles and Practice of Clinical Trials*. London: Livingstone.

Jongh, D. K. de (1954). De betekenis van het placebo. *Ned. T.v. Geneesk.* 98, 1943.

Kerlinger, F. N. (1975). *Foundation of Behavioral Research*. London: Holt, Rinehart, Winston.

Lader, M. H. and P. A. Nicholson (Eds.) (1976). Evaluation of psychotropic drugs. *Brit. J. Clin. Pharmacol.*, suppl. 1.

Leavitt, F. (1974). *Drugs and Behavior*. London: W. B. Saunders Co.

Levine, J., B. C. Schiele and L. Bonthilet (1971). *Principles and Problems in Establishing the Efficacy of Psychotropic Agents*. NIMH, Washington, D.C.: Public Health Service Publication, No. 2138.

Lindemann, E. and W. Malamud (1934). Experimental analysis of psychopathological effects of intoxicating drugs. *Am. J. Psychiat.* 90, 853.

Sainsbury, P. and M. Kreitman (1975). *Methods of Psychiatric Research*. London: Oxford Univ. Press.

Scheving, L., D. Vedral and J. Pauly (1968). A circadian susceptibility rhythm in rats to pentobarbital sodium. *Anat. Rec.* 160, 741.

Shapiro, A. K. (1964). Etiological factors in placebo effect. *J. Am. Med. Ass.* 187, 712.

Wolf, S. (1959). Pharmacology of placebos. *Pharmacol. Rev.* 11, 689.

IV

The Significance of the Monoamines in the Brain

1. MA in the central nervous system

Nearly all psychotropic drugs so far known exert an influence on the central MA metabolism. Psychotropic drugs have greatly stimulated research into the animal and human central MA metabolism; and research into MA in turn is giving productive impulses to research which focuses on the development of new types of psychotropic drugs. Thus, this chapter presents a brief description of the localization and metabolism of the central MA and of the conceivable mechanisms involved in impulse transmission in a central MA-ergic synapse. The relation between MA and psychotropic drugs is discussed in chapters XI and XVI.

In the CNS there are two catecholamines (CA) and one indoleamine (IA) which, although this is yet to be demonstrated with certainty, are generally regarded as neurotransmitters. The CA are dopamine (DA; 3, 4-dihydroxyphenylethylamine) and noradrenaline (NA; norepinephrine). The IA is serotonin (5-hydroxytryptamine; 5-HT). The three are all monoamines (MA) in chemical structure.

Because of their great biological importance they are also known as biogenic amines. The CNS also contains other CA (e.g. adrenaline) and IA (e.g. tryptamine), as well as MA without a catechol or indole group (e.g. phenylethylamine). Their function, however, is still obscure. Neurotransmitters are substances which transmit an impulse from one neuron (nerve cell) to the other via a synapse.

2. Subcellular distribution of MA

Three functionally different components can be distinguished in each nerve cell:

1. The *receptive component*, which receives the (bio-electric) signals and guides them to the axon. This component comprises the dendrite and the cell body.

2. The *conductive component*, i.e. the axon which conducts the signals away from the cell body. Each nerve cell has one axon, which has terminal ramifications. Swellings in these ramifications are known as boutons terminaux, and in Anglo-American literature are referred to as nerve terminals, nerve endings or varicosities. They can be torn from the remainder of the axon by differential centrifugation of homogenized MA-ergic nerve tissue, whereupon the axonal membrane closes so that their contents remain intact. These avulsed nerve endings are called *synaptosomes*. The possibility of isolating them has greatly facilitated the study of impulse transmission.

3. The *transmissive component*, where the signal is transmitted to the next nerve element. The functional contact site between the two nerve elements is called synapse. Morphologically, the two elements are separated by a cleft, the so-called synaptic cleft, with a width of about 200 Å. The membranes which delimit this cleft are called presynaptic and postsynaptic membrane, respectively. Two parts are distinguished in the synapse. The first is the presynaptic part, in which the impulse arrives. Anatomically, it is believed that this is the nerve ending proper, where the synthesis, storage and release of MA take place. The second is the postsynaptic part, being the receptive surface of the next neuron. The word "receptive" can be translated to mean: covered with MA-sensitive receptors.

   An MA-ergic neuron contains a single MA, contained for the most part in the nerve endings. The CA concentration in the nerve endings, for example, exceeds that in the cell bodies and axons by a factor 100-1000. In the nerve ending, the transmitter is found chiefly in vesicular structures—the so-called *synaptic vesicles* which are clearly distinguishable from other cell components such as mitochondria, lysosomes and ribosomes. Only a minute amount is found free in the axoplasm. Synaptic vesicles are formed in the cell body and transported to the nerve endings. They are regarded as stores, where the transmitter is bound to ATP and/or protein (chromogranine). In this form it is physiologically inactive and protected from diffusion from the neuron as well as from the degrading action of the enzyme monoamine oxidase (MAO), for the nerve endings contain a large amount of MAO, bound to the membrane which envelops the mitochondria. MA which "leak" from the synaptic vesicles or cannot immediately be taken up into these vesicles are so immediately degraded that they are prevented from reaching the synaptic cleft at an inopportune moment.

In the literature we frequently encounter the view that the transmitter molecules stored in the synaptic vesicles are distributed over two compartments—one in which the molecules are firmly bound, and one in which they are more loosely bound. The latter pool is believed to be available for immediate use, whereas the former serves to replenish the functional pool, and is directly drawn upon only in extreme conditions. The notion of two pools in a single synaptic vesicle is incompatible with the view that a synaptic vesicle releases its entire contents into the synaptic cleft in response to an impulse (cf. section 4). Should there indeed be exocytosis, then the pools would have to be localized in different morphological structures; these, however, have not (yet) been identified.

3. Cellular localization of MA

The elegant histochemical studies of Hillarp and Falck (Falck et al., 1962) have supplied a wealth of information on the localization of MA-bearing cell bodies and nerve fibres. Their method was based on exposure of thin, freeze-dried slices of brain to formaldehyde vapour, causing CA and 5-HT to be converted to fluorescent compounds which could be visualized with the fluorescence microscope. In a gross, schematic way, the topography of the MA-ergic systems can be described as follows.

The cell bodies of NA-ergic neurons are localized in the medulla oblongata, the pons and the mesencephalon (Fig. 1). The locus coeruleus is a nucleus which almost exclusively contains NA-bearing cell bodies. The axons of the cell bodies in the medulla oblongata descend in the spinal cord. The cell bodies at higher levels extend their

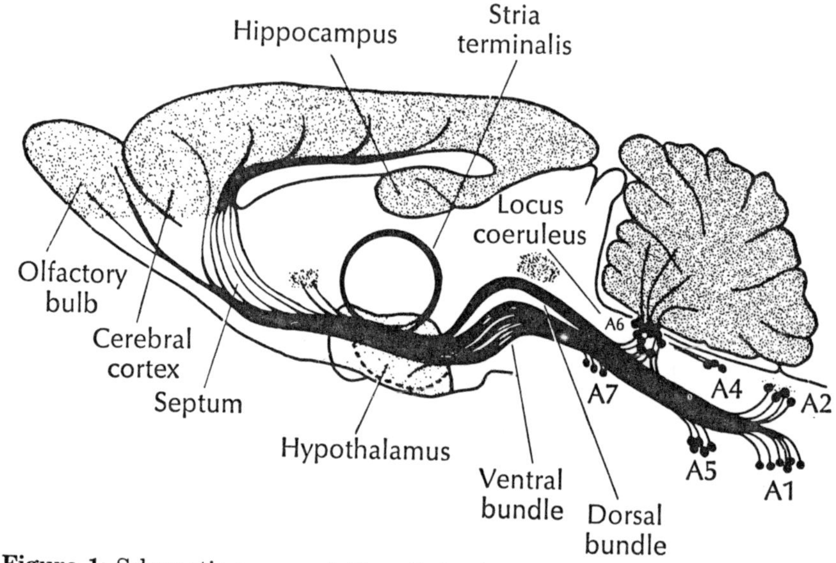

Figure 1: Schematic representation of the distribution of the main ascending central neuronal pathways containing NA. The stippled regions indicate the major nerve terminal areas. The cell groups are named according to the nomenclature of Dahlström and Fuxe (From: Cooper et al., 1974).

axons to the hypothalamus, the limbic system and, to a lesser extent, the neocortex.

The cell bodies of DA-ergic neurons are chiefly localized in three area. : the zona compacta of the substantia nigra, the ventral tegmental region and the arcuate nucleus in the hypothalamus (Fig. 2). The axons of the firstmentioned area extend to the caudate nucleus and the putamen of the corpus striatum (nigro-striatal DA system). From the tegmentum, axons extend to the nucleus accumbens and olfactory tubercle (meso-limbic DA system) and to the cerebral cortex (meso-cortical DA system) (Fig. 3). The DA-bearing cells in the arcuate nucleus innervate the medial eminence and are involved in the regulation of release of pituitary hormones (tubero-infundibular DA system).

The nigro-striatal system of the rat contains about 70-75% of

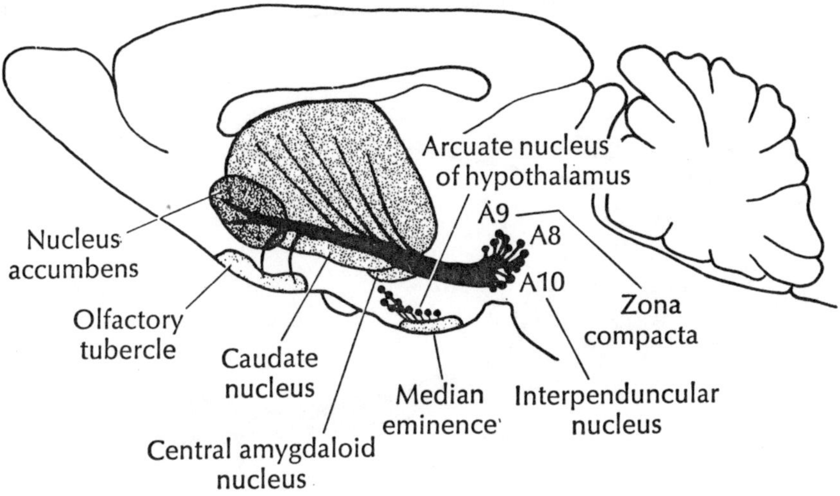

Figure 2: Schematic representation of the distribution of the main neuronal pathways containing DA. The stippled regions indicate the major nerve terminal areas. The cell groups are named according to the nomenclature of Dahlström and Fuxe (From: Cooper et al., 1974).

the total amount of DA in the brain. The meso-limbic and meso-cortical systems rank a fair second with about 20-25%. The tubero-infundibular system is by far the smallest.

The cell bodies containing 5-HT are to be found chiefly in the raphe nuclei localized in the mesencephalon and the cranial part of the medulla oblongata. The latter nuclei (nuclei raphe pallidus and obscurus) extend fibres to the medulla oblongata and spinal cord. The mesencephalic nuclei (nuclei raphe dorsalis and medianus) extend fibres rostrally to the hypothalamus, corpus striatum, neocortex (particularly frontal and parietal cortex), and many other areas: 5-HT terminals are found in varying density at numerous sites in the brain.

Cell bodies containing DA and 5-HT thus form fairly well-defined "nuclei" which are relatively readily accessible to techniques of traumatization and stimulation. This has greatly facilitated the study of the function of these systems.

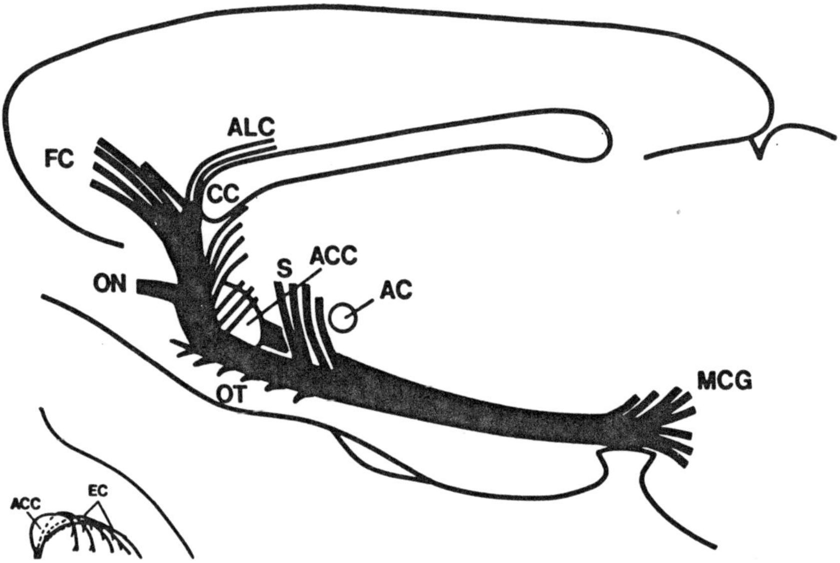

Figure 3: Schematic representation of the presumed dopaminergic mesolimbic and mesocortical systems in a sagittal projection (From: Lundvall and Björklund, 1974).

AC = anterior commissure; ACC = nucleus accumbens; ALC = anterior limbic cortex; CC = corpus callosum; FC = frontal cortex; MCG = mesencephalic CA cell groups; ON = olfactory nuclei; OT = olfactory tubercle; S = septum.

4. MA-ergic transmission in the CNS

Impulse transmission in a MA-ergic synapse is probably effected as follows (Fig. 4 and Fig. 5).

1. An impulse reaches the receptive part of a nerve cell and generates an action potential by depolarization of the axon membrane. The action potential is conducted to the nerve ending and, in response to the depolarization process, transmitter substance is released into the synaptic cleft.

In principle, the transmitter can originate from the cytoplas-

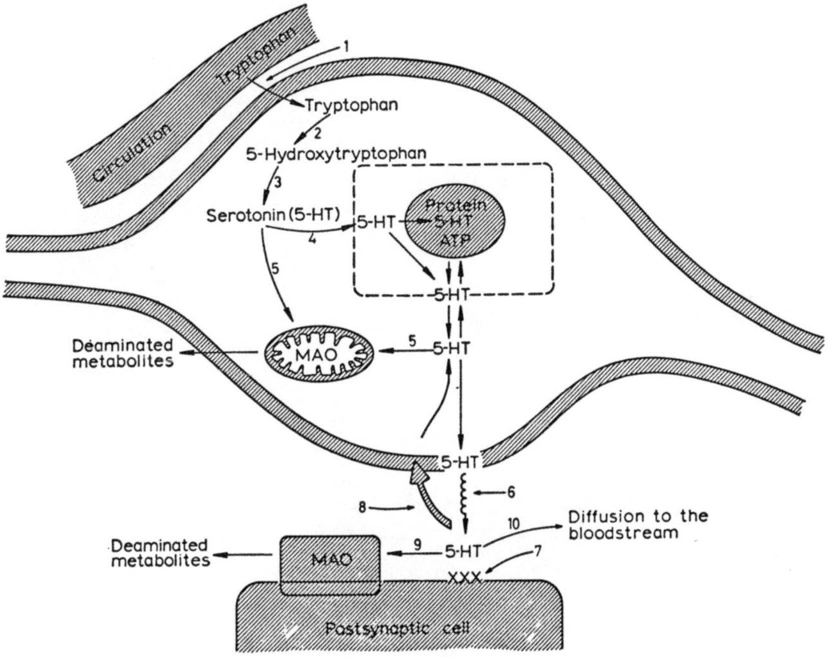

Figure 4: Schematic representation of serotonergic synapse (Modified after Cooper et al., 1974).

1: Active uptake or transport of tryptophan in the CNS; 2 and 3: biosynthesis of 5-HT; 4: uptake of 5-HT in synaptic vesicles and binding with ATP and protein; 5: degradation of unbound ("free") 5-HT by the enzyme MAO, localized largely in the outer membrane of mitochondria; 6: release of 5-HT in the synaptic cleft; 7: interaction of the transmitter with the postsynaptic receptors; 8: re-uptake of 5-HT in the synaptic vesicles; 9: extraneuronal degradation of 5-HT, presumable by MAO, but its extraneuronal localization is unknown; 10: diffusion of 5-HT to the circulation.

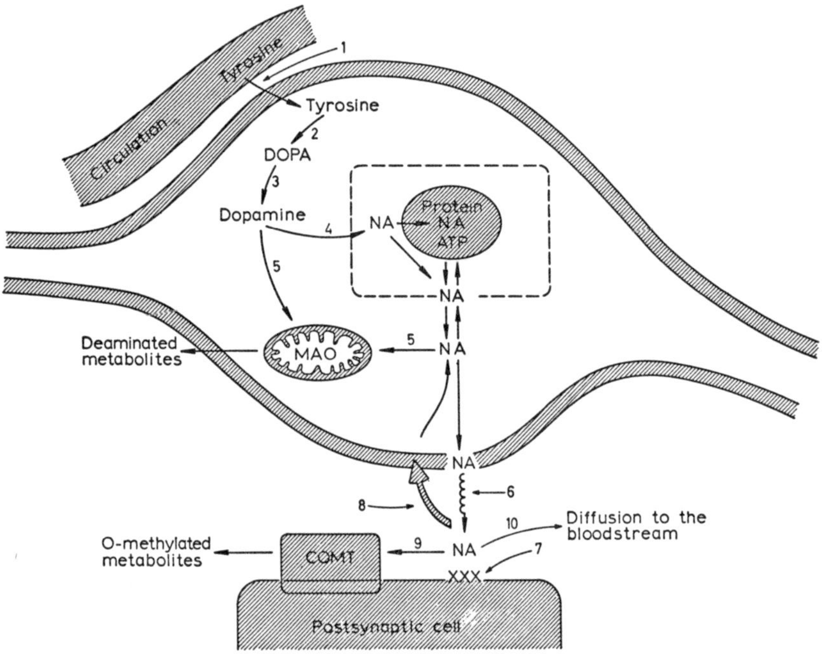

Figure 5: Schematic representation of a noradrenergic synaps (Modified after Cooper et al., 1974).

1: Active uptake or transport of tyrosine in the CNS; 2 and 3: biosynthesis of DA; 4: uptake of DA in synaptic vesicles, transformation in NA and binding with ATP and protein; 5: degradation of unbound ("free") DA and NA by the enzyme MAO, localized largely in the outer membrane of mitochondria; 6: release of NA in the synaptic cleft; 7: interaction of the transmitter with the postsynaptic receptor; 8: reuptake of NA in the synaptic vesicles; 9: extraneuronal degradation of NA, presumably largely by COMT; 10: diffusion of NA to the circulation.

In a dopaminergic synapse DAß-hydroxylase is not available. Therefore DA is not transformed in NA, but stored as such. For the rest structure and functioning of both types of synapses are considered to be similar.

matic or from the vesicular fraction. In the former case we must assume either that the presynaptic membrane's permeability for the transmitter increases in response to the impulse or that the binding of the transmitter to ATP becomes less stable, as a result of which the transmitter concentration in the cytoplasm increases and leakage to the synaptic cleft occurs. This, however, is improbable in view of the results of histochemical studies which cannot be discussed in detail here. This implies that the transmitter must originate from the synaptic vesicles. On this point there are three theories: 1) the vesicle is released in its entirety to the synaptic cleft, where it disintegrates; 2) the vesicle comes into contact with the presynaptic membrane and an aperture forms at the site of contact between the two membranes, whereupon the contents of the vesicle are released into the synaptic cleft—a process known as *exocytosis*; 3) a synaptic vesicle releases its contents in the immediate vicinity of the presynaptic membrane, and the transmitter diffuses through this membrane into the synaptic cleft. The lastmentioned mechanism is the least plausible. In the periphery, after excitation of an NA-ergic nerve, not only NA is found extraneuronally but also other vesicle constituents such as ATP, chromogranine and certain enzymes. In view of the dimensions of these molecules, their ability to pass through the presynaptic membrane is questionable. On the basis of morphological and histochemical findings, exocytosis is now being regarded as the most plausible release process, although there are some indications that there can be extraneuronal (synaptic?) vesicles also.

The mechanism by which depolarization of the axon membrane causes migration of synaptic vesicles to the presynaptic membrane, and the exact mechanism of exocytosis, are ill-known. The influx of calcium ions from the extracellular space into the nerve ending probably plays a role in this respect.

2. Transmitter substance released into the synaptic cleft diffuses to the postsynaptic membrane, where it binds with the postsynaptic receptors. Via a mechanism as yet unknown, this leads to a change in the ion permeability of the postsynaptic membrane. Cyclic adenosine monophosphate (cyclic AMP) possibly plays a role in this respect, for CA activate adenylcyclase in the postsynaptic element, and this is the enzyme which converts ATP into cyclic AMP. Local accumula-

tion of cyclic AMP leads to phosphorylation of membrane proteins, and this might alter the ion permeability of the membrane.

Be this as it may, when the transmitter increases the sodium ion permeability, the membrane depolarizes and the postsynaptic element becomes subject to a state of excitation which is conducted on to the axon. The reverse happens when the transmitter increases the chloride ion and possibly the potassium ion permeability. The postsynaptic system is then hyperpolarized: it is less readily excitable or, in other words, it is inhibited. Biochemists and biophysicists are now focusing considerable efforts on isolation and identification of postsynaptic receptors.

The principal groups of neuroleptics now in use—the phenothiazines, thioxanthenes and butyrophenones—block the postsynaptic receptors in central DA-ergic and NA-ergic neurons. Consequently, impulse transmission in these synapses diminishes. This phenomenon is probably of importance in the mechanism of action of the neuroleptic effects.

3. Once the signal has been transmitted to the next neuron, the transmitter substance disappears from the synaptic cleft, partly by extraneuronal degradation and diffusion to the blood stream, but for the most part by re-uptake into the nerve ending and hence into the synaptic vesicles. This (re-)uptake also takes place against a concentration gradient. For example, brain slices concentrate NA from an incubation medium which has a 5-8 times higher NA concentration. This means that an active, energy-consuming process is involved: a true pump mechanism.

Antidepressants interfere with the removal of MA from the synaptic cleft. Tricyclic compounds block their re-uptake into the neuron, and inhibitors of the degrading enzyme monoamine oxidase (MAO) impede the degradation of MA inside and outside the neuron. Inhibition of intraneuronal MAO causes MA to accumulate in the cytoplasm, as a result of which "leakage" to the synaptic cleft can occur. All these mechanisms lead to an increase in the amount of MA available at the postsynaptic receptors, and therefore possibly also to an increase in neuronal activity in these systems.

Reserpine produces the opposite of the effect of antidepressants. It inhibits uptake of MA into the synaptic vesicles. The MA are therefore degraded by MAO to an increased extent, even before they can reach the synaptic cleft. Their concentration diminishes, and transmission in MA-ergic synapses is inhibited. The well-known antihypertensive reserpine plays a role in psychiatry for two reasons: 1) it has neuroleptic properties, and 2) it is able to induce vital depressions, particularly in patients with a history of such depressive phases. There are indications that the psychological effects of antidepressants and reserpine are related to their influence on central MA.

As already pointed out, the transmitter function of MA in the CNS—although quite plausible—has not been demonstrated with certainty. A transmitter, and the enzymes involved in its synthesis and elimination, ought to be localized in the presynaptic element of a synapse. The MA meet this criterion. A transmitter ought to be released upon excitation of a nerve and, guided to the postsynaptic receptor, it ought to produce the same effect as excitation of the presynaptic nerve fibre. Owing to the enormous complexity of the central neuronal network, it has not been established with certainty whether MA meet these criteria. Release processes have been studied by such means as the use of a so-called push-pull cannula and by perfusion of the lateral ventricles. For the study of the postsynaptic effect of MA, micro-iontophoresis has proved to be a valuable aid. It is in view of results thus obtained that the transmitter function of MA is plausible; but these results are not conclusive, for the techniques used merely give an impression of events which take place in groups of neurons. They are far too crude to give information on events within a given individual synapse.

5. Metabolism of CA

It is difficult for CA to enter the brain from the blood stream. They must therefore be *produced* locally (Fig. 6). The mother substance is the amino-acid tyrosine which, via an active transport mechanism, is taken up into the brain and then into CA-ergic neurons. Several aromatic amino-acids compete for the same transport system and consequently the uptake of tyrosine (and tryptophan, mother substance of 5-HT) into the brain diminishes in the case of, say, phenylketonuria, with high plasma phenylalanine levels. Tyrosine is involved in numerous metabolic reactions, and only a very small amount is utilized for CA synthesis. For this pur-

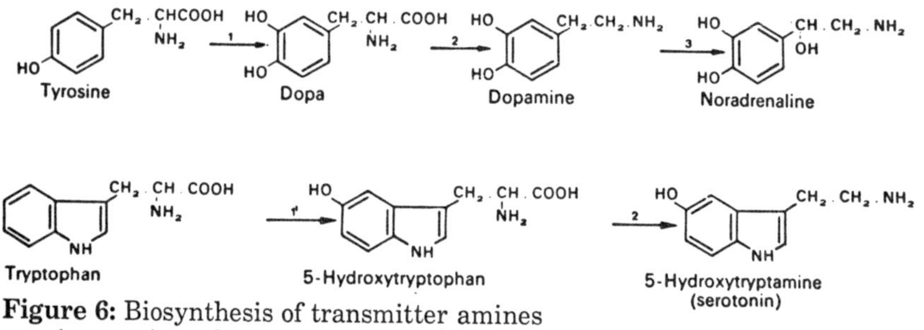

Figure 6: Biosynthesis of transmitter amines
1: tyrosine hydroxylase: 2: DA (5-HT) decarboxylase; 3: DA-ß-hydroxylase; 1′: tryptophan hydroxylase

pose tyrosine is hydroxylated at the 3-site by the enzyme tyrosine hydroxylase, in which process DOPA is produced. This reaction is rate-limiting in the synthesis of CA. With the aid of DOPA decarboxylase, CO_2 is withdrawn from DOPA and DA results. Tyrosine hydroxylase has a high substrate specificity, but DOPA decarboxylase has not: it decarboxylates all natural aromatic 1-amino-acids such as histidine, tyrosine, tryptophan and phenylalanine, as well as 5-hydroxytryptophan (5-HTP) and DOPA. A more appropriate designation for this enzyme would therefore be: 1-aromatic amino-acid decarboxylase. Next, DA is oxidized in the side-chain by DA-ß-hydroxylase, and NA is formed in this process. DA-ß-hydroxylase is localized in the synaptic vesicles, whereas the other enzymes are contained in the cytoplasm of the nerve endings.

The enzyme phenylethanolamine-N-methyltransferase, which converts NA to adrenaline via N-methylation and which is found in abundance in the adrenal medulla, occurs also in the mammalian brain, particularly in areas involved in the olfactory functions (olfactory bulbus and olfactory tubercle); however, its activity is low and the adrenaline concentration similarly. Moreover, the function of central adrenaline is unknown.

CA are *degraded* (Fig. 7) by oxidation and methylation, under the influence of monoamine oxidase (MAO) and catechol-O-methyltransferase (COMT). Contrary to what is often contended, the former enzyme is not exclusively found intraneuronally, bound to the mitochondrial membrane, but mainly outside neurons, for after denervation the MAO activity in the sympathetically innervated end-organ shows only a moderate decrease. It is plausible, on the

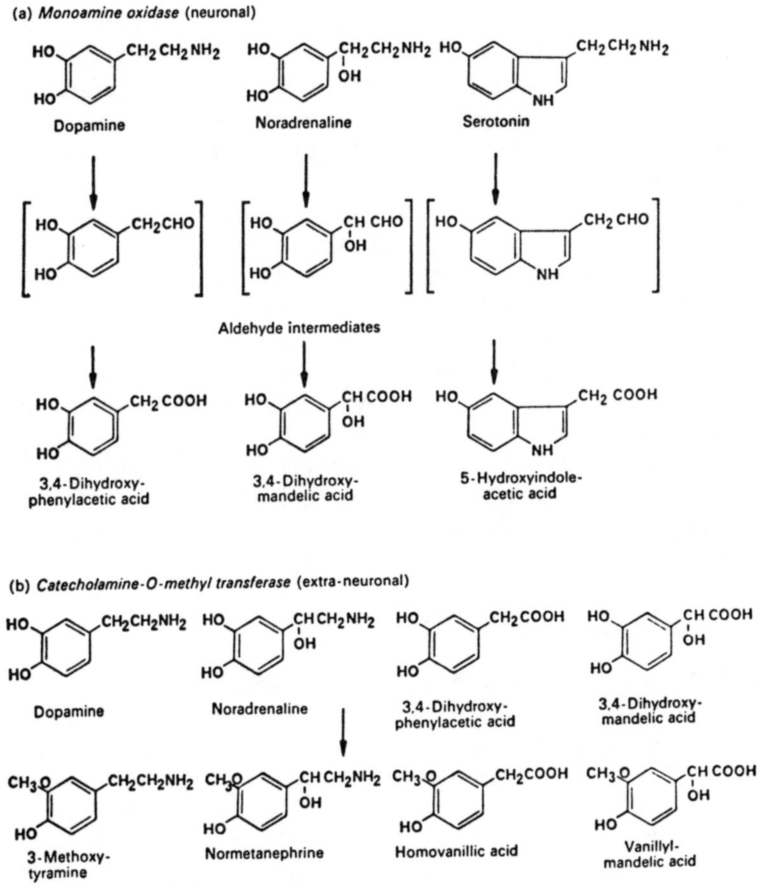

Figure 7: Degradation of 5-HT, DA (peripheral and central) and NA (peripheral) (From: H. S. Bachelard, 1974).

other hand, that mainly intraneuronal MAO is involved in MA degradation. COMT functions chiefly extraneuronally, although its exact localization remains obscure. MAO converts CA to aldehydes, which are immediately further degraded either to the corresponding acid (by the enzyme aldehyde dehydrogenase) or to the corresponding alcohol or glycol (by the enzyme aldehyde reductase). It has recently been demonstrated with the aid of electrophoresis that MAO is not a simple enzyme but occurs in at least two different types. These are called isoenzymes but, strictly speaking, this is an inappropriate name because they differ in substrate specificity (which means that a given type of MAO acts on a given MA and is less active in relation to other MA), and susceptibility to MAO inhibitors. In actual fact they are different (if related) enzymes.

COMT catalyses the transmission of a methyl group from the methyl donor S-adenosylmethionine to the 3-hydroxyl group of the CA. In the CNS the principal degradation product of NA is a glycol: 3-methoxy-4-hydroxyphenylglycol (MHPG) (Fig. 8); this is in contrast to the periphery, where NA is largely converted to an acid (vanillylmandelic acid).

Human central DA is chiefly converted to an acid: homovanillic acid (HVA). The corresponding alcohol (3-methoxy-4-hydroxyphenylethanol; MOPET) is quantitatively of subordinate importance.

6. Metabolism of 5-HT

For the production of 5-HT, too, the brain must rely on itself; it is difficult for this amine to enter the brain from the bloodstream. The mother substance of 5-HT is the essential amino-acid tryptophan (Fig. 6). This is first of all hydroxylated to 5-HTP. The activity of the enzyme tryptophan-5-hydroxylase which is involved in this is low in the brain; this has greatly impeded its detection and identification. It is a cytoplasmic enzyme of high specificity—different from, say, tyrosine hydroxylase and phenylalanine hydroxylase (which forms tyrosine)—which probably occurs exclusively in serotonergic neurons.

Next, 5-HTP is decarboxylated to 5-HT with the aid of 5-HTP decarboxylase—an enzyme of low specificity which is identical to DOPA decarboxylase. Given the presence of a sufficient amount of

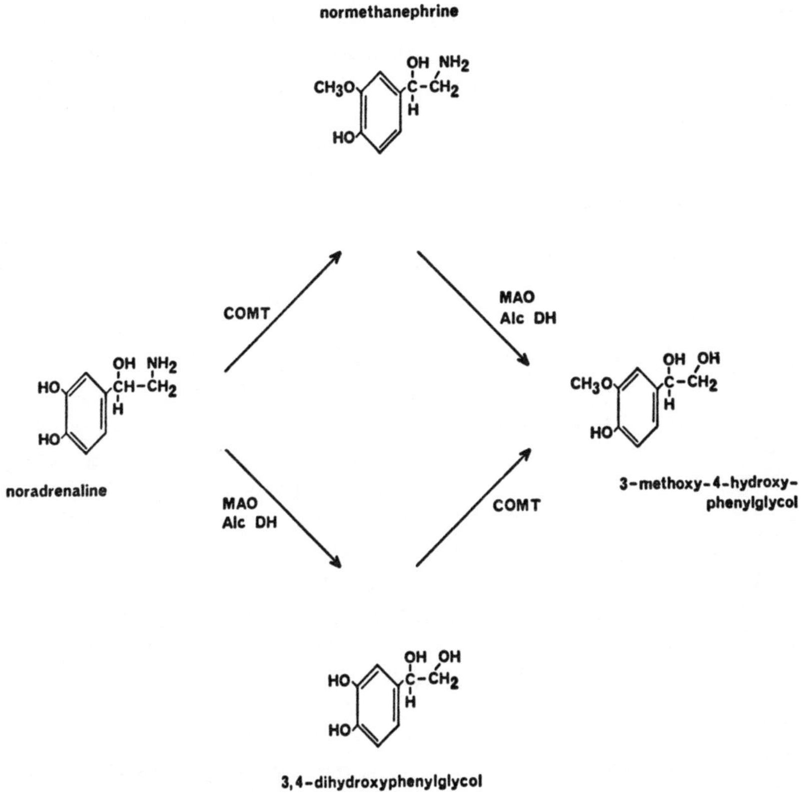

Figure 8: Major catabolic pathways of NA in the CNS
MAO = monoamine oxidase; AlcDH = alcohol dehydrogenase; COMT = catechol-O-methyltransferase.

tryptophan, conversion of tryptophan to 5-HTP is the rate-limiting factor in 5-HT synthesis.

The principal route of 5-HT degradation is: deamination to 5-hydroxyindoleacetaldehyde in response to MAO, and further oxidation to 5-hydroxyindoleacetic acid (5-HIAA) with the aid of aldehyde dehydrogenase (Fig. 7). In principle, the aldehyde can also be reduced to 5-hydroxytryptophol. Whether this conversion is of any importance in the CNS is unknown. The brain contains enzymes able to convert 5-HT directly (without deamination) to the 5-sulphate ester. Under normal conditions, however, this reaction is probably of minor importance.

7. False transmitters

DOPA (= 5-HTP) decarboxylase and DA-ß-hydroxylase have a low substrate specificity. Consequently, numerous compounds capable of being taken up into the MA-ergic cell are converted by these enzymes and then taken up into the synaptic vesicles. In this way they can come to function as a so-called false transmitter. In response to an impulse they are released into the synaptic cleft, but they are incapable of exciting the postsynaptic receptor. An example: when a large amount of 1-DOPA is administered, part of it is taken up into serotonergic neurons and converted by DOPA (= 5-HTP) decarboxylase to DA, which in these neurons probably starts to function as false transmitter. Another example: α-methyldopa (Aldomet, a hypotensive) is converted by DOPA decarboxylase and DA-ß-hydroxylase to α-methyl-DA and α-methyl-NA—potential false transmitters in DA-ergic and NA-ergic neurons, respectively.

8. Regulation of the release and synthesis of MA

Many publications have been devoted to this subject in the past few years. It is impossible to give a concise outline of this literature. I shall merely mention a few possibilities. Whether they are all really active as regulatory mechanisms and, if so, under which conditions, is uncertain.

The amount of NA released into the synaptic cleft is probably regulated via α-receptors in the presynaptic membrane. These are believed to be excited when the NA concentration in the synaptic cleft exceeds a given critical level, with cessation of the release process as a result. Possibly not only the release of NA but also its synthesis is inhibited. Whether a similar mechanism exists in the case of the other MA is unknown. It is assumed that neuroleptics of the receptor-blocking type block both postsynaptic and presynaptic NA receptors.

An obvious possibility for the regulation of transmitter synthesis is so-called end-product regulation. CA inhibit tyrosine hydroxylase activity in vitro. It is therefore assumed that an increase in the concentration of CA in the neuron inhibits their synthesis, and vice versa. In view of the probably inconsiderable changes in the concentration in the nerve endings, it is doubtful whether this mechanism is active under normal conditions.

Another synthesis-regulating factor is the impulse flow in the presynaptic system. This has long been known with regard to NA. In the peripheral sympathetic nerves, the NA concentration is constant within narrow limits, and independent of neuronal activity over a wide range. Consequently there must be a homoeostatic mechanism which keeps the transmitter concentration constant, even though a fraction of this is lost at each impulse transmission. It is likely that the activity of aromatic amino-acid hydroxylases (tryptophan hydroxylase and tyrosine hydroxylase) is indeed influenced by nerve impulses. Whether this is a direct influence or an indirect one, for example via the availability of a cofactor, is unknown.

It is possible, moreover, that postsynaptic receptors exert an influence on transmitter synthesis. The presence of such a mechanism became a probability when it was found that stimulation of postsynaptic CA and 5-HT receptors reduces the synthesis of the corresponding transmitter, and vice versa. The (humoral or neuronal) mechanism of transmission of such a signal is still obscure. With regard to the nigro-striatal DA system, there are indications of the presence of a neuronal system; neurons extending from the striatum to the substantia nigra could transmit the feedback inhibition. These neurons make use of gamma-aminobutyric acid (GABA) as transmitter substance.

Finally there can be little doubt that central MA synthesis is subject to hormonal influences as well. For example, the conversion of ^{14}C-labelled tyrosine to ^{14}C-labelled NA is increased following thyroidectomy. This might well be an important future crossroad for a meeting of transmitter chemistry and (neuro-)endocrinology.

9. Measuring MA turnover

The term "turnover" refers to the overall rate at which the entire amine store available in a given tissue is replaced. It is a chemical concept, and supplies no information on the question whether all the amine converted has been utilized for transmission. The turnover rate of an amine must therefore not be simply regarded as an indicator of the functional condition of the system. On the other hand there are indications (cf. section 8 above) that the neuronal activity in MA-ergic neurons is a factor of importance in regulating synthesis. For this reason it is often hypothesized that the reverse also applies—that the chemical turnover is indeed an index of the functional activity in the system. This generalisation, however, is certainly not justified.

There are several methods of measuring central MA turnover; none of them is ideal. First of all there are methods which make use of a drug. We can inhibit tyrosine hydroxylase with the aid of α-methyl-p-tyrosine, and tryptophan hydroxylase with p-chlorophenylalanine; the central concentration of CA and 5-HT, respectively, then begins to diminish, and the rate of disappearance is a measure of the turnover of these substances. It is also possible to inhibit MA degradation (with the aid of a MAO inhibitor), and then to measure the accumulation of the amines as an indicator of their rate of synthesis. Finally, there is the probenecid technique. Probenecid is a substance that inhibits the transport of the acid 5-HT and DA metabolites 5-HIAA and HVA from the CNS to the bloodstream. As a result, they accumulate in the brain and CSF and the rate of accumulation equals the rate of their synthesis (at least during a few hours). Rate of synthesis of 5-HIAA and HVA and rate of degradation of 5-HT and DA, are of identical magnitudes. The rate of accumulation of 5-HIAA and HVA after probenecid administration is therefore a measure of the rate of degradation of the mother amines.

For the purpose of these studies, the abovementioned drugs must be given in large doses, in which they produce unintended effects as well. This is a disadvantage. The former two methods, moreover, lead to marked changes in MA concentration and it is conceivable that this, as such, could influence the normal control mechanisms.

Radioisotope techniques have also been used in measuring MA turnover. To begin with, labeled amine is introduced intracisternally or into the ventricle (intravenous administration is impossible because MA do not readily pass the blood-brain barrier), whereupon the rate of disappearance of the specific activity of the amine in question is measured. This method starts from three assumptions: 1) that the labeled amine is selectively taken up by the corresponding MA-ergic neurons; 2) that the tracer dose of the isotope is so small that the endogenous amine pool is not or hardly enlarged; 3) that the amine lies stored in a homogeneous pool. The fact that these requirements are not entirely met reduces the validity of this method.

An alternative radioisotope technique calls for intravenous injection of labeled precursors—e.g. tyrosine for measuring CA turnover and tryptophan for measuring 5-HT turnover—whereupon the decrease in the specific activity of the precursor and the increase in that of the amine are measured. This technique, too, has its flaws. For example, it assumes that the MA-ergic neuron has no preference for freshly formed amine as against the old store for transmission; in actual fact, however, there are indications that it has such a preference.

10. Studies of the human central MA metabolism

Several strategies have been used to study the MA metabolism in the human CNS:

1. Determination of the concentrations of MA, their metabolites and some of the enzymes involved in their metabolism in peripheral body fluids, specifically urine and blood.

2. Postmortem determination of the concentrations of MA, their metabolites and some of the enzymes involved in their metabolism in the brain. These studies have in particular been made in depressive patients (suicide victims) and patients with schizophrenic psychoses.

3. Determination of the baseline concentration of MA metabolites in the CSF and of their accumulation after administration of probenecid.

4. Studies of the behavioural effects of drugs which either inhibit or stimulate the synthesis of MA.

The information obtained by the first method is limited, for it is unlikely that the overall metabolism of MA and the activity of certain enzymes in the periphery are representative of the situation in the brain. An important exception is probably the renal excretion of MHPG, for this NA metabolite is largely produced centrally and is of subordinate importance in the periphery. Its urinary excretion, therefore, probably gives an indication of NA degradation in the CNS.

The probenecid technique is the only possibility to obtain some information on the turnover of central MA in human individuals. As pointed out, this technique is based on inhibition of the transport of acid MA metabolites, specifically 5-HIAA and HVA, from the CNS to the bloodstream. They consequently accumulate in the CNS, including the CSF, at a rate which is related to their rate of synthesis. Rate of 5-HIAA and HVA synthesis and rate of 5-HT and DA degradation are different terms for the same concept. Under steady state conditions, moreover, the rate of degradation of 5-HT and DA equals their rate of synthesis. This implies that determination of the probenecid-induced accumulation of 5-HIAA and HVA in the lumbar CSF provides an impression of the turnover rate of the mother substances 5-HT and DA in the CNS. This rate is considered to be high if the accumulation is high, and low if the accumulation is low. However, this technique is unsuitable for studies of the NA metabolism because MHPG transport is not probenecid-sensitive.

The snares and pitfalls of postmortem studies are well-known. The value of the pharmacological strategy has so far been limited because there are as yet no substances which exert a really selective influence on one of the central MA. Otherwise I leave the limitations and imperfections of all these strategies undiscussed here; I have discussed them elsewhere (Van Praag 1977). Suffice it to say that, although each of these methods separately gives only limited information, they jointly produce a pattern of data which, in my opinion, is certainly eloquent. I shall revert to this subject in chapters XI and XVI.

11. Conclusions

MA probably play a role as transmitter in a number of fairly well-defined groups of neurons in the CNS, localized in areas traditionally assumed to play a role in the generation and regulation of motor activity (basal ganglia), emotionality and level of motivation (limbic system). This explains the great interest in these compounds displayed by investigators interested in the mode of action of psychotropic drugs and their development.

BIBLIOGRAPHY

BACHELARD, H. S. (1974). *Brain Biochemistry*, London: Chapman and Hall.

COOPER, J. R., F. E. BLOOM AND R. H. ROTH (1974). *The Biochemical Basis of Neuropharmacology*. New York, London, Toronto: Oxford University Press.

COSTA, E., L. L. IVERSEN AND R. PAOLETTI (1972). *Studies of Neurotransmitters at the Synaptic Level*. New York: Raven Press.

FALCK, B., N.A. HILLARP, G. THIEME and A. TORP (1962). Fluorescence of catecholamines and related compounds condensed with formaldehyde. *J. Histochem. Cytochem.* 10, 348.

FRIEDHOFF, A. J. (1975). *Catecholamines and Behavior. Basic Neurobiology (Vol. I)*. New York: Plenum Press.

FRIEDHOFF, A. J. (1975). *Catecholamines and Behavior. Neuropsychopharmacology (Vol. II)*. New York: Plenum Press.

IVERSEN, L. L., S. D. IVERSEN AND S. H. SNYDER (1975). *Handbook of Psychopharmacology. Biochemistry of Biogenic Amines (Vol. III)*. New York: Plenum Press.

IVERSEN, L. L., S. D. IVERSEN AND S. H. SNYDER (1975). *Handbook of Psychopharmacology. Biogenic Amine Receptors (Vol. VI)*. New York, London: Plenum Press.

JONES, D. G. (1975). *Synapses and Synaptosomes. Morphological Aspects*. London: Chapman and Hall.

LUNDVALL, O. AND BJÖRKLUND, A. (1974). The organisation of the ascending catechol-amine neuron systems in the rat brain, as revealed by the glyoxylic acid fluorescence method. *Acta Physiol. Scand.*, suppl. 412.

PRAAG, H. M. VAN (1977). *Depression and Schizophrenia. A Contribution on Their Chemical Pathology*. New York: Spectrum Publications.

PRAAG, H. M. VAN AND J. BRUINVELS (Eds.) (1977). *Neurotransmission and Disturbed Behavior*. Utrecht: Bohn, Scheltema & Holkema.

SNYDER, H. (1975). Opiate receptor in normal and drug altered brain function. *Nature* 257, 185.

YOUDIM, M. B. H. (1976). *Aromatic Amino Acid Hydroxylases*. New York, Toronto, Sydney: John Wiley.

V

Psychiatry, Biological Psychiatry and Psychotropic Drugs: An Analysis of Their Interrelation

1. The triple character of psychiatry

Psychiatry is believed to be the least medical of the medical disciplines. With regard to the origin of psychopathological processes, it is believed to focus mainly on pathogenic influences of a non-material nature and, for their treatment, to prefer psychotherapy to the so-called somatic methods of treatment. This conception, however, entails a reduction which distorts the image of psychiatry.

In actual fact, psychiatry must deal with three groups of pathogenic factors. To begin with, it must deal with disturbed *intra-individual* relations, i.e. with disturbances in the development of and interaction between the various "components" of the human soul. Secondly, it must deal with disturbed *interindividual* relations, i.e. with disturbances in the relations between individuals and those between the individual and the society. Finally, it is concerned with disturbances in the functioning of the *cerebral substrate,* which "carry" deviant behaviour, i.e. which are instrumental in disorganizing behaviour. Only in the past 10 to 15 years have methods been evolved (biochemical, histochemical, electrophysiological and pharmacological) which are suitable for a systematic study of the last mentioned group of factors.

The triple nature of psychiatry is expressed in psychiatric diagnosis, treatment and research.

As regards psychiatric diagnosis: this comprises (so far as analysis of disease causes is concerned, quite apart from a classification of disease symptoms and their course) a "weighing" of the individual conflict situation and its ontogenesis, of pathogenic group interaction and, if already possible, of the cerebral functional changes underlying the psychopathological syndrome.

As regards psychiatric treatment: one may aim at tensions within the individual or within the group; or one may attempt to normalize behaviour by exerting a direct influence on the (dysfunctioning) cerebral substrate, e.g. with the aid of drugs. These three approaches, like the pathogenic mechanisms at which they aim, are not alternatives but complements, which implies that they can be simultaneously used in the same patient.

As regards psychiatric research: the three models on which psychiatry is based (the psychological-psychodynamic, the social-sociological and the medical-neurobiological) are of equivalent importance and cannot be reduced to each other. In other words: it is impossible to ignore one of these models without seriously detracting from the study of disturbed behaviour.

2. The input-machinery-output scheme

It is apparent from section 1 above that the analysis and testing of the medical-neurobiological model start from the presupposition that disease, even psychiatric disease, is of a material nature. Every behaviour disorder is conceived of as having a material correlate in a complex of disturbed brain functions. An interdependence of the two series of disturbances is postulated, in the sense that the material disturbance is regarded as a prerequisite for the occurrence of the behaviour disorder. No behaviour without a functioning brain; no disturbed behaviour without disturbed brain functions. In this conception, therefore, every behaviour disorder—be it cognitive, perceptive, emotional or of any other kind—is ultimately determined organically (cerebrally). This is not a plea for revival of 19th-century materialism. The postulate is *not* that behaviour disorders *are* brain diseases; the postulate is that pathogenic factors exert their influence on behaviour not directly but via alterations in the function of the central nervous system (CNS). In this conception the brain functions as an intermediary. More precisely, it is an intermediary between input and output or, in other words, an intermediary between the assorted influences, on the one hand, which—recently or in a more distant past—have exerted a disturbing influence on the cerebral machinery and, on the other hand, the behaviour changes which manifest themselves to the investigator.

With this in mind, the concept "disease cause" is found to have two components. It encompasses the factor *process*, i.e. the material cerebral substrate believed to underlie the psychopathological symptoms, as well as the factor *aetiology*. The latter is the sum of all noxious influences which have contributed to the occurrence of the disease process.

The aetiological factors can be widely disparate. They can be related to the individual's course of development, his social environment or his cultural background. This is the complex of factors previously referred to as disturbances in intraindividual and interindividual relations. Secondly, they can be genetically determined. An example could be a primordially absent or marginal enzyme system or an enzyme system which functions imperfectly for some other reason. Finally, they can result from a somatic lesion sustained in the course of life, either causing immediate damage or giving rise to a locus minoris resistentiae. In the latter case the disturbance does not become manifest unless other aetiological factors are involved or become involved at some later time.

If it were possible logically to infer the nature of the disease symptoms from the nature and localization of the cerebral disease process, then the *pathogenesis* of the given syndrome would be known. This situation occurs only if there is some understanding of the function which the (now diseased) substrate normally has. The pathogenesis concept can therefore be regarded as the functional analogue of the concept "disease process."

When the term "disease cause" is used without specifying the factor referred to, or when the concept is used now in one and then in another significance, confusion is imminent. Psychiatric pathology has been unable to avoid this confusion. An example of such a persistent confusion on the basis of a careless use of the disease cause concept is implied in such a question as: "Is behaviour disorder A (e.g. schizophrenia) a biochemical or a psychosocial disease?" This question entails a logical inconsistency in that it suggests alternatives which are no alternatives. All behaviour, including disturbed behaviour, is made instrumentally possible by a given functional condition of the brain. Such conditions can be described in biochemical terms, at least in principle. In this sense, all (disturbed) behaviour is biochemically determined. But psychosocial factors can have made an important contribution to the presence of this cerebral condition. If a division is at all to be made, then the dividing line should be drawn as follows (Fig. 9):

1) behaviour disorders based on cerebral dysfunctions to be ascribed largely to psychological and social factors;

2) behaviour disorders based on cerebral dysfunctions to be ascribed largely to factors other than psychosocial factors, e.g. acquired somatic diseases which entail brain damage, and hereditary factors such as a primordially marginal enzyme system.

It is evident that, in the input-machinery-output scheme, the psychiatric tenet of multifactorial causality is fully maintained. It is merely amended by the postulate that the complex of aetiological factors cannot exert its disturbing influence on behaviour and experiencing directly, but only via functional changes in the CNS.

3. Demarcation of the field of biological psychiatry

I define biological psychiatry as that branch of psychiatric research that concerns itself with the medical-neurobiological model. It encompasses the following components.

1) The study of the cerebral substrate thought to underlie disturbed behaviour. In this context the word substrate is not used in the anatomical sense but with reference to a complex of functional changes.

2) The tracing of possibilities of regulating behaviour by direct interference with brain function. For this purpose, it is possible in

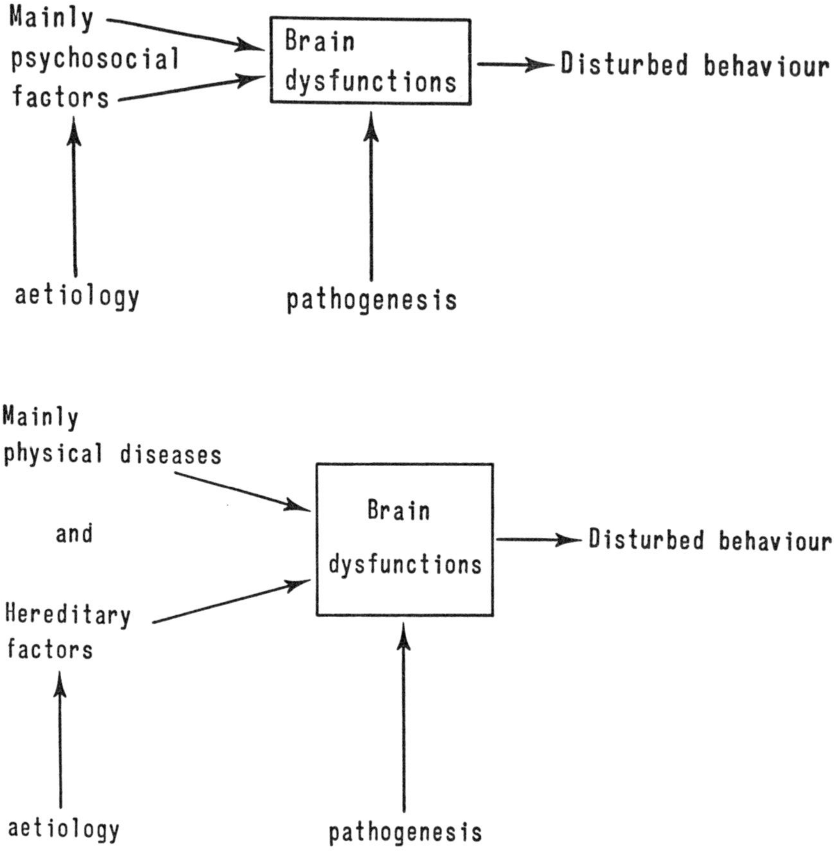

Figure 9: Relationship between biological and environmental factors in the occurrence of behavioral disorders

principle to make use of pharmacological, biochemical, electrophysiological and neurosurgical methods.

3) Since it is the objective of biological psychiatry to correlate neurobiological parameters with variables of behaviour, it will take a close interest in the development of methods which will ensure optimally objective assessment and registration of ele-

ments of human behaviour, according to their nature and severity.

In the context of biological psychiatry, psychopathological manifestations are studied as symptoms, i.e. as signs indicative of another, material reality (the disease process), clarification of which is the ultimate goal of all biological-psychiatric research. This means that, in the field of biological psychiatry, a substantial reduction is applied from two sides. Psychopathology is reduced to an auxiliary discipline, subservient to a psychiatry which is practiced as a medical discipline, i.e. as a discipline of natural science. Moreover, the term biology is reduced to its most limited sense: the physics and chemistry of living matter.

A persistent misconception holds that the starting points of biological psychiatry, on the one hand, and those of psychodynamic and social psychiatry, on the other, should be fundamentally irreconcilable. In actual fact, however, the possibility of disease being primarily provoked by factors of a psychological or a social nature is in no way inconsistent with the views of biological psychiatry. Psychosomatic medicine has shown that the function of a wide variety of organ systems can be severely damaged by psychological tensions. There is no reason to believe that the brain should be an exception in this respect.

The notion that the study of central behaviour-regulating mechanisms and of ways to influence them by pharmacological and electrophysiological interventions is an unalienable aspect of psychiatry is only hesitantly being accepted. Consequently, facilities for applying this notion in practice are still very scanty. Consequently, biological psychiatrists who are capable of translating this notion into terms of actual practice (in other words, psychiatrists who are proficient in clinical psychiatry and combine this proficiency with an adequate knowledge of certain aspects of experimental psychology and neurobiology, sufficient for productive cooperation with the specialists concerned) are few and far between. And this closes the vicious circle.

Half a century ago, biochemistry and physiology rapidly gained significance in internal medicine. The internist of that time understood that, if he were to avoid a dead end as researcher and practitioner, he would have to familiarize himself with the abovementioned preclinical disciplines. It seems to me that the situation in which the psychiatrist finds himself today can be compared with that of the internist a few decades ago.

Far from claiming supremacy, this plea urges nothing more than that biological psychiatry be given an equivalent position beside psychodynamic and social psychiatry. A well-balanced structure of psychiatry would be most advantageous to its scientific development, to the training of its practitioners, and to its practical applications.

I would go even further. I hold that this point of view is valid not only for psychiatry but for the behavioural sciences in general. If it is true that the spirit does not move upon the face of the waters but, like all phenomena of life, is firmly rooted in them, then a type of psychology and a type of sociology which completely abstract themselves from the biological determinants of human behaviour are as limited as a type of medicine which functions as a purely somatic discipline and disregards the pathogenetic significance of environmental and psychological factors. The latter has become a rarity, but the former is unfortunately still the rule.

4. Some semantic questions

Biological psychiatry is not merely a product of the summation of some neurochemistry, neuropharmacology, neurophysiology and neuro-anatomy, combined with experimental behaviour research. Biological psychiatry is integrated research into conditional relations between (disturbed) brain functions and (disturbed) behaviour.

Biological psychiatry does not equate to organic psychiatry—an infelicitous term used with reference to the group of behaviour disorders related to demonstrable anatomical brain lesions. Biological psychiatry accepts as basic tenet that all disturbed behaviour is based on cerebral functional disorders which, in principle, can be analysed. The differentiation between cerebral functional disorders with and without demonstrable anatomical brain lesions is of practical importance with a view to possible therapeutic consequences; in principle, however, the difference is an artificial one. This is why I described the term "organic psychiatry" as infelicitous.

Biological psychiatry does not equate to neuropsychiatry if the latter term is understood as some sort of alloy of neurology and psychiatry. Neurology supplies information on the motor and sensory consequences of brain damage. Biological psychiatry focuses on behaviour disorders which may result from such damage. Neurology and biological psychiatry share an interest in the functioning of the brain, but their objectives differ.

Biological psychiatry does not equate to psychosomatic medicine. The latter encompasses research into the influence of psychological factors on somatic functions; biological psychiatry encompasses research into the cerebral substrate which is "intermediary" in the production of psychological (dys)functions.

The term psychobiology is approximately synonymous to biological psychiatry but, in my view, less suitable. It is an analogue of the term neurobiology—the current collective name for all specialities which concern themselves with the structure and functions of the nervous system. I dislike using this term because it might give the impression that the study of the material "foundation" of psychological dysfunctions requires neurobiological methods other than the conventional; of course, this impression is wrong.

So much for a few semantic problems (not exactly of subordinate importance in a field so strewn with terminological misunderstandings). I only wish to emphasize in addition that, by definition, the biological psychiatrist is not a scientific loner. His maxim par excellence is: to work together (with "pure" neurobiologists on the one hand, and with "pure" experimental behaviour researchers on the other) or not to work at all. It is precisely this middle-man position that gives him his identity.

5. The aims of psychotherapy and pharmacotherapy

The input-machinery-output scheme can elucidate the relation between psychotherapy and somatotherapy (the latter term can be roughly replaced by pharmacotherapy, which is by far the most important type of somatotherapy). Within this scheme, the aim of psychotherapy (or sociotherapy) can be defined as the attenuation or, if possible, elimination of aetiological factors of a psychogenic (or sociogenic) nature. Extending this theoretical line: If in a given case psychogenic factors have already caused irreversible changes in the (cerebral) machinery, then one cannot expect to obtain lasting results by psychotherapy alone. In that case, efforts must be made also to exert a direct influence on the dysfunctioning substrate, e.g. by means of drugs. Another possibility is to "re-program" the cerebral machinery via a learning process (behaviour therapy).

Drugs can be used for two reasons. First of all, in order to exert a direct influence on the cerebral machinery. However, so little is yet known about the nature of central dysfunctions that underlie disturbed behaviour that pharmacological manipulations are of necessity still somewhat unspecific. However, even in the theoretical case of complete knowledge of the dysfunctions and, consequently, optimal correction by pharmacotherapy, psychotherapy would still be indispensable in the majority of cases. In order to avoid a relapse, after all, such psychogenic factors as have contributed to the occurrence of the dysfunction (and most cases involve such factors) will have to be dealt with. And for this purpose, only the psychotherapeutic approach seems suitable. Even in a pharmacotherapeutic Utopia, therefore, we would not be able to do without psychotherapy.

Some psychopathological symptoms—e.g. delusions, compulsions, hallucinations—can be accompanied by violent emotional upsets which, as such, have a disorganizing effect. The need to subdue such emotional reverberations provides another reason for using psychotropic drugs. When they are prescribed for this indication, their effect on the dysfunctioning substrate is a secondary one.

I conclude that the aims of psychotherapy and pharmacotherapy are disparate. The one focuses on the aetiology and the other on the pathogenesis of the syndrome. It would therefore be a fallacy to regard pharmacotherapy not as a different but as an inferior form of treatment, as a second choice, or as an approach to be seriously considered only if psychotherapy has failed. The two methods are equally valuable, and are complements. This implies that they can be simultaneously used in the treatment of the same patient. It is logically tenable and therefore useful to attempt to combat a given pathological condition by simultaneous efforts via different approaches.

The sharp dichotomy between psychotherapy and somatotherapy is a vestige of the long-standing and still not entirely decided controversy between the "psychicists" and the "somaticists"; and as such it can serve only to maintain the fire of this unproductive controversy. Its replacement by less tainted terms (e.g. verbal and non-verbal forms of psychotherapy) seems to merit consideration for this reason. Used in this context, the term psychotherapy would mean "therapy applied to the psyche" rather than "therapy applied by psychological means."

6. The significance of psychotropic drugs in somatic substrate research

The view that psychiatry is the least medical of the medical disciplines is widely accepted, and this is not surprising. The latter half of the 19th century marked the heyday of an orthodox materialism (summarized in Griesinger's maxim: "Mental diseases are diseases of the brain"), which raised the expectation that the enigma of the origin of mental diseases might be solved with the aid of neuroanatomy. During the first half of this century, on the other hand, psychiatry assumed much more spiritualistic overtones. Phenomenology and anthropology were in fashion especially in the German-speaking countries and The Netherlands, and depth psychology was popular in the United States. Phenomenology, with its exclusive focus on the experiential quality of psychopathological symptoms, and anthropology with its marked philosophical tenor, are explicitly a-biological; this is to say that they study behaviour apart from its material substrate. Depth psychology (including psychoanalysis) was not originally a-biological but gradually came to focus more and more on the psychogenicity, and somatic thinking was superseded in actual fact if not in principle.

After the fifties, the enchantment of phenomenology and anthropology has unmistakably waned. At the same time (thus indicating a chronological, not a causal relation) the evolution of another a-biological trend—social psychiatry—rapidly gained momentum. This had a variety of causes: 1) the rise of the social sciences; 2) an increasing awareness that the psychiatrist should place himself *in* the society rather than seclude himself in a soundproof office or a mental hospital; 3) the rise of active political groups of the radical left, who regarded imperfections in the social structure as the pathogen par excellence of the human psyche. Important nuclear groups in this movement are not so much a-biological as clearly antibiological. They reject biological substrate research in psychiatry as "socially irrelevant" and consider biological methods of treatment, specifically psychopharmacotherapy, as evil or, at best, as "sops." Whenever their therapeutic efficacy is undeniable, they are disposed of as "a forcible form of adaptation to a sick and therefore sickening social situation and in fact, therefore, anti-therapeutic."

Likewise in the course of the fifties, biological psychiatry entered its second heyday and flourished in spite of oppression. Psychotropic drugs greatly contributed to this. These agents are effective on two levels: the level of metabolism and the level of behaviour. This raised the question of the possible relation between the two effects. Modern brain and behaviour research would be unthinkable without psychotropic drugs. Inversely, brain and behaviour research has stimulated the development of compounds with a more or less specific effect on the metabolic level and therefore, it is hoped, on the behaviour level as well. In this respect, therefore, biological psychiatry and psychopharmacology stimulate each other. The following examples to demonstrate this.

1) The currently used antidepressants are unrelated in chemical structure, but nevertheless show two similarities. In biochemical terms: They increase the amount of monoamines (MA) available at the central MA-ergic receptors, albeit via different mechanisms. In psychopathological terms: They have a beneficial effect on vital depressions. This has prompted two questions: 1) Is the therapeutic effect related to the MA-agonistic effect, and 2) is there a central MA deficiency in vital depressions? These questions are the core of current biologically-oriented depression research.

When indications were found that the central MA metabolism can indeed be disturbed in depressions, attempts were made to evolve drugs which influence one of the central MA as specifically as possible. The agents resulting from these attempts are now being tested in depressive patients.

2) A similar situation prevails with the neuroleptics. They, too, differ in chemical structure, but nevertheless show two similarities. In biochemical terms: Via different mechanisms, they reduce the transmission of stimuli via DA-ergic and NA-ergic synapses. In psychopathological terms: They have a beneficial effect on psychomotor unrest and psychotic disorders of thinking and experiencing. This has prompted questions similar to those considered in depression research. Is reduced activity in CA-ergic systems an antipsychotic principle, and can the

CA-ergic system be dysregulated in psychoses? Indications that at least the first question should be answered in the affirmative stimulate the development of drugs with a high degree of selectivity for DA-ergic or CA-ergic transmission, respectively.

3) The last example: methylated MA derivatives with a hallucinogenic action, e.g. mescaline and bufotenine. The close relatedness of these compounds to serotonin and dopamine, respectively, raises two questions: Are there human enzymes capable of in-vivo formation of these methyl derivatives and, if so, are they formed during periods of disintegration? The first question must be answered in the affirmative; the second represents a fascinating but still to be concluded chapter in biological psychiatry.

These three examples are all related to the central MA metabolism, and this is no coincidence. The MA have so far had a central place in human and animal brain and behaviour research, but certainly not because MA-ergic systems were believed to play a more or less exclusive role in behaviour regulation. The preference is not fundamental, but technically determined. It is relatively easy to determine concentrations of MA and their metabolites. Moreover, the MA metabolism is a linear process: there is a mother substance and there are end-products, and this means that turnover measurements can be established without undue difficulties. This cannot be said of other central transmitters such as acetylcholine and γ-aminobutyric acid. Nevertheless, the relation between MA-ergic and other transmitter systems will undoubtedly be the subject of intensive research in the next decade.

7. The significance of psychotropic drugs in experimental behaviour research

Psychotropic drugs are pacemakers of biological psychiatric research. Their scientific significance, however, extends further. To begin with, there is the fact that psychopathology owes much to psychopharmacology.

Towards the end of the forties, the field of psychiatric syndrome identification and differentiation seemed to have been fully explored. Then came the psychotropic drugs. Of patients with apparently related syndromes, some did and others did not respond to a given type of compound. This observation led to an unheard-of revival of psychopathological research, but this time with the aid of sophisticated statistical techniques. This brings us to a third field in which psychotropic drugs have served as pacemakers—that of psychometrics. A therapist who administers a drug wants to know (i.e. to measure) what it does and does not do. For this purpose, various instruments have been evolved, e.g. questionnaires, self-rating scales and standardized interviews. These are not ideal measuring methods, but they are suitable to ensure a degree of desubjectivation of psychopathological research and to enhance the transferability and reproducibility of results.

This is an essential step forward, for psychiatric diagnosis has been notoriously unreliable. No two psychiatrists, it is said (and not entirely without justification), make the same diagnosis when confronted with a given patient. An important reason for this lies in the strong resonance, in psychiatric diagnosis, of theoretical (mostly depth psychological and sociological) concepts concerning the origin of behaviour disorders. The psychiatrist is thus tempted to observe whatever fits the theory, and to ignore all that seems inconsistent with it. Psychometric instruments, however, force the investigator to assess the entire range of symptoms in accordance with strictly defined rules. Experience has shown that, with these instruments, a fair level of agreement in diagnostic evaluation can be attained, at least so far as the disease symptoms are concerned; with regard to aetiology agreement is unfortunately less readily reached as yet.

Psychometric research as it is now being carried out in psychiatry is no longer an esoteric pastime for clinical psychologists but an applied psychiatric auxiliary discipline; and this it owes largely to the psychotropic drugs.

In psychiatric circles, it is true, psychometric methods have been received with mixed feelings. They have been described as crude and impersonal, and neither charge can be denied. These methods are relatively crude, but it should be borne in mind that they are still young and will be further developed and sophisticated. They are impersonal also, but then that is precisely what they are meant to be. After all, their principal area of application is within the limits of psychopharmacology or, to be less restrictive, within the limits of the biological psychiatric experiment. As we have pointed out, biological psychiatric research is characterized above all by the features of natural science and experiment. In this context the psychiatric patient is studied, not as an individual, unique, inimitable entity, but as an instance of general variables. The focus is not on what distinguishes him from other patients with related syndromes, but precisely on what he has in common with them. Such an approach calls for diagnostic aids which to some extent are "depersonalized." In actual practice, these methods cannot (and therefore must not) replace strictly individualized diagnosis; very often, however, they are able to provide valuable supplements to this diagnosis.

The biologically-oriented psychiatrist thus follows a path which in some psychiatric circles has for years been regarded as rather unfashionable. He generalizes and schematizes in an effort to objectify mental illness. His orientation is largely descriptive and presentative, more "static" than "dynamic." He wants to explain rather than understand. He renounces the totality in favour of a few component parts, and he is therefore deliberately limited—that is to say, fully aware of the fact that his man-image is an incomplete, reduced image. He is motivated not by philosophical pretense but exclusively by the need to find an adequate test arrangement.

After the brief digression in the above paragraph, let us revert to the subject. The rapid rise of psychopharmacotherapy has revived the interest in a problem too much neglected since the thirties: the problem of psychiatric diagnosis and nosology. Obviously, the psychiatrist closely cooperates with the experimental clinical psychologist in this respect. The latter occupies an indispensable place in the psychopharmacological team, along with the psychiatrist, biochemist, physiologist and pharmacologist.

Some psychiatrists have expressed the fear that the evolution of psychopharmacotherapy will inevitably lead in the long run to an attenuation of psychiatric diagnosis. It follows from the above discussion that this fear is without justification. What characterizes the clinical psychopharmacologist is precisely his dual character of "naturalist" and "alienist." Not only does his problem definition stimulate research in a purely somatic direction, but it equally demands of him a renewed orientation (a renewed experimental orientation) on psychopathological description and differentiation. It is this dual character that I consider to be typical of psychopharmacological research. It is its principal characteristic, and its hallmark.

8. Conclusions

Psychiatry is based on three models: the psychological/psychodynamic, the social/sociological, and the medical/neurobiological. Biological psychiatry is that branch of psychiatry that concerns itself with the last mentioned model.

Psychotropic drugs have played an important role in the rapid scientific exploration of this field in the past 20 years. They have played this role in several ways. Because they produce demonstrable effects on the molecular as well as on the behaviour level, they could serve as crystallization point for various hypotheses on relations between brain function and behaviour. Because research into the effects of psychotropic drugs on human behaviour is impossible without instruments for standardized registration of human behaviour, these drugs have lent strong impetus to the introduction of psychometric techniques in the psychiatric clinic. Because it was found that psychotropic drugs of a given group, e.g. antidepressants and neuroleptics, were not equally effective in all patients of the same nosological category, e.g. depression or schizophrenia, they revived the (experimentally oriented) interest in psychopathological description and differentiation. Psychotropic drugs, therefore, are of significance not only in practical therapeutic terms but also in purely scientific terms.

So far in the course of this century, a-biological trends—phenomenological, anthropological, psychodynamic and sociological—have dominated psychiatry. It is of great importance that the triple character of psychiatry be restored—that biological psychiatry be given an equivalent position beside psychodynamic and social psychiatry. A well-balanced distribution of attention would seem to be of advantage for psychiatric training, for the practical application of psychiatry, and for its further evolution.

BIBLIOGRAPHY

Abel, E. L. (1974). *Drugs and Behavior. A Primer in Neuropsychopharmacology*. New York: John Wiley.

Brown, H. (1976). *Brain and Behavior*. New York: Oxford University Press.

Mendels, J. (1973). *Biological Psychiatry*. New York: John Wiley.

Praag, H. M. van (1969). The complementary aspects in the relation between biological and psychodynamic psychiatry. *Psychiat. Clin.* 2, 307.

PRAAG, H. M. VAN (1971). The position of biological psychiatry among the psychiatric disciplines. *Compr. Psychiat.* 12, 1.

PRAAG, H. M. VAN (1972). Biologic psychiatry in perspective: The dangers of sectarianism in psychiatry. *Compr. Psychiat.* 13, 401.

PRAAG, H. M. VAN (1974). New developments in human psychopharmacology. *Compr. Psych.* 15, 389.

PRAAG, H. M. VAN (1977). *Depression and Schizophrenia. A Contribution on Their Chemical Pathology*. New York: Spectrum Publications.

PRAAG, H. M. VAN: The Scientific Foundation of anti-psychiatry. *Acta Psychiat. Scand.* In Press.

ROSE, S. (1976). *The Conscious Brain*. London: Penguin Books.

SMYTHIES, J. R. (1970). *Brain Mechanism and Behavior*. Oxford, Edinburgh: Blackwell.

WARBURTON, D. M. (1975). *Brain, Behaviour and Drugs*. New York: John Wiley.

WATTS, G. O. (1976). *Dynamic Neuroscience*. New York: Harper and Row.

PART TWO

Pharmacotherapy of Psychoses

What I fully savoured was the wave of optimism and hope which the psychotropic drugs produced when the first of them were introduced into the clinics while I was still a resident.

The patients could be free. One went along with them to another hospital for a football match. One was very busy organizing these events: Delta Boys against Schakenbosch Wanderers, or something. There were older psychiatrists who addressed us. They were moved and said: how marvellous that we have lived to see this; that this is possible. I heard psychotropic drugs being discussed in this vein. With emotion and affection.

J. Van Londen, Maandblad Geestelijke
Volksgezondheid, June 1976.

VI

Diagnosing Psychoses, Particularly Schizophrenia

1. Psychoses and their classification

Neuroleptics combine a sedative with an antipsychotic effect, deriving their identity from the latter. Psychoses are defined as conditions in which the stability of the ego structure is seriously affected—in which the various psychological functions which constitute the psyche are no longer adequately matched. Often an element is added to this definition, namely that the patients make serious errors in evaluating their life situation (disturbance in reality testing). They are no longer able adequately to test ideas and conceptions against earlier experiences in order to estimate their reality value. This definition of the term psychosis is a very general one. It is not surprising that widely diverse symptoms can be placed in this context: delusions, hallucinations, disorientation with regard to time, place and person, anxiety, various motor disorders, and many other symptoms. It is therefore the more surprising that the symptomatology is hardly "weighed" in the classification of psychoses, let alone the criterion prognosis. Exactly as in the classification of depressions, efforts are confined to an indication of the principal aetiological factors:

1. Psychoses caused by acquired somatic diseases. Within this category, a further distinction is made between organic and symptomatic psychoses. The former involve a demonstrable morphological lesion in the brain (e.g. cerebral arteriosclerosis), and the latter involve a somatic disease which has not demonstrably affected the morphology of the brain (e.g. psychoses associated with endocrine disorders).

2. Psychoses which develop in response to severe intrapsychic tensions, which in turn are the product of a combination of intrapsychic conflicts and pressure from the environment. These psychoses are known as psychogenic psychoses—a category widely used in The Netherlands and Scandinavian countries but not in Anglo-American literature.

3. Psychoses of unknown aetiology in which familial-hereditary factors are sometimes demonstrable. Kraepelin called them "endogenous," but Anglo-American literature refers to them as "functional" psychoses. This category comprises the manic-depressive psychoses and schizophrenia.

Such an exclusively aetiological classification would be justifiable only if the factor aetiology would determine the nature of the syndrome to a high degree of probability. But this is not at all the case. Let us take the random example of the delirious syndrome. This can be due to "organic" factors (e.g. cerebral arteriosclerosis), but can also be "symptomatic" (e.g. in febrile diseases); or it can occur in response to severe emotional stress. I therefore regard the current classification of psychoses as hopelessly deficient.

All over the world the "functional" psychoses have received more attention than the "organic" psychoses. It can in fact be safely stated that the latter group has been scientifically neglected as to aetiology, pathogenesis and therapy. More than the manic-depressive psychoses, schizophrenia has on the other hand held an almost mysterious attraction for investigators. There have been innumerable publications on schizophrenia, but nevertheless the concept cannot be said to have been clarified. In spite of this, I intend to add yet another essay to the long list. This does not claim to abolish confusion, but merely aims to highlight a few points which have caused it. Identification of these points could perhaps indicate a way out of the confusion.

The concept of manic-depressive psychoses will be discussed in chapter XII.

2. Questions about schizophrenia

In 1896, in the fifth edition of his "Psychiatrie," Kraepelin used the designation *dementia praecox* to refer to a group of syndromes which had in common "a peculiar destruction of internal connections of the personality and a marked damage of emotional and volitional life." This conception encompassed three diagnostic categories of an earlier time: *démence précoce* (Morel, 1860), *hebephrenia* (Hecker, 1871) and *catatonia* (Kahlbaum, 1874). Kraepelin differentiated between dementia praecox and a group of syndromes with paranoid symptoms but without severe defects in emotional life and volitional functions, which he called *paraphrenia.* In the sixth edition of his textbook, he brought dementia praecox and manic-depressive psychosis together under the heading "endogenous psychoses"—a conception which has held its own in the diagnosis of psychoses to this very day.

In his monograph on schizophrenic psychoses, published in 1911, Bleuler rejected the designation dementia praecox because, he maintained, the disease need not inevitably lead to overall deterioration of the personality and does not necessarily start at an early age. He regarded the loss of coherence and interaction between the various psychological functions as the crucial disturbance, and therefore proposed the term "schizophrenia."

The term schizophrenia has been generally accepted. Yet the syndrome referred to by this name has remained a persistent source of controversy and uncertainty. The crucial question was and still is: Does schizophrenia exist? In fact this is a composite question which has two components. The first question is whether schizophrenia is a classical disease entity with a more or less unequivocal "morphology," or rather a collective name which covers a whole range of subtypes. This is not a controversial question—it is unanimously answered in favour of the latter alternative. The second question is: Do these subtypes have common characteristics in terms of symptomatology, pathological mechanisms or clinical course? If so, then they can be brought under a single denominator and the collective designation schizophrenia has its justification. If not, then the schizophrenia concept has no justification and there is every reason to view the so-called subtypes as independent disease entities and to study them as such.

There has been no unanimous answer to this question. In fact, very few empirical studies have been done on which a conclusion could be based. This has been an enormous handicap to biological schizophrenia research, for we do not know whether the patients in whom this diagnosis has been made are, in fact, a somewhat homogeneous group. In spite of all this, research into biological determinants of schizophrenic behaviour has not been unproductive in the past five years. This has been possible because biochemical psychopharmacology has provided such vigorous impulses as to compensate for the paucity of creative psychopathological research.

In the following sections of this chapter I shall briefly discuss the symptomatology, aetiology and course of schizophrenic psychoses. The intention is not to present a comprehensive review but primarily to demonstrate how unsettled the diagnosis of schizophrenia is and how sorely this concept needs revision on the basis of empirical psychopathological studies. Possible pathogenetic mechanisms will be discussed in chapter XI. Finally I shall describe a simple system of classifying patients with schizophrenic psychoses and selecting, very tentatively, a subgroup which I shall call *nuclear schizophrenia*. Until more solid diagnostic parameters become available, this type of classification can perhaps be useful in coping with the worst of the prevalent confusion.

3. Schizophrenic syndromes

Several different syndromes have been described under the heading schizophrenia. To begin with, there is *hebephrenia*, an exuberant psychiatric syndrome with massive hallucinations and/or delusions, loss of contact with the environment, and loss of initiative, which usually starts at an early age, i.e. during puberty or early adolescence. Next comes *paraphrenia*, in which the patient develops systematized but encapsulated paranoid delusions but shows no overall disintegration of the personality (which is why some psychiatrists do not regard this syndrome as schizophrenic). Unlike paraphrenia, *dementia paranoides* is characterized by barely systematized paranoid delusions and progressive deterioration of the entire personality. The predominant features in *dementia simplex* are loss of initiative and autism, while delusions and hallucinations are not very pronounced. *Catatonia*, finally, is a psychotic syndrome characterized by predominance of motor disorders such as stereotypes, stupor, grimacing, etc.

Not by any stretch of the imagination can these syndromes be brought under the same denominator. They are as dissimilar as circulatory shock and the syndrome of an inflamed gall bladder. But this is not all. Bleuler, for example, has continually expanded the schizophrenia concept. He rejected the independent existence of presenile paranoid states, alcoholic dementia, schizophreniform syndromes associated with brain lesions, infections, and intoxications. All these he regarded as latent schizophrenia becoming manifest. Latent schizophrenia, moreover, he believed to be more common than manifest schizophrenia; and with this the schizophrenia concept loses all boundaries. Kraepelin did not show this tendency. On the contrary, he tried to define the schizophrenia concept more and more exactly; yet he did not abandon his conception of the many subtypes.

4. Schizophrenic symptoms

A second question is whether there exist symptoms characteristic of schizophrenia—symptoms which, regardless of the other components of the syndrome, can be encountered in any type of schizophrenia.

Pathognomonic symptoms?

Kraepelin listed the principal symptoms of schizophrenia as: poor insight, decline of mental flexibility and performance, blunting of affect, and a loosening of internal unity. As features of more or less secondary diagnostic importance he listed: hallucinations, delusions, depressive mood, motor pathology, volitional disturbances, negativism and "Befehlsautomatie" (automatic response to commands). Bleuler considered loosening of associations and "splitting of the personality" essential for the diagnosis of schizophrenia. Splitting means dissociation: dissociation of emotions from ideas, of expression from emotion, of conduct from intentions, and so on. He regarded these symptoms as direct consequences of a supposed brain disease. He dismissed such symptoms as hallucination, delusion, confusion, twilight states, manic and depressive changes of mood, and catatonic symptoms as subordinate and not essential to the diagnosis.

Both Kraepelin and Bleuler showed little finesse in operationalizing the diagnostic criteria for schizophrenia. Moreover, several of the symptoms they deemed characteristic cannot be diagnosed without a fair amount of subjective interpretation; this impedes their transferability. The most carefully elaborated attempt to describe symptoms pathognomonic for schizophrenia was made by Schneider (1959). He described 11 of them, which he called symptoms of the first rank. The presence of any of these symptoms was sufficient to warrant a diagnosis of schizophrenia, unless gross anatomical abnormalities were present in the brain. The first three are specific types of auditory hallucinations:

1) the patient hears voices which say his thoughts aloud;
2) the patient hears voices which talk about him;
3) the patient hears voices which describe his activities.

The fourth symptom is that of delusional percept: a normal perception is followed by an erroneous interpretation with a very special, patient-oriented significance. Symptoms 5 through 11 are expressions of gradual effacement of the boundary between self and environment:

5) the patient is a passive recipient of exogenous physical influences which he cannot resist; they are associated with physical (hallucinatory) sensations (somatic passivity);
6) the patient experiences his own thoughts as introduced into him from outside (thought intrusion);
7) the patient's thoughts are taken away from him by some outside agency (thought removal);
8) the patient believes that he can transfer his thoughts to others by magic means (thought broadcast).

Symptoms 9 through 11 encompass the patient's belief that his affects, impulses and motor activities are imposed on him by some external agency which also controls him in these respects. These ideas are not accompanied by hallucinatory physical sensations.

Subjective criteria

Schneider's choice of the symptoms of the first order was not based on theoretical considerations, but was entirely pragmatic: they could be most readily diagnosed in a patient. On the other hand, there are psychiatrists whose diagnostic preference is for symptoms which it is difficult to objectify, i.e. those which can be established only in communicative contact with the patient. They focus primarily on the patient's ability to enter an affective relationship with another person, and on the extent to which he shows affective "resonance" in such a contact. Disturbances in this ability are regarded as "highly suspect." Conclusions concerning these phenomena are largely based on subjective interpretation, and this is why different evaluators often reach different conclusions. Moreover, the psychiatrist's own ability to establish contacts is, of course, also involved. Last but not least: in actual practice one is often confronted with the question: Is the patient really suffering from restrictive affect or does he suppress his feelings; is this contact really deficient or does he keep at a safe distance due to (neurotic) fear? To put it in diagnostic terms: Are we dealing with a neurotic reaction with serious repression, or indeed with a schizophrenic syndrome?

Rümke (1967) introduced a purely subjective criterion. He maintained that there are actually no symptoms specific to schizophrenia. The diagnosis is in fact made on the basis of a feeling which the patient evokes in the investigator—the so-called praecox feeling. He tried to define this as a sense of estrangement—one senses that one's own overtures meet an obstacle. The patient accepts nothing of what the investigator offers: contact, warmth, understanding. Recognition of this praecox feeling in oneself requires a well-developed empathic ability on the part of the investigator. Since the phenomenon is so difficult to explicate, it is hardly transferable.

Empirical studies

The Schneider criteria prompt two questions. The first is: Are symptoms of the first rank sufficiently common in schizophrenia to have diagnostic value? The second is: Are they truly pathognomonic, i.e. do they differentiate between schizophrenia and other syndromes? Research results in connection with the first question are not unequivocal. Mellor (1970) examined 166 patients diagnosed as schizophrenic for symptoms of the first rank, and found one or several of these symptoms in 119 (72%). He then studied the frequency distribution of these symptoms in "Schneider-positive" patients. Auditory hallucinations were found in 13% of the patients. Delusional perception and the feeling that emotions and impulses are influenced by others were relatively rare: 6%, 6% and 3% of cases, respectively. The frequency of the other symptoms ranged from 9% to 21%.

Taylor (1972) studied the case histories of 78 patients diagnosed as schizophrenic, and found the abovementioned symptoms in 22 (28%). A study by Carpenter et al. (1973) revealed first-rank symptoms in 51% of 103 schizophrenic patients. Thought removal was the least frequent symptom (15%) and thought broadcast was the most common (33%).

Not only the diagnostic but also the discriminative value of the first-rank symptoms is rather limited. For example, one or several of these symptoms proved to be present also in 23% of patients diagnosed as manic-depressive.

My conclusion is that a wide variety of syndromes have been described under the heading schizophrenia, and that empirical studies have failed to reveal clearly pathognomonic symptoms. In symptomatological terms, therefore, there are no grounds to bring the various syndromes described as schizophrenic under a common denominator.

5. Aetiological views: hereditary factors

Kraepelin included dementia praecox among the chiefly hereditary psychoses. Genetic research in subsequent years has demonstrated that hereditary factors are indeed involved. The arguments derive from three types of research. The first is pedigree studies. Schizophrenia is much more frequent among close relatives of schizophrenic patients than in the total population; and the frequency is as much higher as the blood relationship is closer, i.e. higher in brothers, sisters, children and parents of schizophrenic patients than in uncles, aunts, nephews and nieces. In second-degree relatives, too, the incidence is higher than that in the total population (if not much higher). The marked accumulation of schizophrenic pathology in certain families has also been used as an argument by protagonists of family theories on schizophrenia. They argue that, rather than parent-child transmission of genes, family pathology is responsible for the disease: the chaotic, confusing climate in which the child is brought up and in which it learns irrational ways of reacting.

The second type of research involves twin studies. The concordance rate of schizophrenic psychoses is substantially higher in monozygotic than in dizygotic twins. This phenomenon, too, need not necessarily be interpreted genetically. The ties between identical twins are often very close, and the tendency to identify is very strong. If one of the twins becomes psychotic, then the other is very likely to develop a similar pattern of behaviour. This is a psychological interpretation, which is not entirely plausible. In identical twins brought up separately, the concordance rate of schizophrenia was likewise high, and comparable with that in twins brought up together.

The third type of research involves studies of children born from one or two schizophrenic parents but brought up, not by the biological parents but in foster families. So far, all these studies have led to the same conclusion. The incidence of schizophrenic psychoses was much higher in these children than in the children of their foster parents, with whom they were jointly brought up.

Transmission is probably not by a single gene but by a number of genes, each of which adds a given element, or dimension, to the schizophrenic behaviour pattern. The variability of schizophrenic symptomatology; the often irrefutable significance of environmental influences; the frequent impossibility of establishing or excluding the diagnosis with certainty; the gradual transitions between what is called normal if somewhat eccentric behaviour and schizophrenic symptoms—all these are more readily explained by a polygenic theory than by a theory which postulates a single active gene. In genetic terms, a variable number of pathological genes carried could readily explain the variability of symptoms and clinical courses within the group of schizophrenic psychoses.

6. Aetiological views: exogenous factors

Schizophrenia, however, proved not exclusively to be linked to endogenous factors. The syndrome was observed also in patients with demonstrable anatomical brain damage. The widely discussed question has been whether these cases involved "genuine" schizophrenia (the quotation marks are mine) which had been latent prior to the brain injury and was made manifest by it, or really organic schizophrenia. Since the concept "latent schizophrenia" has hardly been operationalized (although it is certainly multi-interpretable), and empirical studies were consequently omitted, the question was never answered and continued to serve as a favorite subject of learned discussions.

On the basis of my own clinical, but not systematized, experience, I would say that the label "provoked latent schizophrenia" is unsuitable in quite a few cases of schizophrenia associated with organic cerebral lesions. I reach this conclusion in view of an untainted family history, a "clean" psychiatric history, and a more or less normal premorbid personality structure in these cases. On this basis I suspect that organic schizophrenia does exist. An argument against my suspicion is that the anatomical lesion in organic (?) schizophrenia has no specific characteristics as to type or localization. It can be of an inflammatory, degenerative or neoplastic type and, so far as we know, schizophrenic syndromes can be observed in association with virtually any localization. Given a direct causal relation, one would expect schizophrenic behaviour disorders to occur only in association with particular lesions of a particular localization. What can be concluded is that the problem of organic schizophrenia is yet to be solved.

The term "organic" invites a few additional remarks in passing. In psychiatry, the term is used with reference to a group of psychoses which occur in the presence of a demonstrable anatomical brain lesion. The psychoses in which this is not the case are sometimes referred to as "functional." This has gradually led to the misconception that only organic psychoses have a cerebral substrate. I have pointed out the untenability of this view in chapter V. If this terminology is to be maintained, then the two types of psychosis should be defined as follows. Organic psychoses are psychoses in whose aetiology anatomical brain damage plays an important role. Their pathogenesis, i.e. the complex of cerebral functional disorders which enables the psychotic behaviour disorders to occur, is unknown. In functional psychoses there are no demonstrable anatomical lesions in the brain; of their pathogenesis we possibly know a few features (chapter VII) and in their aetiology the emphasis seems to be on hereditary and/or psychosocial factors.

7. Aetiological views: psychological and social factors

Bleuler's "reactive schizophrenia" and what this conception has brought about

More frequently than anatomical lesions of the brain, disorders of the (premorbid) personality structure were observed in patients with schizophrenic symptoms, and the period preceding the manifest psychosis was found to have been coloured by intrapsychic and/or more relationally determined tensions. In the fourth edition of his textbook, Bleuler differentiated between "process schizophrenia" and "reactive schizophrenia"—forms which overlap in symptomatological terms but differ in that the former should have a chiefly organic aetiology, whereas the latter should be largely psychogenic. This distinction has given rise to numerous obscurities in classification, symptomatological hair-splitting, and aetiological misunderstandings which have continued to burden psychiatric diagnosis to this very day. Let me discuss a few; any attempt at comprehensiveness would produce a whole book on the evolution of diagnostic thinking in psychiatry.

1) Many followed Bleuler's example and divided the schizophrenias into two groups. As to nomenclature, everyone followed his own taste. This led to such categories as true schizophrenia versus schizophreniform psychoses (Langfeldt, 1959); true schizophrenia versus pseudo-schizophrenia (Rümke, 1967), and many others. As the number of dichotomies increased, the criteria were watered down. The dichotomy was made on the basis of aetiology (psychogenic versus non-psychogenic), course (poor versus good prognosis), and symptomatology (presence or absence of so-called essential symptoms), as such or in various combinations.

2) New categories of psychoses were distinguished and differentiated from schizophrenia. By way of example I mention psychogenic and degenerative psychoses. Psychogenic psychosis was differentiated on the basis of aetiological considerations. This category encompassed psychoses interpreted as the catastrophic

nadir of a neurotic development, as the extreme consequence of unsolved psychological problems. The differentiation of a category of degenerative psychoses was justified with reference to symptomatology and aetiology as well as course. This type of psychosis was described as one with frequent relapses, without a distinct psychogenic cause, and complete remission to the premorbid level after each phase. Moreover, the syndrome varied markedly from phase to phase. In recurrent forms of schizophrenia, the syndrome was believed to be much less variable.

How valid are these differentiations? For example, is the course of a psychogenic psychosis essentially changed by psychotherapy, or does the syndrome tend to relapse nevertheless, the psychogenic provocation becoming less and less evident? Such a course of events is repeatedly seen in "true" schizophrenia. Is it really true that the personality structure remains undamaged in degenerative psychosis, or do these patients come to resemble chronic schizophrenics after all? In the absence of empirical studies, these questions must remain moot.

In any case, genetic findings do not justify these differentiations. Conditions known as schizophreniform psychosis, symptomatic schizophrenia, psychogenic psychosis, degenerative psychosis, atypical or reactive schizophrenia, schizo-affective psychosis, or borderline schizophrenia—all are genetically linked to "true" schizophrenia. They seem to be members of the same genetic family.

3) The introduction of the psychogenic schizophrenia concept also caused partial effacement of the boundaries between schizophrenia and non-psychotic behaviour disorders. A wide variety of strange, inexplicable character traits; a tendency towards reticence; relational deficiencies (to mention only a few phenomena)—these were all labeled "schizoid" or, worse, diagnosed as pseudoneurotic schizophrenia, and given a room in the vast mansion called schizophrenia. This is one of the reasons for the fact that statistics on the incidence of schizophrenia in different countries and institutions show differences which ridicule the concept of scientific classification.

So much for the diagnostic confusion caused by the concept of reactive (psychogenic) schizophrenia. Let us now revert to the concept itself.

The aetiological weight of psychosocial factors

Few psychiatrists will maintain that the psychopathology of the schizophrenic patient as a rule begins with the manifestation of the psychosis. In many cases the life history reveals such factors as: an unhappy parental marital life; a youth during which patient was exposed to excessive expressions of aggressivity and hostility among the parents; abnormalities in the personality of one or both parents, and so on. Family theorists such as Lidz, Bateson, Laing and many others have rightly emphasized that mutual relations in the home of a schizophrenic patient can be very disturbed, "schizophrenic." There is no question about this. Questions arise when we consider the aetiological weight of these factors. Can they constitute a principal cause, or is their significance limited to provocation of latent schizophrenia? As with organic schizophrenia, an unequivocal answer to this question cannot be given. On the one hand, every clinician regularly sees cases in which psychogenic problems are inextricably entangled in the manifestation and in the content of the psychosis. This is an argument in favour of the psychogenic schizophrenia concept. An argument against this concept is the absence of any specificity. Psychodynamic mechanisms described in schizophrenia are also encountered in a variety of non-schizophrenic, non-psychotic psychiatric disorders.

The same applies to family tragedies. There is not a trace of evidence that the communication pathology described is specific to the family life of schizophrenic patients, or that this pathology accumulates within this category of patients. Authors in this corner of the field, moreover, tend to think somewhat naively in analogues. They discern a direct causal relation between irrationalities which they discover in the patient's family relations and irrationalities in the patient himself. Their conclusions: the disturbed behaviour, e.g. patient's conviction that his thoughts are literally removed from him, is directly provoked by the domineering mother; his incoherent line of thoughts is derived, or rather learned, from the sadomasochistic associations between his parents. For the sake of convenience it is overlooked that the mother is not suffering from delusions and that the parents are capable of coherent communication (unless they suffer from schizophrenic psychoses). This is reminiscent of an attempt to explain the excretory functions of the body directly from the ingestion of food, ignoring such factors as digestion and metabolism. Moreover, but this in passing, family theorists have tended to disregard the notion that schizophrenic family tragedies could develop secondarily, i.e. in response to the patient's disturbed (and disturbing) behaviour.

Be this as it may, the aspecificity of the psychodynamic and psychosocial mechanisms reduces their aetiological weight and necessitates introduction of a factor x, which renders the psychosis manifest. This is why of the two concepts—psychogenically provoked schizophrenia and psychogenic schizophrenia—the former seems to me to be the most plausible.

To avoid misunderstandings, it should be pointed out that my use of the word aspecificity with regard to the psychodynamic mechanisms described refers to the *form* of the disturbed behaviour. When the same mechanism can lead to, say, a delusional syndrome, a hallucinatory syndrome or a compulsive syndrome, then it is inadequate as a mode of explanation. A different matter is that this mechanism can indeed be specific with regard to the *content* of the disturbed behaviour. A delusion of sin, the hearing of threatening voices, and a washing ritual can each give expression to unassimilated guilt feelings rooted in the individual course of development. Very often, psychodynamic and psychosocial mechanisms do indeed have a high degree of specificity with regard to the substance of disturbed thinking and experiencing, and they can give a modicum of insight into the sense of the psychotic "nonsense."

8. Aetiological views: conclusion

The aetiology of schizophrenic psychoses involves, not a single factor but a pattern of factors; so much seems certain. However, we do not know what this pattern looks like, nor whether one pattern underlies all types of schizophrenia or whether a given pattern of factors is required for a given syndrome to become manifest. For the time being, therefore, there is no reason to bring schizophrenic syndromes under a common denominator on the basis of aetiological criteria.

9. The course of schizophrenic psychoses

In Kraepelin's definition of dementia praecox, the poor prognosis was a central feature. The patient would either show gradual deterioration without evident remissions, or an intermittent course with incomplete remission after each phase, finally leading to a chronic defect state. Let me mention in passing that the diagnosis "chronic schizophrenia" is very ill-defined. In actual practice the designation serves as a receptacle for numerous serious but possibly diverse personality defects which markedly impede the patient's social adjustment and in which there is no demonstrable interference with the anatomical integrity of the brain.

In his monograph, Bleuler made a rather half-hearted effort to attack the prognostic criterion. In one place he stated that schizophrenia is incurable, or at least that *restitutio ad integrum* does not occur, but elsewhere he maintained that the disease can recede or be arrested in any stage.

In subsequent years the prognostic criterion has been used entirely at will. Some authors have remained faithful to Kraepelin, using the term schizophrenia only if the prognosis is obviously unfavourable and considering complete recovery to be inconsistent, by definition, with a diagnosis of schizophrenia. In the case of complete recovery they speak of schizophreniform psychosis or pseudoschizophrenia, or classify the syndrome in a separate diagnostic category, e.g. that of psychogenic or degenerative psychoses (see section 7 above). Others regard the prognostic criterion as inconclusive, and diagnose schizophrenia mainly on symptomatological grounds. They belong to the group of psychiatrists who have claimed therapeutic, especially psychotherapeutic, success and who vehemently refute the incurability of schizophrenia. This may seem to be a battle of principles; in reality it is a semantic conflict. If we define the term carcinoma as a collective name for all (benign and malignant) tumours, then we can claim a high cure rate; if we confine the term carcinoma to malignant tumours, then the cure rate is low. Let me add immediately, however, that the emphasis on the curability of schizophrenia has been beneficial in a practical sense: types of schizophrenia with in principle a favourable prognosis received adequate (psycho)therapy; and schizophrenic patients bound to show an unfavourable prognosis were treated more humanely than in the past.

The controversy intensified with the introduction of the neuroleptics. Many patients regarded as schizophrenic made a rapid recovery in response to these agents. Is this a reason to revise the diagnosis, or are there two types of schizophrenia—one that is curable and the other that is not (yet) curable? The answer to this question is of necessity an arbitrary one. Our present knowledge warrants no well-argued decision. We are waiting for a decision *ex cathedra* by a psychiatric council, or for empirical studies. I definitely prefer the latter.

In all, we find that the syndromes called schizophrenic can apparently take any conceivable course: rapid complete recovery; recovery with residual personality damage; a chronic recurrent course with or without personality damage after each active phase; and a chronic course. The prognostic criterion, therefore, is unsuitable to unite all the syndromes characterized as schizophrenic.

10. Three-dimensional classification of schizophrenic psychoses

Aetiological aspecificity of psychiatric syndromes

In psychopathology, there is no predictable relation between aetiology and syndrome. For example, psychogenic factors can be responsible for neurotic symptoms, involved in the development of psychoses, and causative of dissocial behaviour. Inversely, it is impossible to infer the aetiology from the nature and course of a given syndrome. Example: a vital depression can be of chiefly hereditary determination; it can occur in response to severe psychosocial stress; or it can be provoked by somatic diseases such as a viral infection, e.g. infectious hepatitis.

The fact that psychiatric syndromes are aetiologically aspecific has an important implication. The implication is that these behaviour disorders must always be classified on the basis of three criteria: *symptomatology, aetiology* and *course*. This means that one-word diagnoses such as neurosis, depression and schizophrenia are futile. There are two possibilities: either they suggest something about symptomatology, aetiology and course simultaneously, but not explicitly, giving these concepts the diagnostic depth of focus of a poor photograph (e.g. the schizophrenia concept); or they are used sometimes in the symptomatological and at other times in the aetiological sense, thus creating chaos rather than diagnostic order (e.g. the neurosis concept).

In the following I shall apply the principle of three-dimensional classification to the group of psychoses which generally involve no clouding of consciousness, in which there is usually no severe anatomical brain damage, and which are commonly referred to as schizophrenic. This procedure makes it possible to form groups of patients which tend to be homogeneous and are recognizable to other investigators. These are prerequisites for reduplication studies. Moreover, this is the only way to distinguish, within the group of schizophrenic psychoses, subgroups which differ from other categories in, say, response to therapy, pathogenesis or prognosis. This method of classification is primarily intended for research purposes, but I believe that it is useful also in daily practice and enhances the precision of diagnostic evaluation.

Symptomatological typology of schizophrenic psychoses

A system of diagnostic classification is not a catalogue. It does not encompass all conceivable symptoms but only those which are often prominent. In the classification of each individual patient I propose to mention which of the following symptoms are present.

1) *Lowered level of consciousness*. The old rule that consciousness is unclouded in schizophrenia seems to be generally correct, although in acute psychoses which occur in response to marked psychological stress, the level of consciousness can be lowered during the first few days or weeks. In the more chronic schizophrenic psychoses, consciousness is always unclouded.

2) *Delusions, defined as ideas whose content is probably incompatible with reality but which nevertheless cannot be corrected*. The content of these ideas is indicated whenever paranoid delusions or delusions of influence are involved. The former category comprises ideas of being in some way wronged by external agencies; the latter category comprises ideas that external agencies influence one's thinking, feeling or physical functioning, or that one has the power so to influence others. The suggestion to note specifically whether a delusion is paranoid arises from the uncertainty whether paranoid states do or do not come under the heading schizophrenia. This uncertainty is upheld by two data: the fact that the personality structure outside the paranoid foci is often quite intact, and the fact that the course is often not progressive. The suggestion to note specifically whether a delusion is one of being influenced is based simply on the fact that this phenomenon has of old been regarded as "typically schizophrenic."

3) *Hallucination and delusional percept*. A true hallucination in-

volves sensory perception without sensory stimulation. If there is sensory stimulation but evidently faulty interpretation (e.g. the patient regards a glass bowl in his room as a functioning television screen), then the term delusional percept applies. In schizophrenic psychoses, auditory and tactile hallucinations (illusions) are believed to be predominant; the latter are often associated with delusions of being influenced. In organic psychoses, visual hallucinations are believed to be predominant.

4) *Emotional flattening*. A certain chilliness characterizes contacts with the patient. There is little evidence of (adequate) emotions at appropriate moments. The investigator consequently has a sense of difficulty in establishing a relation with the patient. There is no affective rapport. Attempts at empathy are unsuccessful. This emotional flattening or chilliness is most apparent in schizophrenic psychoses with a chronic course; it is by no means always pronounced in acute forms.

5) *Motor activity*. Schizophrenic psychoses can be accompanied by motor retardation, to the point of stupor, but also with hyperkinesia: grimacing, stereotyped movements, strange movements, etc. In the so-called catatonic stupor there is often more active resistance than passive endurance; this is evident from the high muscle tonus and the resistance encountered when an attempt is made to move, say, the limbs. The abnormal movements often have a symbolic significance for the patient.

6) *Inertia*. Loss of initiative is common in schizophrenic psychoses. The patient can hardly bring himself to meaningful activities. He stops working, stays at home, spends much time in bed. Contacts with the environment become scanty. Sometimes the inertia disappears as the psychosis disappears; in other cases it persists, or even increases, after disappearance of the other symptoms. In this case we have a cure with a residual defect. Inertia is an ominous symptom because it is so difficult to treat, and it can render the patient quite unsuitable for an existence in normal society.

7) *Incoherent train of thoughts*. This symptom is not seen in all types of schizophrenic psychosis. In association with unclouded consciousness, it signifies severe, diffuse disintegration.

Aetiological typology of schizophrenic psychoses

A carefully taken family history gives an impression of the weight of the endogenous (hereditary) factor. This factor is considered to be positive if psychoses are or have been present in first-degree or second-degree relatives. I propose that it be regarded as not positive if the taint exclusively involves manic-depressive manifestations, for there are arguments which indicate that schizophrenic psychoses and the group of manic-depressive syndromes are genetically different. Manic-depressive manifestations are rare in families with schizophrenic psychoses, and vice versa. Moreover, there has been no report on monozygotic twins of whom one was regarded as schizophrenic while the other suffered from a manic-depressive syndrome.

Involvement or non-involvement of pathogenic factors of a physical nature can be established by internal examination and neurological examination. The diagnosis should specify whether a cerebral lesion has been demonstrated, or a systemic disease which can be assumed possibly to interfere with cerebral function.

Finally, the contribution of psychogenic and social factors is to be evaluated. Here lurk dangers of deflation as well as of inflation. It is as confusing to inflate events of little significance to severe psychotraumata as it is to ignore serious frustrations or to wave them away as insignificant. Psychological stress prior to manifestation of the psychosis does not as such warrant the use of the term psychogenic (unless the stress has been excessive, and hardly bearable for a majority of people, e.g. the violence of war, natural disasters, etc.). It should be made plausible why this stress (which is usually assimilated independently) has exceeded the coping capacity of this particular individual. This is the case if:

1) A chronic intrapsychic conflict situation can be traced, which the patient cannot solve unaided and on which the stressful life situation was directly imposed.

2) The patient's (premorbid) personality structure shows weak spots which explain why he was unable independently to solve the conflict.

3) The weak spots in the personality structure can be related to disturbed psychological development.

The use in actual practice of the terms psychogenic and idiopathic as synonyms is a serious devaluation of the former concept.

Aetiologically, therefore, a given psychosis is classified as being of idiopathic, hereditary (endogenous), exogenous or psycho(socio)-

genic origin, or determined by a combination of the last three factors.

Typology of schizophrenic psychoses according to course

On the basis of this criterion, the following categories can be distinguished.

1) First psychotic phase with a duration of less than one year.
2) A history of several psychotic phases, each followed by restoration to the premorbid level. The number of phases is to be stated in the classification.
3) A history of several psychotic phases, with increasing damage to the personality structure after each phase.
4) Chronic schizophrenic psychoses, continuously existing for a year or longer, despite more or less adequate treatment (medication, psycho(socio)therapy).
5) Like 4), but with no or with evidently inadequate treatment. The duration of the psychosis is to be stated for categories 4) and 5).

Proposed nomenclature

I regard psychoses which take their course without clouding of consciousness as schizophrenic psychoses. The diagnosis is made exclusively on symptomatological grounds: presence of psychotic symptoms, or whatever type, while consciousness remains unclouded. The diagnosis is qualified as follows: schizophrenic psychosis characterized by . . . (follows an outline of the principal symptoms), provoked by . . . (follows an outline of the principal aetiological factors) and with a . . . (follows specification) course.

I deliberately use the term schizophrenic psychosis rather than schizophreniform (schizophrenia-like) psychosis because there is no agreement on what "true" schizophrenia really is. I do want to maintain the concept behind the designation "true schizophrenia," but on the basis of the considerations already presented I prefer the designation *nuclear schizophrenia*. I use the course as *sole* criterion for this diagnosis, describing a schizophrenic psychosis as nuclear if its course is unfavourable: chronic or chronic recurrent with personality deterioration. The deterioration should occur in spite of therapy which can be considered adequate, with both pharmacological and nonpharmcological means. Nuclear schizophrenia is symptomatologically a schizophrenic psychosis because consciousness remains unclouded during its course. Otherwise this concept has been entirely detached from symptomatological considerations and from the factor aetiology. I propose this unlinking because neither clinical features nor premorbid personality structure or presence or absence of precipitating factors warrant a reliable prediction about the prognosis of a schizophrenic psychosis.

Tentatively, I should like to circumscribe one group within the schizophrenic psychoses: that of the *psychogenic psychoses*. Apart from the fact that a disturbance of consciousness *may* occur during the first days or weeks, this category does not fundamentally differ symptomatologically from that of the schizophrenic psychoses. The diagnosis is based mainly on aetiological grounds: 1) evident involvement of psychosocial factors; 2) fading of the syndrome soon after removal of the patient from the situation which has become unbearable; 3) emergence of a neurotic personality structure after recession of the psychosis; 4) the investigator has reason to expect that psychotherapy will lead to stabilization of the personality and so to reduction of the risk of a relapse.

The psychogenic psychosis concept does not coincide with the category described by Robins and Guze (1970) as schizophrenia with a favourable prognosis. Criteria for the latter category include: acute onset, relatively undisturbed premorbid personality structure, and a family history which is untainted or tainted only by manic-depressive manifestations. In the group of psychogenic psychoses, however, neurotic problems of adjustment in the premorbid life situation are the rule, and the family history does include psychoses. Cases in which disintegration is gradual, over several weeks, are not uncommon.

Psychogenic psychosis is a provisional diagnosis because, not infrequently, the psychosis shows relapse tendency despite psychotherapy, and in subsequent psychotic phases the psychogenic aetiology is less and less apparent, leading to the conclusion that we are after all dealing with a schizophrenic psychosis.

I do not by any means propose this classification system as definitive. It is merely an aid, to be used in an effort finally to find a way out of the labyrinth we call schizophrenia; on the way, it can be adjusted, if necessary.

11. Conclusions

The schizophrenia controversy boils down to two controversial questions. The first is: Does schizophrenia exist as a recognizable disease entity? The second is: Is schizophrenia a biochemically, psychologically or socially determined disease? In other words: Is its main cause to be found in intracerebral metabolic disorders, in intrapsychic conflict situations, or in chronically disturbed family relations?

Kraepelin presented a fairly rigid definition of schizophrenia (although he called it dementia praecox). It was a syndrome with a given symptomatology, of chiefly hereditary determination, and with a poor prognosis. The schizophrenia concept has been more and more loosely used since Kraepelin. Schizophrenia, it was believed, could be caused also by psychogenic factors and by anatomical brain lesions. The prognosis need not be unfavourable; recovery was believed possible. The specificity of the symptoms became a perpetual source of dispute. Which symptoms are characteristic, which are secondary? Empirical studies were not started until half a century after Kraepelin's time, and have so far failed to reveal any pathognomonic symptoms, i.e. symptoms which are characteristic of schizophrenia and only sporadically found in other syndromes. For the time being, neither clinical features nor aetiology or course justify attempts to bring all the syndromes described as schizophrenic under a common denominator. This means that "schizophrenia" is a completely inadequate diagnosis. One should diagnose a schizophrenic psychosis with a given symptomatology, a given aetiology and a given course. The term schizophrenic psychosis is simply a collective name for psychoses which take their course without clouding of consciousness. The available empirical data do not permit a more exact definition. This is why a three-dimensional diagnosis of schizophrenic psychoses—i.e. their consistent classification according to three criteria: symptomatology, aetiology and course—is an indispensable requirement if ever we are to find our way out of the labyrinth of the schizophrenic psychoses.

The primary requirement today is empirical research in an effort to chart the schizophrenia concept. Such charting efforts should start from carefully defined syndromes and then consider whether, apart from the symptoms, there are other features which characterize the syndrome, e.g. aetiology, pathogenetic factors, course, or response to therapy. The more characteristic features, the greater the chance that we are dealing with a separate entity. Research of this kind has been in progress since the early seventies—having started some 70 years after the introduction of the schizophrenia concept. This seems to be characteristic of the rate of scientific development in psychiatry, and therefore is rather depressing.

The question of whether "schizophrenia" (the quotation marks naturally arise from the above considerations) is a biochemical or a psychosocial disease poses a spurious problem. Behavior is unthinkable without corresponding cerebral substrate. Disturbed behavior, therefore, presupposes a disturbed cerebral substrate. At least in principle, this disturbed cerebral substrate can be described in biochemical terms. In this sense, the schizophrenic psychoses, like any other behavior disorders, are biochemical diseases. A different question is whether the behavior disorders, including their cerebral substrate, are determined chiefly by psychosocial or (acquired or hereditary) somatic factors. It seems likely that both groups of factors play a role, but in varying relations of importance.

As long as pathogenesis and aetiology are not consistently differentiated in psychiatry, biologically and psychosocially orientated psychiatrists will face each other across a chasm; and consequently, theorization about and research into the causes of disturbed behavior must stagnate.

BIBLIOGRAPHY

Arieti, S. (1974). *Interpretation of Schizophrenia*. New York: Basic Books.

Bleuler, E. (1911). Dementia Praecox oder die Gruppe der Schizophrenien. In: G. Aschaffenburg (ed.) *Handbuch der Psychiatrie*. Leipzig: Euticke.

Bleuler, E. (1923). *Lehrbuch der Psychiatrie*. Berlin: Springer.

Carpenter, W. T., J.S. Strauss and S. Muleh (1973). Are there pathognomonic symptoms in schizophrenia? *Arch. gen. Psychiat.* 28, 847.

Faergeman, P. M. (1963). *Psychogenic Psychoses*. London: Butterworth and Co.

Falek, A. and H. M. Moser (1975). Classification in schizophrenia. *Arch. gen. Psychiat.* 32, 59.

Hecker, E. (1871). Die Hebephrenie. *Arch. Path. Anat. Physiol. Clim. Med.* 52, 394.

Hirsch, S. R. and J. P. Leff (1975). *Abnormalities in Parents of Schizophrenics*. London, New York, Toronto: Oxford University Press.

Kahlbaum, K. L. (1874). *Clinische Abhandlungen einige Psychische Krankheiten; I. Katatonia oder das Spannungsirresein*. Berlin: Springer.

Kendell, R. E. (1975). What are our criteria for a diagnosis of schizophrenia? In: H. M. van Praag (ed.) *On the Origin of Schizophrenic Psychoses*. Amsterdam: Erven Bohn.

KETY, S. S. (1975). Mental illness in the biological and adoptive families of adopted individuals who have become schizophrenic. In: H. M. van Praag (ed.) *On the Origin of Schizophrenic Psychosis*. Amsterdam: Erven Bohn.
KRAEPELIN, E. (1896). *Psychiatrie. Ein Lehrbuch für Studierende und Artzte*. Leipzig: Barth.
KRAEPELIN, E. (1899). *Psychiatrie. Ein Lehrbuch für Studierende und Arzte*. Leipzig: Barth.
LANGFELDT, G. (1959). *The Schizofreniform States*. London: Oxford University Press.
MELLOR, C. S. (1970). First rank symptoms of schizophrenia: I. The frequency in schizophrenics on admission to hospital; II. Differences between individual first rank symptoms. *Brit. J. Psychiat.* 117, 15.
MOREL, B. (1860). *Traité des maladies mentales*. Paris: Masson.
REICH, W. (1975). The spectrum concept of schizophrenia. *Arch. gen. Psychiat.* 32, 489.
REID, A. A. (1973). Schizophrenia—Disease or Syndrome? *Arch. gen. Psychiat.* 28, 863.
ROBINS, E. and S. B. GUZE (1970). Establishment of diagnostic validity in psychiatric illness: Its application to schizophrenia. *Amer. J. Psychiat.* 126, 983.
ROSENTHAL, D. (1970). *Genetic Theory and Abnormal Behavior*. New York: McGraw-Hill.
RÜMKE, H. C. (1967). Uber die Schizophrenic. In: H. C. Rümkc (ed.) *Eine blühende Psychiatrie in Gefahr*. Berlin: Springer.
SCHNEIDER, K. (1959). *Klinische Psychopathologie*. Stuttgart: Georg Thieme Verlag.
SEDGWICK, P. (1975). The social analysis of schizophrenia. Theories of Laing, Cooper etc. In: H. M. van Praag (ed.) *On the Origin of Schizophrenic Psychoses*. Amsterdam: Erven Bohn.
SERBAN, G. AND C. B. GIDYNSKI (1975). Differentiating criteria for acute-chronic distinction in schizophrenia. *Arch. gen. Psychiat.* 32, 705.
STRÖMGREN, E. (1975). Genetic factors in the origin of schizophrenia. In: H. M. van Praag (ed.) *On the Origin of Schizophrenic Psychoses*. Amsterdam: Erven Bohn.
TAYLOR, M. (1972). Schneiderian first-rank symptoms and clinical prognostic features in schizophrenia. *Arch. gen. Psychiat.* 26, 64.

VII

Neuroleptics I: Development, Therapeutic Effects, Indications

1. Concept definition and systematics

Neuroleptics are compounds which mainly act subcortically and, in human individuals, lead to various symptoms which are summarized as "neuroleptic syndrome." This syndrome comprises symptoms of three different types: psychological, extrapyramidal and vegetative. By slightly schematizing the complex influence of neuroleptics on the psyche, these compounds can be characterized as follows. They are strong sedatives with a not very pronounced hypnotic effect. In addition they have a series of effects which are called "antipsychotic"; the nature of these effects will be defined in section 4 of this chapter. The neuroleptic syndrome is largely a brain stem syndrome; it can be roughly reproduced in test animals.

Neuroleptics, therefore, are by no means exclusively psychotropic, even though they are used mainly in the treatment of mental disorders. They produce a whole range of effects, and many of these effects are not psychological but somatic. There are indications (chapter XI) that psychological and somatic, more specifically motor, effects of neuroleptics are closely related. It therefore seems advisable, for the time being, to interpret the latter as accompanying symptoms rather than as side effects. This does not mean that these somatic effects should not be regarded as undesirable from a practical therapeutic point of view. In the next chapter they will be separately discussed.

The group of the neuroleptics comprises compounds of different chemical structure:

1) Phenothiazine derivatives. Prototype: chlorpromazine (Largactil, Thorazine).
2) Thioxanthene derivatives. Prototype: chlorprothixene (Truxal, Taractan).
3) Butyrophenones. Prototype: haloperidol (Serenace, Haldol).
4) Diphenylbutylpiperidines. Prototype: pimozide (Orap).
5) Dibenzazepines. Prototype: clozapine (Leponex).
6) Indole derivatives. Prototype: oxypertine (Opertil, Integrin).
7) Rauwolfia alkaloids. Prototype: reserpine (Serpasil).
8) Benzoquinolizine derivatives. Prototype: tetrabenazine (Nitoman).

Phenothiazine derivatives are characterized by a core which consists of two benzene rings, linked by a sulphur and a nitrogen atom—the so-called phenothiazine skeleton (Fig. 10). At R_1, groups of a widely different nature are substituted, e.g. halogens, an acetyl group, a methoxy-group or other organic radicals. A side chain is located at R_2. According to its structure, the phenothiazine derivatives can be divided into three subgroups:

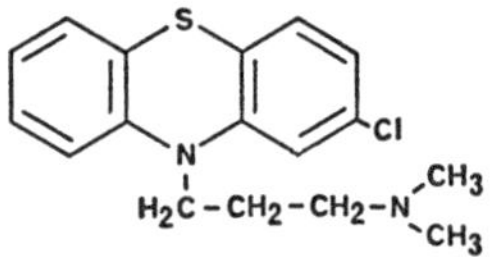

Figure 10. Phenothiazine nucleus. The fact that the distance between the two nitrogens atoms equals three carbon atoms proved to be of essential importance for the neuroleptic activity of all phenothiazine derivatives known so far.

1) Compounds with an amino-alkyl group in the side chain: $N(CH_3)_2$.
2) Compounds with a piperidine ring in the side chain: 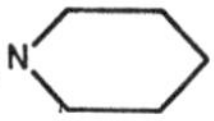

3) Compounds with a piperazine ring in the side chain: 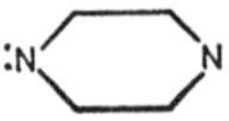

Despite their disparate chemical structure, neuroleptics show so many clinical and pharmacological similarities that it seems justifiable to discuss them as one group in a single chapter. Intra-group differences, which of course exist, will also be discussed, but no particulars on individual preparations will be given. For these, I refer the reader to chapter X.

2. Why neuroleptics?

There are two motives for using neuroleptics. To begin with, they *reduce the duration* of most psychotic disorders, as an extensive literature indicates. Klein and Davis (1969) collected 118 placebo-controlled studies, in 101 of which the neuroleptic was superior to the placebo used. By way of illustration I discuss one particular study, made in 1964 by the National Institute of Mental Health. It comprised 400 acutely psychotic patients in nine different hospitals. In a double-blind study over a period of six weeks, several phenothiazines were compared with a placebo. Moderate-to-marked improvement was observed in 75% of the patients treated with a phenothiazine derivative, versus only 25% of those given a placebo (Figs. 11 and 12). After 6 weeks, 48% of the patients in the phenothiazine group were regarded as symptom-free, versus 15% of those in the placebo group.

A study by Goldberg et al. (1965) in which the action *profile* of neuroleptics was analysed, showed that there is no ground for the theory that neuroleptics can do no more than "brick up the cat." The improvement obtained with these compounds concerns not only the factors agitation and anxiety but certainly also prototypical psychotic symptoms such as delusion, hallucination, contact deficiency and emotional effacement.

Another reason to prescribe neuroleptics is that, in long-term medication, they *reduce the risk of a relapse*. Many psychotic disorders tend to relapse. In principle, there are several reasons for this tendency. One can imagine that the ego structure is habitually unstable due to primary flaws in its "carrier," the cerebral machinery. These flaws in turn can be genetically determined, or caused by somatic influences in the course of life, or caused by early psychological factors which have prevented optimal maturation of the brain. Another possibility is that the ego structure, although originally

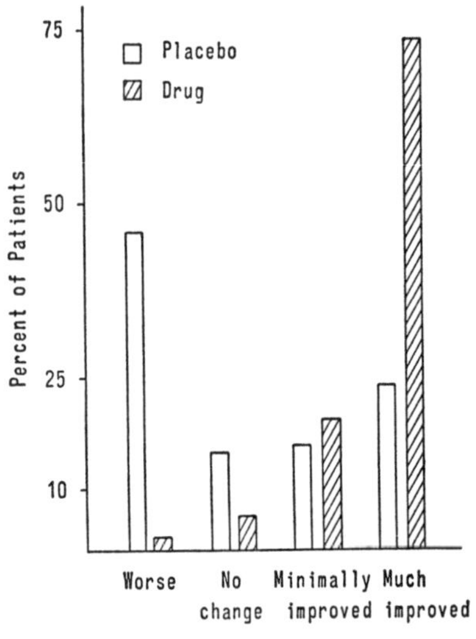

Figure 11. Global evaluation by the attending physician of the effect of 6 weeks' (double-blind) medication with a phenothiazine neuroleptic or a placebo in patients suffering from acute psychoses (NIMH Collaborative Study 1964; Davis 1976).

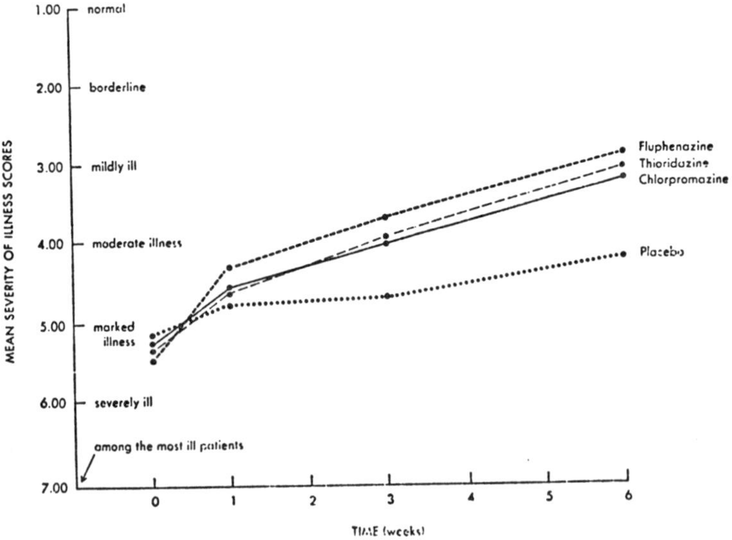

Figure 12. The influence of phenothiazine neuroleptics on the prognosis of acute types of schizophrenia as compared with that of a placebo (NIMH Collaborative Study 1964; Klein and Davis 1969).

normal, is subject to chronic stress as a result of unsolved inner conflicts and/or environmental pressures. In either case even minor factors—psychological or somatic—can upset the precarious mental balance.

Be this as it may, the risk of relapse can be substantially reduced with the aid of neuroleptics. A survey of 24 controlled studies of the effect of long-term neuroleptic medication of high-risk patients (Davis 1975) revealed the following. Of 1068 patients given a placebo, 698 (65%) relapsed, versus 639 of 2127 patients given an antipsychotic agent (30%). In these studies, not only long-acting but also short-acting neuroleptics were used. Walking patients (with whom these studies were concerned) are known often to be careless about taking the drugs prescribed. This is why long-acting neuroleptics are far preferable in maintenance therapy.

A comparison between long-acting neuroleptics and a placebo reveals considerably more striking differences. By way of example I mention the study by Hirsch et al. (1973). This covered a one-year period and concerned patients who had been hospitalized with psychotic disorders and, after discharge, were treated with either a placebo or fluphenazine decanoate. The relapse rate in the former group was 66%, versus 8% in the latter group (Table 2).

Table 2. Relapse rate in a group of 74 patients who, after discharge from hospital where they had been treated for an acute type of schizophrenia, were followed up over a period of 1 year and treated by injections of either fluphenazine decanoate or a placebo (Hirsch et al. 1973).

	Number of patients	Relapse	No relapse
fluphenazine	36	3 (8%) } *	33 (92%)
placebo	38	25 (66%) }	13 (34%)

*p <0.001

Hogarty et al. (1974) demonstrated just how indispensable maintenance therapy with neuroleptics can be. They made a follow-up study over a period of two years of 374 walking patients discharged from hospital after treatment for acute forms of schizophrenia. Maintenance therapy consisted of chlorpromazine or placebo medication, with or without intensive psychosocial guidance, so that four groups were formed:

1) chlorpromazine alone;
2) chlorpromazine with intensive psychosocial guidance;
3) placebo alone;
4) placebo with intensive psychosocial guidance.

The relapse rate (re-admission necessary) was 80% in the placebo group and 48% in the chlorpromazine group (Fig. 13)—an impressive difference particularly in view of the fact that the neuroleptic was not given in a long-acting form so that a number of "irregular users" must be accounted for. The relapse rate in groups 3 and 4 was the same, social guidance apparently having no effect on the relapse rate. This does not mean that this guidance is useless. Its value was apparent in the improved "quality of life" in the intervals between the psychotic phases; the social adjustment and integration of the patient were facilitated by this guidance.

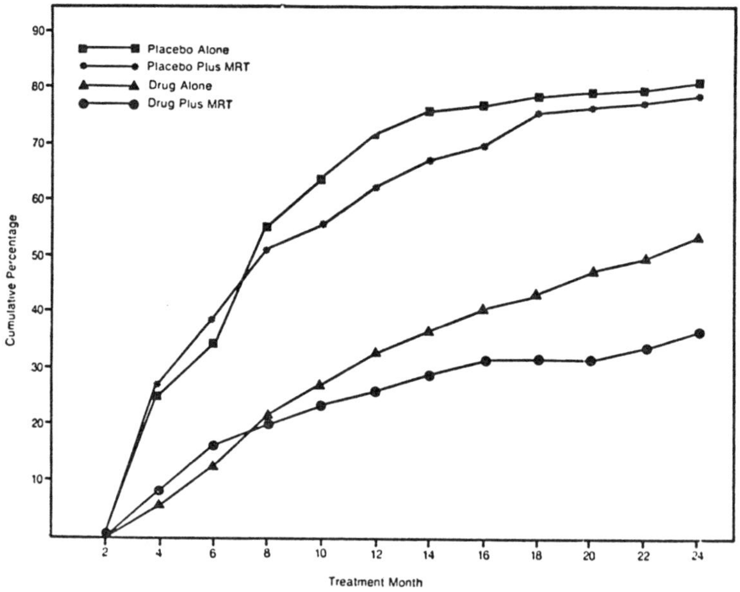

Figure 13. Cumulative relapse rates in a group of 374 patients who, after discharge from hospital where they had been treated for an acute type of schizophrenia, were followed up over a period of two years and treated in four different ways. MRT stands for Major Role Therapy, defined by the authors as a combination of intensive social casework and vocational rehabilitation counselling (Hogarty et al. 1974).

These findings confirmed an old maxim: you fight more effectively with both hands than with one hand behind your back.

3. Development of neuroleptics

The rise of psychiatric pharmacotherapy commenced in 1952 with the discovery of the neuroleptic effect of chlorpromazine, the prototype of the group of phenothiazine derivatives.

Phenothiazine derivatives were first synthesized in 1883 by Bernthsen, an investigator who concerned himself with the synthesis of methylene blue. Phenothiazine itself had been used for a while as antihelminthic agent and urinary disinfectant, but was abandoned in view of its toxic properties. In the forties of this century, however, both France and the USA showed a revival of interest. On the basis of the phenothiazine skeleton, efforts were made to evolve compounds effective against protozoal infections. It was in the context of this research that promethazine (Phenergan) was evolved in the laboratories of Rhône-Poulenc-Specia. Although this product lacked chemotherapeutic properties, it proved to be an effective antihistamine. This line of research was continued and, in 1950, led to the synthesis of chlorpromazine—a compound with a structure closely related to that of promethazine. Although not without histamine-antagonizing potency, it was for different qualities that chlorpromazine would become famous.

The first clinical reports were submitted in 1951 by the anaesthetist Laborit and the surgeon Huguenard, who swept chlorpromazine to the very front of general attention. Chlorpromazine was characterized as "stabilisateur végétatif" and, together with pethidine and promethazine, included in Laborit's famed "cocktail lytique." This cocktail effected what Laborit described as "artificial hibernation," and was used in shock and as an adjuvant in anaesthesia. More or less casually, Laborit and Huguenard made mention of a phenomenon which was later to prove quintessential in their observations. They found that patients treated with chlorpromazine, although alert, were striking indifferent with regard to their environment. In fact they tolerated minor surgery without anaesthesia, although completely aware of the procedure. The notion that chlorpromazine might be of importance in the treatment of psychiatric conditions thus derived from a surgeon's experience.

Shortly afterwards, in 1952, the first reports from clinical psychiatry came forth. Hamon et al. described a maniacal patient who rapidly improved in response to chlorpromazine and pethidine. In the same year Delay and Deniker reported spectacular results in psychotic agitation of widely different origin. Their description of the therapeutic activity of chlorpromazine is a classic example of sharp, unbiased clinical observation. The patients in question, they reported, became quiet, less active and more or less indifferent to experiences and situations which had previously made them very emotional. Intellect and level of consciousness were hardly influenced. It is Delay and his staff who should be honoured for having immediately recognized the significance of chlorpromazine. Their names are rightly associated with the introduction of this compound in psychiatry.

The structure of *thioxanthene compounds* is closely related to that of phenothiazine derivatives. They, too, have a tricyclic core, the difference being that the central nitrogen atom is substituted with a carbon atom. Thioxanthene derivatives, therefore, should also be regarded as a product of phenothiazine research.

Shortly after the introduction of chlorpromazine, clinical psychiatry made the acquaintance of a related compound called *reserpine*. The compound was related only in terms of effect, not in chemical structure. Reserpine is an alkaloid from the root of Rauwolfia serpentina, a plant found in many tropical regions of Asia and Africa. India had known for centuries that an extract from this root has a tranquillizing influence. It was a popular remedy sold in local markets as "pagal-ka-dawa" (insanity herb). In 1930 Sen and Bose introduced Rauwolfia serpentina in official medicine as a "drug for insanity and high blood pressure"; the extract was then used on a moderate scale as a hypotensive. Its possible psychotherapeutic properties, however, were still disregarded. In 1973 Gupta et al. published a report largely confirming the findings of Sen and Bose, but this communication elicited virtually no response. Interest was not aroused until 1952, when Müller et al. succeeded in isolating the principal Rauwolfia alkaloid, reserpine, from the root extract. Two years later Weber reported that the effect of reserpine on psychotic patients largely corresponds with that of chlorpromazine—a fact which was to be corroborated by many other investigators. With the rise of the phenothiazine derivatives, however, reserpine as neuroleptic was completely superseded.

The *benzoquinolizine derivatives* are synthetic compounds which form a highly interesting group—interesting because they closely resemble reserpine in clinical effect and influence on monoamine metabolism in spite of the difference in chemical structure. Only one representative of this group—tetrabenazine—was introduced in clinical psychiatry but, although the compound has been available since 1959, it has been used only sparsely in the treatment of psychoses; the reason for this has remained obscure.

The *butyrophenones* are likewise synthetic compounds, derived from the analgesic pethidine. Their neuroleptic potency was accidentally discovered by Janssen et al. (1967) in the course of a study of the analgesic activity of a series of pethidine derivatives. The first member of this group—haloperidol—was introduced in clinical psychiatry about 1960. The *diphenylbutylpiperidines* were derived from the butyrophenones, to which they are closely related in chemical structure.

Dibenzazepines are tricyclic compounds like the phenothiazines and thioxanthenes, but centrally they have an asymmetrical 7-ring. Their principal representative, clozapine, was introduced in 1962. This group has also yielded an antidepressant: dibenzepine.

There are two neuroleptics with an *indole core*: oxypertine and molindone. They were independently evolved in different laboratories, and few studies have so far been made either of their clinical aspects or of their influence on a molecular level. This is remarkable, because the suspected but still totally obscure role of serotonin (a monoamine with an indole core) in the pathogenesis of psychoses should have stimulated such research.

4. Therapeutic activities of neuroleptics

The complex influence of neuroleptics on disturbed mental life can be reduced to two principal effects: sedation and antipsychotic effect.

Sedation

In response to neuroleptics, feelings of anxiety, inner restiveness and tension decrease in intensity. This subduing effect, however, is not confined to affective life but also comprises impulses, initiative and activity. The agitated patient calms down, and the hyperactive patient becomes quieter. Aggressiveness and destructiveness abate, to be replaced by a degree of passiveness. The loss of initiative can be so marked as to approach in fact a state of (often undesirable) apathy.

Does the agitation really abate or is it suppressed? Either the one or the other can be the case. A majority of patients really feel relieved, but others are hardly satisfied with the result of treatment. The latter feel "flattened" or, on the other hand, have a sensation of being under restraint—the brake pedal has been kicked down, but the pressure on the throttle has hardly diminished. The latter possibility is more prominent in syndromes largely determined by psychogenic or neurotic factors. The dosage, of course, also plays a role in this respect. It should be borne in mind that the optimal range of neuroleptics is not sharply defined. The optimal dosage varies from patient to patient, even within the same diagnostic category, and should therefore be determined individually. This is a golden rule which cannot be emphasized enough.

Neuroleptics are sedatives with two special features. To begin with, they are the strongest sedatives available. Secondly, they sedate without producing pronounced hypnotic effects, and in this respect they differ from the conventional sedatives. Complaints about dullness, drowsiness, diminished concentration and a sensation of numbness in the head are really heard only during the first few weeks of medication, and they rarely reach a serious level. This is, of course, an important advantage. However, neuroleptics do potentiate the hypnotic effect of conventional sedatives.

Antipsychotic effect

Neuroleptics have their tranquillizing effect in common with all sedatives. It is their antipsychotic effect that makes them a unique group of compounds. The meaning of the word "antipsychotic" is not sharply defined; it could not be because the term psychosis is itself a collective name for a wide range of disparate behaviour disorders. The term antipsychotic indicates that neuroleptics can exert a beneficial influence on such prototypical psychotic symptoms as delusion, hallucination, incoherent thinking and disorientation. The exact profile of therapeutic activities is not expressed in the term. Although this is not the same with all neuroleptics, but we are ill-informed about inter-agent differences.

Neuroleptics differ not only in therapeutic action profile but also in efficacy. A neuroleptic can cause total disappearance of all psychotic symptoms, quickly (within a few days) or less quickly (in a few weeks). In other cases the psychotic symptoms change but do not disappear. In these cases we have a de-emoting rather than an antipsychotic effect. The affective response to the psychotic disorders of thinking and experiencing diminishes, and thus their penetration diminishes.

For some understanding of this de-emoting effect, it should be borne in mind that the human brain not only registers but also evaluates the stimuli it receives. What we perceive of our outer and inner world is often not neutral but coloured by emotional overtones, be they positive or negative. It is these emotional overtones that are attenuated by neuroleptics. In other words: the perception and registration of stimuli remain unaltered but their emotional reverberations (the emotional "tone") diminish. The impressions and experiences pass through a neutralizing filter (so to speak). In actual fact, this means a marked reduction of the impact of various pathological experiences, and more specifically those of a delusional or hallucinatory nature. Without disappearing, these are now experienced as if from some distance, ego-alien to some extent, and therefore less agonizing and less anxiety-provoking. The patient no longer lives *in* the world of his delusions and hallucinations, but instead lives *with* these symptoms. This effect also becomes manifest with regard to situations which used to frustrate the patient. He is to some extent armoured against them and can meet them more or less unmoved. Not without some justification, this complex of effects has sometimes been characterized as "chemical leucotomy."

As a result of this de-emoting complex of actions, adjustment of the mentally disturbed patient to his environment and his interest in the environment may show substantial improvement.

Behaviour effects in animals

Not only in clinical terms but also in animal experiments, neuroleptics have a number of characteristics in common, regardless of their chemical structure.

1) They effect a reduction of spontaneous motor activity, sometimes to the point of akinesia, but leave reactivity to stimuli intact (catalepsy).
2) They potentiate the hypnotic effect of barbiturates and antagonize the motor activating effect of amphetamines.
3) Wild animal species show reduced aggressiveness in response to neuroleptics (taming effect).
4) They inhibit conditioned reflexes. Example: animals taught to avoid a danger zone (e.g. an electric stimulus) upon a given acoustic signal (e.g. a buzz) lost this conditioned reflex in response to neuroleptics. The unconditioned reflex (flight reaction upon application of an electric stimulus) is not or hardly influenced by neuroleptics.
5) Neuroleptics inhibit emotional defaecation, i.e. defaecation which occurs when a test animal (usually a rat) is placed in a situation of anxiety and tension.

There is an unmistakable similarity, therefore, between human and animal behaviour effects of neuroleptics. Only with regard to their antipsychotic effect can no adequate animal model be found.

5. Indications for neuroleptics

Indications

The psychiatric syndromes which, generally speaking, can be considered for neuroleptic medication, can be deduced from the data discussed in section 4 above. They are the following:

1) Syndromes with anxiety, aggression, motor hyperactivity or inner restiveness as prominent features. For example:
   Maniacal syndromes (as they occur in the context of manic-depressive psychosis but also in other psychoses, e.g. organic, psychogenic and schizophrenic psychoses).
   Delirious syndromes (which may be conditioned by a variety of usually somatic noxae such as cerebral ar-

teriosclerosis, head injury, operation, abstinence after chronic abuse of alcohol, drugs, etc.).

States of agitation (as observed, for example, in certain types of psychopathy, in oligophrenia, and on the basis of severe organic cerebral defects).

2) Syndromes characterized by severe disturbances in thinking and experiencing, particularly those in which delusions and hallucinations are prominent, regardless of whether they are mainly endogenous, exogenous, or psychogenically determined. The anxiety which so often accompanies such psychotic syndromes likewise usually shows a favourable response to neuroleptic medication.

Contraindications

Neuroleptics are not indicated in the following syndromes:

1) Syndromes characterized by inactivity and apathy. Neuroleptics can nevertheless be indicated in such cases if delusions and hallucinations are likewise present (e.g. in certain types of chronic schizophrenia). Not infrequently, however, the former symptoms show exacerbation in such cases. The groups of neuroleptics to be preferred in such cases are discussed in section 9 below.

2) Depressive syndromes. Neuroleptics exert no primary influence on the mood (they do exert a secondary influence, via their beneficial effect on the abovementioned series of psychopathological symptoms). It is therefore useless (even though it is still often done) to prescribe neuroleptics for patients suffering from a depression (unless possible agitation is to be controlled).

3) Neurotic disorders—e.g. neurotic anxiety states, phobic neuroses, psychosomatic diseases—are generally also outside the range of indications for neuroleptics (unless these compounds are given in very small doses, which practically equates their effect to that of the ataractics). Of course it is possible in these patients, too, to reduce the outward signs of anxiety and inner tension (although often only transiently); but their source—the partly subconscious conflict situation—remains unaffected. The disease symptoms are masked rather than controlled, and the patient is generally not well served in this way. It is especially the neurotics who show poor tolerance to neuroleptic medication. They feel restricted under this medication: "bricked up," as one of

my patients expressed it. The lack of initiative, the emotional indifference, the "damper" put on the possibilities of motor expression, are all experienced by these patients as inconveniences.

Neuroleptics are always to be avoided with patients considered to be suitable subjects for a systematic psychotherapeutic approach. The affective flattening produced by these compounds is at odds with the objectives of the psychotherapist: to activate possibilities of emotional experience and expression. If in a certain phase of psychotherapy a degree of relaxation is considered desirable, then ataractics are more suitable than neuroleptics, for ataractics sedate without subduing emotional resonance. Unlike the classical sedatives, moreover, they have hardly any hypnotic effect.

Limits of the range of indications

The effect of neuroleptic medication is usually disappointing in the following cases:

1) Syndromes accompanied by compulsive symptoms or sensations of derealization (e.g. profound neurotic disorders, certain types of schizophrenia and some cases of organic cerebral damage).

2) Behaviour anomalies based on organic cerebral damage (e.g. in oligophrenia, epilepsy and acquired cerebral lesions, for example after a head injury).

   If in the lastmentioned cases medication is to produce any result, then the doses required are generally so large that various troublesome side effects develop. The phenothiazine derivative periciazine may be an exception to this rule, but careful (comparative) studies have not yet been made.

   In this context it should be pointed out that brain-damaged children who are hyperirritable and hyperactive can show a favourable response to such stimulants as dextro-amphetamine and methylphenidate. There are also reports on good results obtained in these patients with ataractics, particularly hydroxyzine (chapter XXV).

Neuroleptics are generally superior to ataractics in psychotic syndromes. So far only one exception to this rule has been demonstrated: high-dosage parenteral administration of chlordiazepoxide or diazepam in patients with imminent or already manifest delirium tremens (alcoholic delirium). The ultimate therapeutic result is not superior to that obtained with neuroleptics, but it is obtained more rapidly, and that is a great therapeutic advantage in such cases.

Neuroleptics in normal test subjects

Kraepelin was the first to make a systematic study of the influence which drugs exert on the mental life in healthy subjects. In 1892 he reported on his experiments in a publication entitled *Ueber die Beeinflussing einfacher psychischer Vorgänge durch einige Arzneimittel*. It was likewise Kraepelin who introduced the term pharmacopsychology for this branch of research. Unfortunately, research into the influence of modern psychotropic drugs on behaviour in normal or little-disturbed individuals has been badly neglected.

6. Determining indications for neuroleptics and the duration of medication

Determining indications

It is apparent from section 5 that neuroleptics are prescribed on the basis of symptomatological considerations, i.e. guided by the most prominent disease symptoms. This observation warrants two conclusions. The first is that, in terms of their effects, neuroleptics do not respect the boundaries of the conventional nosological entities. A patient is given neuroleptics, not because he is suffering from schizophrenia, dementia paralytica, or alcoholic delirium, but because he shows (for example) delusions, hallucinations, anxiety or agitation. Syndrome or symptom determine the indication; whether it is set in a schizophrenic, or infectious or an alcoholic context is irrelevant. The second conclusion is that the factor aetiology appears to play no role in determining indications for neuroleptic medication. This is not surprising in view of the fact that aetiology and pathogenesis of the vast majority of psychotic disorders are still virtually obscure. This also implies that we do not know whether we are giving causal or symptomatic treatment when we prescribe neuroleptics. In most cases we are probably giving symptomatic therapy, as indicated by the fact that early discontinuation of treatment—even in cases in which it seems to be completely successful—often leads to a relapse. This means that the symptoms are being controlled but their cause remains unaffected.

Duration of medication

The probably non-causal character of neuroleptic medication has two practical implications:

1) In psychoses with a phasic course (more generally in psychoses in which the prognosis is regarded as favourable in principle), neuroleptic medication should be continued until the disease period has reached its natural end. This time is not predictable. In actual practice, therefore, one starts reducing the dosage when the patient has been in good condition for some time. This is done gradually and under constant supervision. If nothing untoward happens, medication is finally discontinued. Otherwise, the former dosage is resumed.
2) In psychoses with a chronic course, which include the large group of the chronic types of schizophrenia, and in those with a marked tendency to relapse, it is nearly always necessary to continue medication for a long time, and possibly for life, uninterrupted and at the lowest dosage at which an optimal condition can be maintained.

Once released from hospital, many patients tend to be careless about their medication: due to lack of disease insight, resistance to the representatives of illness, or simply due to indifference. In some cases the family doctor approves, misguided by a condition which seems fair. This situation is almost bound to lead to a relapse. For these patients, long-acting neuroleptics proved to be a boon. These compounds need be given only once per 1-4 weeks, by injection or orally. When a physician takes care of these administration, the risk of negligence is minimized.

"Depot outpatient clinics"

There is still another way in which long-acting neuroleptics have contributed to a better prognosis of chronic and chronic recurrent psychoses. They have ensured regular contacts between the patient and the therapeutic agency which administers the medication (usually by injection). And this ensures regular psychotherapeutic contact with the patient as well as regular evaluation (and necessary correction) of his situation in life. Whenever the patient fails to report as agreed, efforts are made immediately to establish the reason for his absence. Such an approach functions best if centralized, in a so-called depot outpatient clinic. This is entirely comparable with the lithium outpatient clinic for patients with bipolar and unipolar depressions (chapter XVIII). It, too, can well be run by a general practitioner or by a nurse with a physician (or psychiatrist) as supervisor. A social worker is an indispensable figure in such outpatient clinics.

Long-acting neuroleptics have substantially improved the prognosis of chronic and chronic recurrent psychoses. This does not mean that this medication should be automatically continued year after year. From time to time (by gross rule of thumb, every 2-3 years), efforts should be made to establish whether a smaller dose will do, or whether the patient can be entirely without this medication.

7. Pharmacokinetic aspects

It has been established with several neuroleptics that a given dosage produces quite different blood concentrations in different patients. The plasma chlorpromazine values, for example, can differ by as much as factor 100. An important reason lies in individual differences in turnover rate. There are slow and fast metabolizers. In the former, the effective dose of a neuroleptic is larger than that in the latter. Another obvious inference is that, given a particular dosage, the slow metabolizers show more side effects than the fast metabolizers. This, however, remains to be investigated. After oral administration, moreover, the amount of a neuroleptic taken up differs, partly due to differences in absorption and partly because neuroleptics can also be metabolized in the intestinal wall and because the turnover rate, as pointed out, shows individual variations.

There is still another factor which contributes to the marked interindividual differences in plasma levels. After being used for some time, neuroleptics induce an increase in the microsomal liver enzymes which break them down; the degree and speed of this enzyme induction are subject to individual variations.

For all these reasons it is of primary importance to determine neuroleptic dosages individually. The only reliable guide in this respect is the ratio between therapeutic efficacy and side effects. Routine assays to determine the plasma concentration of the various types of neuroleptics are not yet available. Once they are, they might substantially optimize neuroleptic medication.

8. Use of neuroleptics outside clinical psychiatry

Phenothiazine derivatives and reserpine are used also for nonpsychiatric purposes. Reserpine has long been used on a large scale as antihypertensive agent. The affective flattening which phenothiazine derivatives produce can be very useful in cases of intractable pain. Their anti-emetic effect can be utilized in hyperemesis gravidarum, uraemia, radiation disease and other diseases associated with violent vomiting. Specifically, prochlorperazine is a strong anti-emetic. Like the antipsychotic and extrapyramidal activity of neuroleptics, their anti-emetic activity is believed also to be based on block of DA receptors in the brain, and more specifically of those in the so-called chemoreceptor trigger zone in the area postrema.

Chlorpromazine, finally, has been successfully used to control singultus. Beckman (1961) described this compound as "the most effective agent ever introduced into the therapy of intractable hiccup."

9. Inter-agent differences in effect

In section 4 above, the therapeutic activites of neuroleptics were roughly divided into two categories: sedative and antipsychotic activities. It would be a fallacy, however, to put all neuroleptics on a par in this respect. It is certain that inter-agent differences in the clinical action profile exist, and therefore also inter-agent differences in indications. The difficulty is that our information on this point is still very incomplete. We are dealing here with the consequences of the bottleneck mentioned in chapter VI: that in the diagnosis of psychoses insufficient justice is done to syndrome differentiation and symptom definition, and that in the analysis of neuroleptic effects the total score on a rating scale is decisive, rather than possible changes in the *profile* of psychopathological symptoms. This lack of psychopathological differentiation explains why comparative studies of neuroleptics often fail to yield the desired information or cannot corroborate earlier results. The subject of differentiated determination of indications for neuroleptics, therefore, will be discussed only briefly, disregarding all controversial and often not readily verifiable details. Even these broad outlines are not presented without some reservation. I certainly do not claim that they are all documented by hard experimental facts.

Starting from their two principal categories of activity, neuroleptics could be differentiated as follows. Phenothiazine derivatives are the most universal neuroleptics. Their antipsychotic effect is probably superior to that of the other neuroleptics. Their sedative component is likewise vigorous, but in this respect they are inferior to the butyrophenones and reserpine. Thioxanthene derivatives are very similar to phenothiazines, both in activity and in chemical structure.

The antipsychotic effect of butyrophenones may be slightly less marked than that of phenothiazines. Their sedative effect, however, is remarkably strong; even marked psychotic agitation can often be quickly and effectively controlled with these agents. The same applies to reserpine, but this is definitely inferior to the other neuroleptics as an antipsychotic agent. The benzoquinolizine derivatives are little used and therefore not readily classifiable as to their activity. However, this seems to be largely comparable to that of reserpine.

On the whole, severity and frequency of extrapyramidal side effects increase in this order: phenothiazines, butyrophenones and reserpine, apart from a few exceptions in the phenothiazine series (e.g. thioproperazine, with its exceptionally marked affinity for the extrapyramidal system). In this context it is to be noted that reserpine frequently provokes Parkinson symptoms and akathisia, but rarely dyskinesia.

Within the phenothiazine series, further differentiation of activity is possible on the basis of the structure of the side chain at R_2 (section 1 above). The compounds with a terminal dimethyl group in the side chain have a pronounced sedative effect, associated with more or less strong suppression of drive and initiative. They may lead to a state of apathy which can only very partly be controlled by means of stimulants such as caffeine. The sedative effect of phenothiazine derivatives with a piperazine ring in the side chain is less pronounced, and they are much less de-activating. Not infrequently, in fact, they cause some activation. These compounds are therefore preferable to the dimethyl derivatives in the treatment of psychotic disorders in which lack of initiative is predominant. We need hardly say that this is often the case in chronic types of schizophrenia.

Finally, the two groups of phenothiazine derivatives differ in their affinity for the extrapyramidal system. Piperazine compounds more frequently lead to motor disorders than dimethyl compounds, the difference being most manifest in hyperkinetic and dyskinetic changes. Finally, the piperazine phenothiazines have the strongest anti-emetic effect of all phenothiazines. Because of this property they can impede the diagnosis of processes in the cranium or the abdominal cavity.

The third group of phenothiazine derivatives—those with a piperidine ring in the side chain—are therapeutically placed between the dimethyl and the piperazine phenothiazines. They hardly stimulate, nor do they induce a state of apathy. Their influence on the extrapyramidal system is small and less pronounced than that of the other two groups.

Of the dibenzazepines, clozapine is the compound so far most thoroughly studied. It is a very strong sedative in psychotic agitation. Views on its antipsychotic activity differ. Some authors maintain that in this respect it equals the phenothiazines; others regard it as inferior in this respect.

Oxypertine is a moderately strong antipsychotic, distinguished by a relatively marked activating effect; it is therefore to be considered in the treatment of inert psychotic patients.

The above classification of neuroleptics according to activity is based on the ratio between sedative and antipsychotic activity. It is a very superficial one. One would wish for a classification according to the nature of the antipsychotic activity, but the necessary data are not available.

BIBLIOGRAPHY

Ayd, F. J. Jr. (1975). The depot fluphenazines: a reappraisal after ten years' clinical experience. *Amer. J. Psychiat.* 132, 491.

Beckman, H. (1961). *Pharmacology*. Philadelphia and London: Saunders.

Blackwell, B. (1972). The drug defaulter. *Clin. Pharmacol. Ther.* 13, 841.

Clark, M. L., W. K. Huber, K. Sahota, D. C. Fowles and E. A. Serafetinides (1970). Molindone in chronic schizophrenia. *Clin. Pharmac. Ther.* 11, 680.

Davis, M. D. (1975). Overview: Maintenance therapy in psychiatry I. Schizophrenia. *Amer. J. Psychiat.* 132, 1237.

Davis, J. M. (1976). Recent developments in the drug treatment of schizophrenia. *Amer. J. Psychiat.* 133, 208.

Delay, J. and P. Deniker (1952). 38 Cas de psychoses traités par la cure prolongée et continuée de 4568 RP. *Ann. méd. psychol.* 110, 364.

Fann, W. E. and C. R. Lake (1976). Amantidine versus trihexyphenidyl in the treatment of neuroleptic induced parkinsonism. *Amer. J. Psychiat.* 133, 940.

Forrest, I. S., C. Jelleff Car and E. Usdin (Eds.) (1974). *Phenothiazines and Structurally Related Drugs*. New York: Raven Press.

Goldberg, S. C., G. L. Klerman and C. O. Cole (1965). Changes in psychopathology and ward behaviour as a function of phenothiazine treatment. *Brit. J. Psychiat.* 3, 120.

Groves, J. E. and M. R. Mandel (1975). The long-acting phenothiazines. *Arch. gen. Psychiat.* 32, 893.

Gupta, J. C., A. K. Deb and B. S. Kahali (1973). Preliminary observations on use of rauwolfia serpentina benth in treatment of central disorders. *Ind. Med. Gaz.* 78, 547.

Hamon, J., J. Paraire and J. Velluz (1952). Remarques sur l'action du 4560 RP sur l'agitation maniaque. *Ann. méd. psychol.* 110, 331.

Hirsch, S. R., R. Gaind, P. D. Rhode, B. C. Stevens and J. K. Wing (1973). Outpatient maintenance of chronic schizophrenic patients with long-acting phenothiazines. *Brit. med. J.* 1, 633.

Hogarty, G. E., S. C. Goldberg, N. R. Schooler and R. F. Ulrich (1974). Drugs and sociotherapy in the aftercare of schizophrenic patients: II. Two-year relapse rates. *Arch. gen. Psychiat.* 31, 603.

Hogarty, G. E., S. C. Goldberg and N. R. Schooler (1974). Drugs and sociotherapy in the aftercare of schizophrenic patients: III. Adjustment of non-relapsed patients. *Arch. gen. Psychiat.* 31, 609.

Janssen, P. A. J. (1967). Haloperidol and related butyrophenones. In: *Psychopharmacological Agents*. Vol. 2, 199, New York: Academic Press.

Klein, D. F. and J. Davis (1969). *Diagnosis and Drug Treatment of Psychiatric Disorders*. Baltimore: Williams and Wilkins.

Kraepelin, W. (1892). Über die Beeinflussung einfacher psychischen Vorgänge durch einige Arzneimittel. Experimentelle Untersuchengen. Fischer, Jena.

Laborit, H. and P. Huguenard (1951). L'hibernation artificielle par moyens pharmacodynamiques et physiques. *Presse méd.* 59, 1329.

Leff, J. P. and J. K. Wing (1971). Trial of maintenance therapy in schizophrenics. *Brit. Med. J.* 2, 599.

May, P. R. (1974). Treatment of schizophrenia: I. A critique of reviews of the literature. *Compr. Psychiat.* 15, 179.

Müller, J. M., E. Schittler, and J. Bein (1952). Reserpin-der sedative Wirkstoff aus Rauwolfia Serpentina Benth. *Experientia* 8, 338.

National Institute of Mental Health (1964). Phenothiazine treatment in acute schizophrenics. Psychopharmacology Service Center Collaborative Study Group. *Arch. gen. Psychiat.* 10, 246.

Praag, H. M. van, L. C. W. Dols and T. Schut (1975). Biochemical versus psychopathological action profile of neuroleptics: a comparative study of chlorpromazine and oxypertine in acute psychotic disorders. *Compr. Psychiat.* 16, 255.

PRAAG, H. M. VAN, J. KORF AND L. C. W. DOLS (1976). Clozapine versus perphenazine or the value of the biochemical mode of action of neuroleptics in predicting their therapeutic activity. *Brit. J. Psychiat.* 129, 547.
QUITKIN, F., A. RIFKIN AND D. F. KLEIN (1975). Very high dosage vs standard dosage fluphenazine in schizophrenia. A double-blind study of non-chronic treatment-refractory patients. *Arch. gen. Psychiat.* 32, 1276.
SEN, G., AND K. C. BOSE (1930). Rauwolfia serpentina: a new Indian drug for insanity and high blood pressure. *Indian Med. World* 2, 194.
WEBER, E. (1954). Eine Rauwolfia alkaloid in der Psychiatrie: seine Wirkungsähnlichkeit mit chlorpromazin. *Schweiz. med. Wschr.* 84, 968.
ZIRKLE, G. L. AND C. KAISER (1974). Antipsychotic agents. In: *Psychopharmacological Agents*. Vol. 3, 39, New York, San Francisco, London: Academic Press.

VIII

Neuroleptics II: Side Effects

1. Psychological side effects

Delirium

All known neuroleptics are capable in principle of provoking delirious changes: the patient becomes restive and disoriented, with more or less incoherent thoughts. The level of consciousness is lowered, if often only intermittently, with periods of clouded consciousness alternating with clear periods. Visual and/or auditory hallucinations occur. This development should, of course, be identified and differentiated from the syndrome for which therapy was instituted. Otherwise the dosage of the medication might be erroneously increased.

This complication has proved to be dose-dependent. When it was still customary to increase dosages rapidly and to combine several neuroleptics—the presumption being that an optimal therapeutic effect could not be expected until gross extrapyramidal disturbances of motor activity developed—toxic syndromes of this type were regularly observed. They have become rare since greater restraint is, rightly, observed. Great prudence remains necessary in the treatment of elderly patients with symptoms of cerebral arteriosclerosis. They are to some extent predisposed to states of confusion. In the actual cases, the contribution of the drug and that of the cerebrovascular disease are indistinguishable.

In accordance with its exogenous nature, the state of confusion usually rapidly disappears after reduction or discontinuation of the medication. When the complication takes a more protracted course, one may consider the possibility of prescribing a different type of neuroleptic or a sedative (e.g. paraldehyde or chloral hydrate).

Depression

Depressions, often with the typical features of a vital depression (chapter XII), can develop in response to reserpine. In most cases discontinuation of treatment is not sufficient to control the depression, but antidepressant medication is required. The risk of reserpine-induced depression is gravest in patients with a history of depressive phases.

The reserpine-induced depression was discovered outside the psychiatric clinic, among the numerous patients who were given reserpine to combat their hypertension. Neuroleptics of other types lack such an extensive area of non-psychiatric indications and the question whether they, too, have depressogenic activity is still moot. One might expect them to have this activity because: 1) *all* known neuroleptics probably reduce the activity in central CA neurons (chapter IV), and 2) there is an acceptable theory on the relation between a central CA deficiency and the development of depression (chapter XVI). Some authors maintain that neuroleptics other than reserpine can indeed lower the mood level, but there is no absolute certainty in this respect. The symptomatology of a psychosis, after all, is not necessarily constant but can vary within the course of a single phase. This is the case with patients who in the USA are diagnosed as schizo-affective, while in Europe they are more likely to be included in the category of psychogenic or degenerative psychoses. Complications of a depressive type are frequently observed in these cases, but in the individual patient it cannot be decided whether they are due to the medication or constitute a feature of the "natural history" of the disease.

Akathisia

This condition can be a source of confusion. It is characterized by marked motor unrest, usually brought under the heading of extrapyramidal side effects of neuroleptics and discussed in detail in section 4 below. It can be interpreted as a symptom of the psychosis rather than as an effect of the medication, and consequently the dosage can be increased instead of reduced, so that the akathisia increases.

Inertia

Finally, neuroleptics can so suppress impulses and initiative as to lead to a state of inertia. Particularly, phenothiazine derivatives with an amino-dimethyl group in the side chain can produce this effect. Of course, such a state of inertia is undesirable and demonstrates that the margin between the therapeutic and the untoward effects of neuroleptics is fairly narrow.

2. Neuroleptics and the extrapyramidal system

Affinity of neuroleptics for extrapyramidal systems

All neuroleptics have a certain affinity for the extrapyramidal system. The degree of their influence on this system depends both on the dosage and on the type of compound used. In this respect there are substantial differences between the groups of neuroleptics, as well as between individual neuroleptics within the same group. The patient's sex is also of importance in this respect: the incidence of (gross) motor disorders is about twice as high in women as in men. The individual disposition, finally, also plays a role. One patient develops extrapyramidal changes in response to a given drug in a given dose, whereas another does not.

Psychological and motor effects of neuroleptics are probably related. At least there are no known neuroleptics which are therapeutically effective but leave the extrapyramidal system entirely unaffected. Moreover, Haase (1965) demonstrated in a series of ingenious experiments that successful neuroleptic medication is always accompanied by slight impairment of fine motor activity. He regarded these inhibitory symptoms as a *conditio sine qua non* for therapeutic success. It has been established, however, that the relation between the therapeutic potency of neuroleptics and their affinity for the extrapyramidal system is certainly not a proportional one. This fact has three practical implications.

1. The degree of affinity of neuroleptics for the extrapyramidal system is not in any way predictive of their therapeutic efficacy.
2. Gross motor disorders are not an indispensable prerequisite for obtaining an optimal therapeutic result—contrary to what was supposed during the first few years after the introduction of neuroleptics. This statement is not inconsistent with the abovementioned findings reported by Haase. While he demonstrated that the therapeutic effect of neuroleptics is always accompanied by slight motor impairment, he also established that an increase of dosage to the level at which gross motor disorders appeared did not improve the therapeutic result. Such gross disturbances are therefore clearly undesirable and should be avoided.
3. Extrapyramidal symptoms which occur in the course of neuroleptic medication can be combated with anti-parkinson drugs without difficulty. According to the majority of clinicians, this has no unfavourable effect on the therapeutic result. Only one research group reached the opposite conclusion (Singh and Kay 1975), but I would wait for corroboration of their findings before changing the existing guideline.

The extrapyramidal symptoms produced by neuroleptics can be roughly divided into two categories: *hypokinetic/hypertonic* and *hyperkinetic/dyskinetic syndromes*. Although they may be observed in combination, they will be separately discussed in the following sections.

Relation between psychological and extrapyramidal effects

These become to some extent understandable if we bear in mind that all conventional neuroleptics inhibit transmission in central dopaminergic neurons (chapter XI). Dopamine (DA) is localized in several different systems in the brain. Two important localizations are the following: neurons whose body is localized in the substantia nigra and whose axons extend to the caudate nucleus of the corpus striatum (nigro-striatal DA system); second, neurons whose body is localized in the ventral tegmental region and whose axons extend to certain nuclei which are part of the limbic system (nucleus accumbens and olfactory tubercle) and to the cerebral cortex (mesolimbic and mesocortical DA system). There are strong indications that inhibition of the nigro-striatal DA system is responsible for certain motor effects of neuroleptics. A plausible hypothesis is that inhibition in the mesolimbic and mesocortical DA system is a prerequisite for the development of the (or of certain) therapeutic actions of neuroleptics. If these hypotheses are correct, then it would be possible in principle to separate motor from psychological effects in the development of new neuroleptics.

3. Hypokinetic/hypertonic symptoms

These syndromes are by far the most common and can be produced by all groups of neuroleptics. They usually develop gradually in the course of days to weeks. Hypokinesia, in all degrees of severity, is always the initial symptom and sometimes remains the only one.

Nearly always there is some slight motor impairment during neuroleptic medication. Spontaneous motility diminishes, and the same applies to movements which usually accompany walking. Facial expression also loses some details. In more pronounced cases, motor activity is more seriously impaired. The patient takes smaller steps and finally begins to shuffle. He stands slightly stooped, with the arms against the body. Facial expression has stiffened and speech has become monotonous. In this stage, the muscular tonus is nearly always increased, and the cogwheel phenomenon may be provocable. In this way, features may develop which are hardly distinguishable from a Parkinson syndrome, particularly if tremors and hypersalivation are observed in addition. This, however, is not often the case. The tremor can be a classical Parkinson tremor: 4-6 Hz, with "pill-rolling" motions; but other types are also observed, e.g. a fine tremor of high frequency. This drug-induced extrapyramidal syndrome is sometimes described as pseudo-parkinsonism, or referred to by the mellifluous term "parkinsonoid." It need hardly be pointed out that, in pronounced cases, it is experienced as exceedingly inconvenient. The reduced mobility and motility give the patient a sense of being imprisoned in his own body. The term "chemical straitjacket" seems appropriate in some of these cases. As already pointed out, the hypokinetic-hypertonic syndrome does not always occur in its complete form. Several components of this syndrome, e.g. hypokinesia and hypersalivation, can also develop separately.

Parkinson symptoms generally disappear within one to a few weeks of discontinuation of medication. If they persist longer, then the possibility of a neuroleptic-induced "true Parkinson" should be borne in mind. It is often maintained that habituation to the Parkinson symptoms develops in the long run, but this statement has not been convincingly documented. However, it would be consistent with the observation in animals that habituation develops to the influence of neuroleptics on the nigro-striatal DA system, but not to their influence on the mesolimbic and mesocortical DA system.

Dosage is undoubtedly a factor of importance for the development of hypokinetic-rigid symptoms. The larger the dose and the more quickly it is increased, the graver the risk that these symptoms occur. But this is not the only factor. With a particular dosage scheme, some patients do and others do not develop these symptoms. The determinants of this predisposition are not known with certainty. Age plays a role. The risk of neuroleptic parkinsonism increases with increasing age. There are indications, moreover, that the pretherapeutic level of DA turnover also plays a role: the lower this level, the graver the risk of neuroleptic parkinsonism (chapter XI).

4. Hyperkinetic/dyskinetic symptoms

Apart from the tremors already mentioned, neuroleptics can provoke all sorts of dyskinesias. With no attempt at completeness, I mention: torticollis, hyperextension of the neck, carpopedal spasms, spasms of the pharyngeal musculature with dysphagia, trismus, spasms of the facial muscles which give rise to bizarre grimaces, myoclonus, choreatiform movements and oculogyric crises. The musculature of the trunk can also be involved, particularly in children. They develop such symptoms as opisthotonus, scoliosis, lordosis, tortipelvis, etc. A remarkable phenomenon also is the sensation of a swollen tongue, which some patients report. They speak with difficulty, sometimes mumbling, and the tongue often protrudes from the mouth.

The phenomenon known as *akathisia* merits separate mention. It is a motor unrest which manifests itself mostly in the legs. In actual fact there are few reasons to classify the symptom as "extrapyramidal," but this is nevertheless done as a rule. In mild cases the patient is always seen to shuffle. In the case of severe akathisia the patient is in constant motion and hardly able any longer to sit or lie down. If he is forced into a sitting or recumbent position, the activity of the legs persists. Nearly always the restiveness is accompanied by insomnia. Akathisia can occur as an isolated symptom or in combination with other motor symptoms. In some cases it persists for weeks after medication has been discontinued. Akathisia can be mistaken for psychotic unrest and consequently the medication may be erroneously intensified rather than reduced. Psychotic unrest is often "fed" by demonstrable disorders of thinking and experiencing, but akathisia is not. It is experienced more as exogenous, as alien to the ego.

Dyskinetic symptoms are less common than hypokinetic-rigid symptoms, and largely linked to particular groups of neuroleptics (chapter VII). They can occur as isolated symptoms or in combination with features of the Parkinson syndrome. Not infrequently, dyskinetic disturbances occur intermittently, and may then be confused with symptoms of a hysterical nature. Acute overdosage is nearly always involved in these cases; dyskinesias, therefore, are mainly observed during the first days of medication and after an abrupt marked increase in dosage. They develop very quickly, sometimes peracutely. A pronounced Parkinson syndrome, on the other hand, more likely results from chronic overdosage and often does not develop until after several weeks.

Obviously, dyskinetic symptoms can be very alarming for the patient. In purely somatic terms, too, they are not entirely without danger. I once saw a woman aged 23, suffering from hebephrenia, who developed severe deglutition pneumonia based on spasm of the pharyngeal musculature in the course of neuroleptic medication. Dyskinetic disorders, therefore, should be controlled immediately by emergency measures.

5. Tardive dyskinesia

The term tàrdive dyskinesia is used with reference to a dyskinetic disturbance which: a) is caused by protracted administration of usually large doses of phenothiazines or butyrophenones; b) often does not become manifest, or at least more prominent, until after discontinuation or reduction of the medication; c) proves to be irreversible but not progressive after discontinuation of the medication. In the majority of the published cases, the medication had been continued over a period of more than two years.

The orofacial form is the most common type: the tongue executes rolling motions in the mouth and is sometimes protruded. Sucking movements of the lips, chewing movements of the jaws, bulging of the cheeks and smacking sounds are features of the fully developed syndrome. Speech can be impaired. The strange grimaces made by the patient can make him socially "impossible." The upper half of the face is usually not involved: blepharospasms and upward deviation of the eyes are rare features.

Tardive dyskinesia need not be confined to the orofacial region. In elderly patients particularly, the limbs may show myoclonic, choreatiform or athetotic movements. This leads to strange movements and postures of the trunk, spreading of the fingers, heel-tapping, growling sounds, disturbances in respiratory rhythm, etc. These disturbances may resemble those in akathisia, but they differ in that the subjective urge to move is absent. They are intensified by emotions and abate in repose, as is the rule for extrapyramidal kinetic disorders. We have no knowledge of any factors which predispose to tardive dyskinesia.

Mild forms of this syndrome can be transiently observed as so-called "withdrawal dyskinesia" after abrupt discontinuation of protracted neuroleptic medication. In such cases the dyskinetic symptoms disappear gradually in the course of a few weeks.

6. Pathogenesis of extrapyramidal disorders

Parkinson symptoms

Neuroleptics block postsynaptic receptors in central dopaminergic neurons (chapter IV). The increase in dopamine (DA) turnover which they cause is regarded as a compensatory mechanism aimed at breaking the block (which is of a competitive nature). In view of what we know of the causal relation between central DA deficiency and Parkinson's disease, it is assumed that inhibition of transmission in DA neurons of the nigrostriatal system underlies neuroleptic parkinsonism. It is pointed out in chapter XI that there are also direct arguments in support of this hypothesis.

The corpus striatum comprises, in addition to DA, other transmitters: 5-hydroxytryptamine (serotonin; 5-HT), acetylcholine and γ-aminobutyric acid. Phenothiazines and butyrophenones influence not only DA but also acetylcholine in the corpus striatum. They increase its rate of synthesis and promote its release into the synaptic cleft. DA agonists such as apomorphine do the opposite. These observations have led to the hypothesis that the acetylcholine neurons of the corpus striatum carry DA receptors which exert an inhibitory influence. For this reason, it is believed, DA antagonists such as neuroleptics enhance the activity of these acetylcholine neurons. In view of this hypothetical relation, it is understandable why anticholinergic anti-parkinson agents can favourably influence motor side effects of neuroleptics. Moreover, it warrants the expectation that anticholinergics should be contraindicated in conditions caused by DA-ergic *hyper*activity.

Whether other transmitters in the corpus striatum are also influenced by neuroleptics is still unknown.

Hyper(dys)kinesia

The blocking of postsynaptic DA receptors by neuroleptics is reversible; it can be overcome by an excess of DA molecules. Should DA synthesis increase too much in response to receptor block, then it would overshoot its target and could provoke DA-ergic hyperactivity. It is conceivable, but by no means certain, that a mechanism of this kind underlies neuroleptic hyperkinesia and dyskinesia. This hypothesis has not been tested in human individuals and cannot be tested in (lower) animals because in the lower species neuroleptics do not produce such kinetic disorders. An argument against this hypothesis is that anticholinergic anti-parkinson agents do not aggravate but in fact alleviate neuroleptic hyperkinesia.

Tardive dyskinesia

Hypersensitivity of postsynaptic DA receptors has been hypothetically held responsible for tardive dyskinesia. Arguments in favour of this hypothesis are: a) the symptoms occur or show exacerbation when neuroleptics (i.e. DA antagonists) are discontinued or their dose is reduced; b) they show exacerbation in response to 1-DOPA, a DA agonist; c) they resemble the dyskinetic symptoms which Parkinson patients can develop in response to DOPA therapy. DOPA is a DA precursor which is centrally converted to DA. The fact that anticholinergic agents have an unfavourable rather than a favourable effect on tardive dyskinesia is also consistent with what one could expect in a condition of DA hypersensitivity.

The receptor hypersensitivity has been explained on the basis of disuse ("disuse hypersensitivity"). In response to protracted receptor block, new DA receptors are believed to be formed. When the block diminishes, an excess of DA receptors results (or, in functional terms: receptor hypersensitivity). If tardive dyskinesia should indeed by a direct consequence of DA receptor block, then it could be expected that parkinson symptoms should always have preceded. This has not been demonstrated, and the hypothesis is weakened as a result.

Another possibility is denervation hypersensitivity: the postsynaptic DA receptors could become hypersensitive (i.e. increase in number) as a result of damage inflicted on the presynaptic element. This would explain the irreversibility of the dyskinetic symptoms. In animals, however, no consistent morphological changes in the brain have been demonstrated after chronic phenothiazine medication. Nor has this so far been done in human subjects. This means that a convincing explanation of tardive dyskinesia is not yet available. Pathogenetic studies are impeded by the fact that these symptoms cannot be provoked in test animals.

7. Treatment of motor side effects

The treatment of extrapyramidal disorders caused by neuroleptics should consist of reduction (if only temporarily) of the dosage and administration of classical anti-parkinson drugs. *Hypokinetic-rigid symptoms* usually respond well to, say, orphenadrine (Disipal, 3 × 50-100 mg per day) or trihexyphenidyl (Artane, 3 × 2-5 mg per day) or benzatropine (Cogentin, 3 × 0.5-2 mg per day). A long-acting anticholinergic anti-parkinson drug is dexetimide (Tremblex), of which only 0.5-1 mg need be given orally once every 24 hours. *Acute dyskinesia and hyperkinesia* respond well to intramuscular injection of 40 mg orphenadrine or 2-5 mg biperiden (Akineton). The injection can be repeated several times at intervals of a few hours, whereupon treatment is continued by mouth.

1-DOPA is not indicated in neuroleptic parkinsonism because it can aggravate psychotic symptoms. Amantadine (Symmetrel, 100-200 mg per day), a new anti-parkinson drug believed to promote release of DA into the synaptic cleft, is effective also in drug-induced extrapyramidal disorders. A major advantage of this compound is the absence of anticholinergic effects, for there are indications that reduction of central cholinergic activity is a disintegration-promoting factor.

Persistent tardive dyskinesia is much more difficult to treat, and the results are often disappointing, particularly in the long run. Treatment initially may have some success. Several strategies can be tried:

1) Drugs which exhaust the DA stores. *Tetrabenazine* (Nitoman) is a benzoquinolizine derivative which impedes the uptake of CA into the synaptic vesicles so that it is degraded by monoamineoxidase (MAO) and the stores become exhausted. With a daily dose of 75-200 mg, favourable results have been obtained in tardive dyskinesia. A similar biochemical action have *reserpine* (Serpasil, 1-5 mg per day) and *oxypertine* (Opertil, 100-200 mg per day), and there are reports on the successful use of these compounds also.

   α-Methyldopa (Aldomet) is converted in the brain to α-methyl DA and α-methyl NA—compounds which oust the DA and NA from the stores and come to function as false transmitters. The results obtained with these compounds are very variable.

2) DA receptor-blocking compounds. Both *phenothiazines* and

butyrophenones can be used, and often with some success. They confront the clinician with the peculiar dilemma of having to combat a disorder by prescribing the very type of compound that has caused it.

3) Inhibitors of DA synthesis, e.g. *α-methyl-p-tyrosine*(α-MT), an inhibitor of the enzyme tyrosine hydroxylase. In principle this medication seems rational. Because of the toxicity of α-MT, however, it is impractical except in fully equipped clinics under strict supervision.

4) Acetylcholine-potentiating compounds. If a) DA-ergic systems and cholinergic systems in the corpus striatum are indeed reciprocally related, and b) tardive dyskinesia is indeed based on hypersensitivity of the DA receptors, then cholinergic compounds can be expected to exert a beneficial influence, whereas anticholinergic compounds should have the opposite effect.

   Anticholinergic anti-parkinson agents in fact have either no effect on tardive dyskinesia, or an aggravating effect. A few scattered reports indicate that cholinergic compounds, on the other hand, can be useful. This applies to *2-dimethylaminoethanol* (Deanol, 600-1600 mg per day), a compound which may convert to acetylcholine in the brain, and to *physostigmine*, which inhibits the degradation of acetylcholine. Physostigmine has been given intravenously (1 mg) together with 1 mg methylscopolamine to combat peripheral cholinergic effects. Physostigmine should only be tried under strict control of a specialist. Deanol is allegedly harmless, but experience so far gained with it has been limited. Theoretically, choline, precursor of acetylcholine, would be a suitable candidate. Its efficacy is now under investigation.

8. Prophylaxis of motor side effects

As already pointed out, gross motor changes occur particularly when the dosage is rapidly increased to a high level. From a prophylactic point of view, therefore, booster doses are best avoided. The dosage should be gradually increased on the basis of the patient's psychological condition. If the situation is too serious to permit of this procedure, then it is advisable to combine the neuroleptic from the start with an anti-parkinson drugs, e.g. orphenadrine (Disipal, 3 × 50 mg per day). This is the more urgent if the neuroleptic used is one with a high affinity for the extrapyramidal system. The long-acting anti-parkinson drug dexetimide (Tremblex) also merits consideration. Given by mouth (0.5-1 mg per day), it is effective for 24 hours; the effect of an intramuscular injection of 0.125-0.250 mg lasts 2-3 days.

Some authors have raised objections to the prophylactic use of anti-parkinson agents. They argue that neuroleptics can irreversibly damage the extrapyramidal system in the long run, and tend to interpret extrapyramidal disorders which occur during neuroleptic medication as warning signals which cannot be disregarded without risk. For the time being, this interpretation is no more than an assumption. No definite relation has been demonstrated between tardive dyskinesia and preceding extrapyramidal disorders. Nevertheless, one should avoid unnecessarily protracted neuroleptic medication with large doses under the "umbrella" of anti-parkinson drugs. For this reason, too, it is advisable to reduce to a maintenance dose as soon as possible, whereupon anti-parkinson agents can usually be discontinued.

9. Vegetative symptoms

Antiadrenergic and anticholinergic activity

Most neuroleptic compounds are adrenolytics of the α-receptor-blocking type. In several respects they therefore behave like antagonists of adrenaline and noradrenaline. But not in all respects: the hyperglycaemic effect of catecholamines, for example, remains uninfluenced. On the basis of their adrenolytic activity, neuroleptics can be expected to cause arterial vasodilatation, to reduce the peripheral resistance and therefore to reduce the blood pressure. In fact, hypotension is one of the most common and treacherous cliffs on which neuroleptic medication can be stranded. Both central and peripheral mechanisms are involved here. Moreover, some neuroleptics (e.g. reserpine) have a pronounced anticholinergic, i.e. atropine-like activity. This explains complaints about difficult micturition, blurred vision (due to impeded accommodation), etc.

In view of the influence on sympathetic as well as parasympathetic functions, it is understandable that vegetative syndromes provoked by neuroleptics often show mixed features. But this does not take away the fact that anti-adrenergic activity usually prevails over anticholinergic activity so that the ultimate result is an overall state of parasympathetic hyperactivity or, to use the terminology of Hess, a state of trophotropism.

Circulatory disorders

Systolic as well as diastolic hypotension is the most common complication of neuroleptic medication. It is of a largely orthostatic type. Regular determinations have shown that some decrease in blood pressure occurs in virtually all cases. If the effect is more pronounced, then the patient reports complaints such as a sensation of lightness in the head and palpitations, mainly upon abrupt changes in posture. A sensation of heaviness and dullness in the legs is another common complaint. In serious cases the patient may enter a state of shock, with clouded consciousness. Even acute death has been reported in a few instances; an abrupt decrease in blood pressure probably led to failure of the cardiac or cerebral circulation in these cases.

The decrease in blood pressure is dose-dependent; its severity as well as its frequency increases with increasing dosage. An increased risk exists in the case of elderly patients (particularly if previously hypertensive), alcoholics and individuals suffering from vegetative instability, i.e. sympathicotonic persons.

The cardiovascular system usually adjusts itself spontaneously to the new situation. A decrease in blood pressure is a phenomenon of the first few weeks of medication; gradual recovery usually follows and the symptoms in question disappear.

A troublesome degree of hypotension can nearly always be *prevented* by increasing the dosage gradually. A high "ceiling" can in this way be attained without undue risk. Even so, regular determinations of blood pressure remain necessary during the first month, and this is the more urgent when walking patients receive the medication. Orthostatic hypotension, it should be borne in mind, entails substantial risks in many occupations and professions. If the psychological condition calls for a quickly established effective concentration of neuroleptics, then it is advisable to confine the patient to bed for a few days. In any case, this type of medication is best given in a clinical setting.

The *treatment* of this complication is of necessity restricted to reduction (if only temporarily) of the dosage: more or less harmless agents with a moderate hypertensive effect are unfortunately not yet available. In serious cases medication should be discontinued immediately, and it may be necessary to administer vasoconstrictors. For this purpose, noradrenaline should be used, not adrenaline or one of its synthetic derivatives because the latter's hypertensive effect is significantly reduced (and may even be reversed) by phenothiazine derivatives.

Neuroleptics with anticholinergic properties, such as reserpine and tetrabenazine, can reduce the pulse rate, in rare cases even to a dangerously low level.

Gastrointestinal disorders

Xerostomia and constipation are common complaints during neuroleptic medication. There are even some reports on paralytic ileus probably related to the use of neuroleptics. Hypersalivation—a fairly rare phenomenon—usually occurs in combination with gross motor changes. A few authors have mentioned diarrhoea but this complaint is so infrequent that a relation to neuroleptic medication is doubtful.

Disorders of the urogenital apparatus

Micturition is often impeded, particularly in male patients. The patient has a sensation of voiding against a resistance; the jet of urine is feeble, and the first micturition after sleep is particularly difficult. This phenomenon is probably based on paresis of the detrusor urinae. It is often transient and rarely necessitates discontinuation of treatment. The symptom can be adequately controlled with the aid of cholinergics such as carbachol (Doryl) or neostigmine (Prostigmine).

Pollakisuria can occur in rare cases. For the sake of completeness (the phenomenon is fairly rare), I mention impeded ejaculation, with undisturbed erection and orgasm.

Other vegetative manifestations

Deficient accommodation and mydriasis can give rise to blurred vision. Complaints of hyperhidrosis, hot flushes and nausea are relatively common, but this does not mean that they are directly determined by the medication in all cases. Side effects of psychotropic drugs and hypochondriacal complaints are not readily distinguishable.

Swelling of the nasal mucosa (which the patient describes as a clogged nose) is a common phenomenon particularly in reserpine medication. Whether this should come under this heading or under that of "allergic manifestations" remains uncertain.

10. Allergic manifestations

Under this heading I shall briefly discuss three complications which are probably of allergic origin, although this has not been demonstrated with certainty: liver lesions, blood dyscrasia, and skin lesions.

Liver lesions

The term "Largactil jaundice" is still appropriate for the risk of liver lesions is greater with chlorpromazine than with other phenothiazine derivatives. Thioxanthenes, butyrophenones, reserpine and benzoquinoline derivatives are virtually harmless in this respect. Liver lesions have been described in a few rare cases, but their causal relation to the medication is doubtful.

It was initially believed that, like the mother substance phenothiazine, chlorpromazine might damage the liver directly, by a toxic effect; but this is unlikely, for the development of jaundice was found not to be dose-dependent. Neither the daily dose nor the total dose administered was of importance in this respect. Numerous patients, moreover, have received chlorpromazine for years without any untoward effect on the liver. Similar experience was gained with test animals. Even a massive overdose of chlorpromazine, e.g. in suicidal attempts, seldom leads to demonstrable liver lesions. The principal argument in favour of an allergic origin is the following:

jaundice usually develops, independent of the dose administered, within a given time span—between the second and the fourth week of medication. After the fifth week this complication is rare. The liver lesions, moreover, are often accompanied by blood eosinophilia, and eosinophilic infiltrates are also found in the liver itself.

In the vast majority of cases chlorpromazine jaundice has the characteristics of obstructive jaundice. It is based on intrahepatic bile obstruction. Prodromal symptoms are fever, malaise and gastrointestinal disorders. Primary parenchymal damage is exceedingly rare. Microscopic examination shows that the bile capillaries are swollen and reveals bile thrombi in the central canaliculi. Pericapillary oedema is also observed. The liver cells proper are usually unaffected, although parenchymal lesions can of course develop secondarily, after bile obstruction has become chronic. The latter, however, is unusual. A complete recovery is nearly always made. Cirrhosis of the liver rarely develops.

Data on the incidence of chlorpromazine jaundice differ widely. On the basis of a large material, Keup (1959) estimated the incidence to be about 1%. It should be immediately added, however, that in most clinics the incidence substantially decreased after 1961, perhaps due to an increasing use of other neuroleptics. Better screening may also have played a role; patients with a hepatic history or manifest hepatic disease are preferably not treated with chlorpromazine. It is finally also possible that a second noxa has been active during the period indicated—a circulating hepatitis virus. A subclinical viral hepatitis could have facilitated development of chlorpromazine jaundice. However, this theory is not very plausible because this virus preferably affects parenchymal cells, and chlorpromazine jaundice is usually of a cholangiolytic type.

For the *prophylaxis* of this complication, the following measures merit consideration.

1) Determination of liver functions prior to medication. If they are disturbed or if there is a recent history of liver disease, then chlorpromazine should be advised against. Other phenothiazine derivatives also require restraint. The use of other types of neuroleptic is less ill-advised as long as liver functions are regularly tested.

   A history of chlorpromazine jaundice does not necessarily contraindicate the use of other phenothiazine derivatives, for cross hypersensitivity is rare within this series. Yet in those circumstances one would preferably select one of the non-phenothiazine neuroleptics.

2) Liver functions should be tested regularly (at least once a week) during the first five weeks of chlorpromazine medication. This is less urgent with other types of neuroleptic, but nevertheless advisable.

The most suitable screening procedure is determination of SGPT, SGOT and serum alkaline phosphatase activities. This gives information both on the integrity of the parenchymal cells and on the patency of the bile passages. This procedure is not entirely foolproof. It fails in the case of peracute development of liver lesions (which is rare). It is also to be borne in mind that a slight increase in the activity of the abovementioned enzyme systems occurs repeatedly during neuroleptic medication.

This applies to phenothiazine derivatives as well as to other types of neuroleptics. The increase is generally transient even when medication is continued. Some authors hold that these fluctuations are of central origin and unrelated to the integrity of liver functions. Consequently, they regard the abovementioned screening procedure as meaningless. However, there are hardly any arguments to support this view. For the time being it seems advisable to regard these fluctuations in activity as no more than an indication that neuroleptics frequently interfere with liver functions, albeit usually only slightly and transiently. In my opinion, the phenomenon has only one consequence: intensified testing and discontinuation of medication whenever rapid normalization fails to occur or the increase in activity persists.

The *treatment* of this complication is a matter for the internist.

Haemopoietic disorders

Agranulocytosis is undoubtedly the most serious of these disorders. In the cases described, chlorpromazine and some related compounds were usually the culpit. However, the use of phenothiazine derivatives far exceeds that of the other neuroleptics, so for the latter compounds a prudent attitude also remains imperative. Griffith and Saameli (1975) describe an "epidemic" of agranulocytosis in patients being treated with the new neuroleptic clozapine. Since all cases occurred in one place, it is dubious whether clozapine was indeed the (principal) culprit.

Agranulocytosis in response to phenothiazines develops, regardless of the dose administered, within a well-defined time-span: between the fifth and the tenth week of medication. This raised the suspicion that the bone marrow is not damaged directly, but indirectly, via an allergic mechanism. This suspicion was strengthened by the observations of Hippius and Kanig (1958), who in blood from such patients demonstrated antibodies specifically active against the patient's own leucocytes. Moreover, the occurrence of this complication is not related to the daily or total dose of phenothiazine given. In large series, the incidence of phenothiazine-linked agranulocytosis is 0.07-0.7%. Women are more frequently affected than men. In many cases only the white system is affected, while erythrocytes and platelets remain at a normal level.

The *prophylaxis* of this complication of course consists of regular leucocyte counts in the peripheral blood during the first three months of medication. Unlike other drug-induced agranulocytoses, that due to phenothiazines as a rule develops gradually, so that weekly counts are sufficient (more frequent counts would pose practical problems with walking patients). Acute infections of the oropharyngeal cavity or unexplained pyrexia calls for immediate leucocyte counts. The question of the "critical" value, at which medication should be discontinued, is still controversial. Many investigators accept a limit of 2000 leucocytes per cu mm.

During the first four weeks of neuroleptic medication—i.e. before the period which is critical for agranulocytosis—slight leucocytopenia is repeatedly observed (rarely below 3000/cu mm), without changes in the differential count. This leucocytopenia is usually transient even when medication is continued, but it does call for intensified counts.

The *treatment* of agranulocytosis is entirely a matter for the internist. Once the white blood picture has normalized, neuroleptic medication can be resumed, if necessary with another phenothiazine derivative, for cross-hypersensitivity is rare. Yet it seems a wise policy to select a compound from one of the other groups in these cases.

In rare cases, thrombocytopenia can occur during neuroleptic medication, and it also seems that haemorrhagic diathesis can develop without abnormalities of the various clotting factors. In the latter cases, toxic or allergic damage to the capillaries may be involved. Anaemia (normochromic) of any significance has been observed only in response to prochlorperazine and perphenazine. Eosinophilia (up to 40%) is rarely an isolated finding, but usually occurs in combination with liver lesions or allergic skin lesions.

Dermatoses

Skin lesions usually develop between the second and the fourth week of medication. In rare cases there may be an immediate response, usually accompanied by fever and decreased blood pressure. In view of their predilection for a particular period, their independence of the dose administered and the eosinophilia which frequently accompanies them, these skin lesions are considered to be of allergic origin. Pruritus can be the sole manifestation of sensitization. Some patients in addition develop an exanthema which may show macular, maculopapular or urticarial features. The incidence of these skin lesions is about 5% with chlorpromazine, while that with the other phenothiazines and the thioxanthenes is much lower (about 1%). Butyrophenones and reserpine have remained undiscussed in this respect.

In the early years of treatment with phenothiazine derivatives, allergic dermatoses regularly developed in nurses also, probably after percutaneous sensitization. The complication has been rare since the tablets in question have been sugar-coated.

Treatment of the exanthema with an antihistamine such as promethazine (Phenergan) is usually successful. In persistent cases hydrocortisone derivatives may be indicated (in consultation with the dermatologist). Cross-hypersensitivity is rare, which means that the antibodies formed are generally specific against the compound used. One may therefore switch to a related neuroleptic without undue risk.

A phenomenon even more common than allergic dermatosis is photosensitization—erythema and swelling occurring more quickly than normal in areas exposed to (sun)light. Chlorpromazine produces this effect in some 10% of cases, the incidence with the other phenothiazines and with thioxanthenes being lower. So far as we know, butyrophenones and reserpine do not cause photosensitization. The phenomenon persists as long as medication continues, but rarely attains a degree of severity which necessitates discontinuation of treatment. The patient should, of course, avoid sun bathing.

Oedema of the angioneurotic type is a rare complication, observed only in patients given chlorpromazine.

11. Hormonal disorders

Menstrual disorders—menorrhagia as well as oligomenorrhoea and amenorrhoea—repeatedly occur during neuroleptic medication, but are not uncommon in untreated psychoses as well. However, their incidence substantially increases in response to the compounds in question, and a causal relation is therefore not improbable. There is no relation to the dosage. The complaints often disappear spontaneously in the course of medication, but sometimes persist as long as medication continues. Nothing is known about their pathogenesis.

Independent of any menstrual disorders, engorgement of the breasts can occur even before the menarche or in the menopause. Galactorrhoea is not an uncommon feature in these cases. Rare instances of gynaecomastia have been observed in men. These symptoms could be related to an increased prolactin production in the anterior pituitary, caused by neuroleptics (chapter XI).

Many patients show a significant weight gain during neuroleptic medication. The cause of this weight gain has so far remained obscure, but an improved psychological condition and a corresponding increase in appetite undoubtedly play a role. The increase in appetite may even be excessive and assume the features of real gluttony; yet this is not the only factor. There may be a substantial weight gain even when treatment fails and/or food uptake remains uninfluenced. There is a suspicion that water retention plays a role in this respect. Even though manifest oedema is only sporadically observed during neuroleptic medication, extracellular fluid accumulation cannot be excluded. An increased intracellular fluid compartment is likewise possible, in principle. This touches upon a fascinating question: the significance of the water balance in the development and abatement of psychotic disorders. This question, however, has hardly been systematically studied, if at all.

12. Thrombosis

Thrombosis is a little-known complication of neuroleptic medication. Häefner et al. (1965) reported 49 cases in a series of 1590 patients. Venous stasis as a result of markedly reduced activity of the voluntary musculature is probably a factor of importance in this respect. The thrombosis is often localized in the leg or thigh, but there have also been reports on atypical localizations: axilla, cubital fossa, upper arm and back of the hand. Elderly patients run an increased risk, and this is all the more reason to avoid large doses of neuroleptics in this category.

13. Epileptic manifestations

Changes in the electroencephalogram (EEG) generally do not occur unless the neuroleptic is given in large doses. In these circumstances, synchronization of electrical activity can occur. The amplitude of the alpha-rhythm increases and its frequency diminishes. In addition, theta- and even delta-waves can appear. In some cases, unmistakable epileptic activity becomes manifest (e.g. spikes and after-potentials). The corresponding clinical features are seizures of the generalized type. It was precisely on the basis of this epileptogenic activity that chlorpromazine was used in the past to provoke epileptic EEG changes in patients suspected of epilepsy. This is in striking contrast with the anti-epileptic activity customarily expected of conventional sedatives.

In principle, all known neuroleptics are able to lower the convulsion threshold, but phenothiazines do this more readily than butyrophenones. Manifest seizures, however, are usually a result of an inadequate dosage scheme—daily doses too quickly increased to a very high level. Aivazian and Reese (1959), for example, mentioned occurrence of convulsions in 30 to 65 (non-epileptic) patients treated with promazine. They received 1100-3800 mg daily of this compound!

If epileptic patients are to be given neuroleptics, then an increase in anti-epileptic medication should be contemplated. It is to be noted, in this respect, that the hypnotic effect of barbiturates is potentiated by neuroleptics.

14. Pigment deposits in eyes and skin

In the course of protracted chlorpromazine medication (usually in large doses), pigment can be deposited in the cornea and lens. Visual acuity may diminish as a result, but never to any serious extent. The changes are irreversible. In these circumstances, pigment can also accumulate in the skin, particularly in areas exposed to air. The discoloration is initially brownish and subsequently becomes bluish-grey. The histochemical properties of this pigment are identical to those of melanin. Skin and eye pigmentations not uncommonly occur together, but this does not mean that their causes are identical.

Pigment accumulations in the retina have been described in patients given large doses of thioridazine.

Whether other phenothiazines can produce similar effects is unknown. They have never been described in association with other types of neuroleptics.

15. Other accompanying phenomena

In the initial phase of neuroleptic medication many patients complain of dizziness even though the blood pressure has not significantly decreased. During this period, moreover, slight pyrexia may occur in the absence of any demonstrable inflammation. Both phenomena disappear spontaneously in a short while.

Several authors maintain that the resistance of the organism to infections diminishes during neuroleptic medication, and consequently they consider neuroleptics contraindicated in febrile diseases. This view, however, lacks a firm foundation. There are no indications that infectious diseases are more frequent or take a more serious course in patients treated with neuroleptics than in untreated patients. I therefore consider it justifiable to keep infectiously conditioned psychiatric syndromes within the range of indications for neuroleptics.

16. Somatic contraindications to neuroleptic medication

Phenothiazine derivatives are contraindicated if liver or bone marrow functions are deficient. The hepatotoxicity and haematotoxicity of the other neuroleptics are low, and these can therefore be used in such cases if the indication is urgent and under strict supervision.

Poor heart functions, fixed hypertension and severe hypotension are not absolute contraindications but do necessitate prudence as to dosage and alertness to any changes in blood pressure. Under these conditions, after all, a rapid decrease in blood pressure can easily lead to cerebral or cardiac disaster.

17. Overdosage of neuroleptics

The acute toxicity of most neuroleptics is remarkably low, although there are individual differences in this respect. Hippius (1960) described some patients whose consciousness was only slightly clouded after a single dose of 5 g chlorpromazine, whereas others became comatose in response to much smaller doses.

Massive overdosage, as in attempted suicide, leads to loss of consciousness, hypotension, hypothermia, tachycardia and tachypnoea. Tendon reflexes are absent and convulsions often develop. In principle, the treatment of this state of intoxication is the same as that of intoxication caused by hypnotics. There are no specific measures. After gastric lavage, if necessary, special attention should focus on circulation, pulmonary ventilation and fluid and electrolyte balance. Hypertensive agents (only noradrenaline is suitable as such, as pointed out on page 123) and parenteral fluid administration can be indicated. Seizures, if any, should be combated with chloral hydrate, not with barbiturates because their hypnotic effect is vigorously potentiated by neuroleptics so that the duration of the coma is increased.

The prognosis quoad vitam of this state of intoxication is favourable. Successful suicidal attempts with neuroleptics are rare. Many of these compounds are "suicide-proof" in a high degree, and this is an unmistakable advantage. Residual symptoms, too, are rare. The prognosis is substantially less favourable when hypnotics have been taken as well.

BIBLIOGRAPHY

AIVAZIAN, G. H. AND H. C. REESE (1959). Clinical evaluation of promazine therapy for schizophrenia. *Dis. Nerv. Syst.* 20, 472.

AYD, F. J. (1974). Side effects of depots fluphenazines. *Compr. Psychiat.* 15, 69.

AYD, F. J. (1975). Deanol therapy for tardive dyskinesia. *International drug therapy letter* 10, 37.

BEUMONT, P. J. V., M. G. GOLDEN, H. G. FRIESEN, G. W. HARRIS, P. C. R. MACKINNON, B. M. MANDELBROTE AND D. H. WILES (1974). The effects of phenodiazines on endocrine function. I. Patients with inappropriate lactation and amenorrhoea. *Brit. J. Psychiat.* 124, 413.

BEUMONT, P. J. V., C. S. CORKER, H. G. FRIESEN, T. KOLAKOWSKA, B. M. MANDELBROTE, J. MARSHALL, M. A. F. MURRAY AND D. H. WILES (1974). The effects of phenothiazines on endocrine function. II. Effects in men and postmenopausal women. *Brit. J. Psychiat.* 124, 420.

DEGKWITZ, R., U. CONSBRUCH, S. HADDENBROCK, B. NEUSCH, W. OEHLERT AND R. UNSÖLD (1976). Therapeutische Risiken bei der Langzeitbehandlung mit Neuroleptika und Lithium. *Nervenarzt* 47, 81.

DIMASCIO, A., D. L. BERNARDO, D. J. GREENBLATT AND J. E. MANDER (1976). A controlled trial of amantidine in drug-induced extrapyramidal disorders. *Arch. gen. Psychiat.* 33, 599.

GARDOS, M. D. AND J. O. COLE (1976). Maintenance antipsychotic therapy: Is the cure worse than the disease? *Amer. J. Psychiat. 133*, 32.

GOODWIN, F. K., M. H. EBERT AND W.E. BUNNEY (1972). Mental effects of reserpine in man. In: R. I. Shader, *Psychiatric Complications of Medical Drugs*. New York: Raven Press.

GRIFFITH, R. W. AND K. SAAMELI (1975). Clozapine and agranulocytosis. *Lancet* 2, 657.

HAASE, H. J. AND P. A. J. JANSSEN (1965). *The Action of Neuroleptic Drugs*. Amsterdam: North-Holland Publishing Company.

HÄEFNER, H. AND I. BREHM (1965). Thromboembolic complication in neuroleptic treatment. *Compr. Psychiat.* 6, 25.

HÄEFNER, H., B. HEYDER AND I. KUTSCHER (1965). Undesirable side effects and complications with the use of neuroleptic drugs. *J. Neuropsychiat.* 1, 46.

HIPPIUS, H. AND K. KANIG (1958). Agranulozytose unter neuropsychiatrische Phenothiazin-Therapie. *Arztl. Wschr.* 13, 501.

HIPPIUS, H. (1960). Therapeutisch unerwunschte Wirkungen der modernen Psychopharmaca I. Phenothiazin-Derivate und verwandte Verbindungen. *Internist* 1, 453.

KAZAMATSURI, H., C. P. CHIEN AND J. O. COLE (1972). Therapeutic approaches to tardive dyskinesia. *Arch. gen. Psychiat.* 27, 491.

KEUP, W. (1959). Effect of phenothiazine derivatives on liver function. *Dis. Nerv. Syst.* 20, 161.

KLAWANS, H. L. AND R. RUBOVITS (1974). Effect of cholinergic and anticholinergic agents on tardive dyskinesia. *J. Neurol. Neurosurg. Psychiat.* 27, 941.

KLAWANS, H. L. (1975). Disorders of the extrapyramidal system. In: M. M. Cohen (Ed.) *Biochemistry of Neural Disease*. New York: Harper and Row.

LACOURSIERE, R. B., H. E. SPOHN AND K. THOMPSON (1976). Medical effects of abrupt neuroleptic withdrawal. *Compr. Psychiat.* 17, 285.

MARSDEN, C. D., D. TARSY AND R. J. BALDESSARINI (1975). Spontaneous and drug-induced movement disorders in psychotic patients. In: D. F. Benson and D. Blumer, *Psychiatric Aspects of Neurologic Disease*. New York, San Francisco, London: Grune and Stratton.

MCGLASHAN, T. H. AND W. T. CARPENTER JR. (1976). Postpsychotic depression in schizophrenia. *Arch. gen. Psychiat.* 33, 231-239.

SHADER, R. I. AND A. DIMASCIO (1970). *Psychotropic Drug Side Effects*. Baltimore: Williams and Wilkins.

1.

READ, A. E., J. LAIDLAW AND C. F. MCCARTHY (1969). Effects of chlorpromazine in patients with hepatic disease. *Brit. Med. J.* 3, 497.

SHADER, R. I. AND A. DIMASCIO (1970). *Psychotropic Drug Side Effects*. Baltimore: Williams and Wilkins.

SINGH, M. M. AND S. R. KAY (1975). Therapeutic reversal with benztropine in schizophrenics. Practical and theoretical significance. *J. Nerv. Ment. Dis.* 160, 258.

WEIDEN, P. L. AND C. D. BUCKNER (1973). Thioridazine toxicity: agranulocytosis and hepatitis with encephalopathy. *J. Amer. Med. Ass.* 224, 518.

IX

Neuroleptics III: Practical Guidelines for Neuroleptic Medication

Most of the following points have already been discussed in the two preceding chapters, and are briefly recapitulated here.

1) The therapeutic action of neuroleptics is a dual one: sedative and antipsychotic. The intensity of each of the two components differs in different groups of neuroleptics. Neuroleptics are indicated syndromally, not nosologically, which is to say that they are administered to combat agitation or certain anomalies of experiencing, regardless of the nosological context in which these symptoms occur.

2) Gradually increasing dosage reduces the risk of complications (hypotension, extrapyramidal symptoms) and is therefore advisable in terms of prevention. If the seriousness of the psychological condition calls for rapid neuroleptization, then the neuroleptic should be combined with an antiparkinson agent and the patient should be confined to bed for a few days (with a view to possible hypotension).

3) The blood pressure should be carefully monitored during the first few months of medication. This is particularly urgent in elderly patients whose vascular system can be expected to have lost some of its elasticity. In such patients the hypotensive effect of neuroleptics can have disastrous con-

sequences for the heart and the brain. Although with the majority of compounds this is not absolutely necessary, regular determination of liver functions and leucocyte counts in the peripheral blood can be regarded as desirable during the first few months.

4) In section 9 of chapter VII, an attempt has been made to differentiate the various groups of neuroleptics according to clinical effects. Undoubtedly there are other differences also. How else could one explain that one neuroleptic can fail, whereas another is effective in the same patient. These suspected differences, however, have not yet been adequately studied. In actual practice this means that neuroleptic treatment cannot be considered a failure until it is ascertained that several consecutively given compounds have remained ineffective. This is certainly not meant as a plea for the indiscriminate use of the entire range of neuroleptics. On the contrary, it is advisable to confine oneself to a few compounds from different groups. Only in this way can adequate experience be gained with each of these agents.

5) Neuroleptic medication decidedly calls for individualized dosage. None of these agents has a generally valid optimal dosage. The optimum varies from one syndrome to the other and, within the same diagnostic context, from one patient to the next. One should beware of overdosage (gross extrapyramidal disorders are to be avoided), but underdosage is likewise to be avoided. The dosage should be gradually increased until further psychological improvement fails to develop. The smallest dose with which this optimal condition is maintained should be continued for some time (and certainly not too short a time).

6) Some investigators have stated that very large doses of, say, fluphenazine are more effective than standard doses, and that consequently mega-doses are indicated in the treatment of refractory patients. Experimental findings have so far failed to support this theory. In view of the risk of lesions of the extrapyramidal system, therefore, I consider very large doses to be contraindicated for the time being. By this I do not mean to say that there are no patients who require large doses of a particular neuroleptic. There are such patients: those who metabolize a given neuroleptic unusually quickly. As long as routine determinations of blood concentrations of neuroleptics are impractical, these patients can be identified only by increasing the dosage *gradually* until the desired effect is obtained. Only if attained in this way are mega-doses justifiable.

7) No general guidelines can be given for the duration of treatment. In the case of psychoses in which the prognosis is estimated to be favourable in principle, the time at which medication can be discontinued should be determined in each individual patient by gradually reducing the dosage on the basis of the psychological condition. Emphasis is placed here on the word gradual; only in this way is it possible to establish whether the reduction is tolerated; and only in this way is it possible to intervene in time when a relapse seems imminent. Abrupt discontinuation, moreover, especially after protracted medication, can give rise to withdrawal symptoms such as nausea, vomiting, hyperhidrosis and insomnia.

   In psychoses with a chronic or chronic recurrent course, neuroleptic medication must be continued for a long period, sometimes for life, but never without supervision and regular attempts to establish whether the patient can do with less, or possibly without. Protracted neuroleptic medication can lead to irreversible lesions of the extrapyramidal system, resulting in severe dyskinesia. This risk increases with increasing doses. This is why attempts should always be made to establish the lowest effective dosage. Otherwise the chronic toxicity of neuroleptics is low, and addiction or habituation has seldom been observed.

8) A not uncommon question in chronic neuroleptic medication is whether the compound in question should absolutely be administered in several fractional doses per day, or whether the entire daily dose can be taken at once without undue problems. This question has not yet been adequately studied. For the time being, however, administration in fractional doses seems preferable with a view to a reasonably even blood concentration.

   For patients who cannot be trusted to take their medicine regularly, long-acting neuroleptics may be considered. A major advantage of these compounds lies in the certainty that the patient does receive what is considered to be necessary (at least if one administers the compound personally). A disadvantage is that accurate dosage of long-acting compounds is much more difficult than that of the short acting types. Moreover, problems can arise when the patient needs other drugs in addition (e.g. anaesthetic agents for an operation) or is a user of alcohol.

9) It has been demonstrated for phenothiazines that, after oral administration, a substantial amount is not absorbed and/or broken down in the intestinal wall. This has not yet been

investigated for other types of neuroleptic. Parenteral administration of phenothiazines is therefore more efficient than oral administration, but carries an increased risk of side effects, e.g. hypotension and motor disorders. Parenteral administration, a substantial amount is not absorbed and/or in the case of severe agitation. As soon as the desired effect is obtained, it is advisable to continue treatment by mouth. In view of the grave risk of complications, intravenous injection is not recommended.

10) Even in therapeutic doses, neuroleptics lower the convulsion threshold, and in epileptic patients this can necessitate an increase in anti-epileptic medication.

11) The somnifacient effect of barbiturates and other hypnotics is potentiated by neuroleptics, the more so as the sedative effect of the latter is stronger. The same applies to the sedative hypnotic effect of antihistamines of the promethazine (Phenergan) type. Clinical psychiatry has made grateful use of this fact in prolonged sleep (Dauerschlaf) cures (a more or less obsolete form of treatment). It should finally be mentioned in this context that the effect of alcohol is potentiated by phenothiazine derivatives. Patients should be instructed accordingly.

12) Unless they are administered in small doses, neuroleptics exert an unfavourable influence on reactivity and alertness. Driving an automobile should therefore be discouraged, at least during the first 6-8 weeks of neuroleptic medication.

13) The combination of neuroleptics with electro-shock therapy (EST)—a combination advocated by some authors in acute types of schizophrenia—is not without danger. Severe hypotension with shock symptoms following the EST has been reported. This risk can be substantially reduced by withdrawing neuroleptics during the 12 hours preceding EST, and by confining the patient to bed for a few hours afterwards.

14) So far there have been no reports on incompatibility between individual neuroleptics. Generally, therefore, there is no objection to combining two neuroleptics—a procedure which, of course, aims at enhancement of the therapeutic effect. It is to be borne in mind, however, that the two compounds can potentiate each other's side effects as well. This also applies to a combination of a neuroleptic with an antidepressant. This can be very useful in agitated depressions, but the price to be paid is an increased risk of com-

plications (hypotension!). Combined psychotropic medications, therefore, necessitate intensified monitoring.

15) So far as has been established, neuroleptics have no teratogenic activity. Yet the reticence conventionally observed with regard to medication during pregnancy should also be extended to the psychotropic drugs.

X

Neuroleptics IV: Specific Part

In the preceding three chapters the neuroleptics were discussed as a group. In this chapter the individual compounds will be separately discussed, adhering to the classification presented in section 1 of chapter VII. Deviations from the general action profile, if any, will be mentioned under the heading "Particulars." The dosages indicated are averages, not optima; as already pointed out, neuroleptic medication is decidedly a matter of individualized dosage. The generic name is always followed by a number of trade names, but no attempt at comprehensiveness is made. For a comprehensive survey I refer to the Index Psychopharmacorum of Pöldinger and Schmidlin (1972).

Table 3. Phenothiazine derivatives with an aminoalkyl group in the side chain.

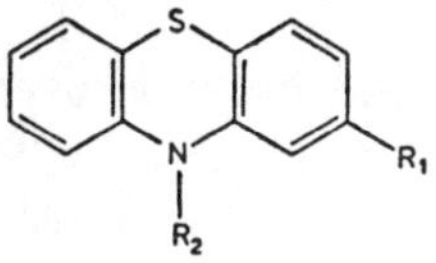

Chemical structure R_1	R_2	Generic name	Trade name	Average dose per day in mg by mouth
—	CH_2—CH—CH_2—$N(CH_3)_2$ | CH_3	Alimemazine	Nedeltran Theralene	50-300
Cl	CH_2—CH_2—CH_2—$N(CH_3)_2$	Chlorpromazine	Largactil Megaphen Thorazine	150-600
OCH_3	CH_2—CH—CH_2—$N(CH_3)_2$ | CH_3	Laevomepromazine	Neurocil Nozinan	150-300
—	CH_2—CH_2—CH_2—$N(CH_3)_2$	Promazine	Prazine Protactyl Sparine	300-1000
CF_3	CH_2—CH_2—CH_2—$N(CH_3)_2$	Triflupromazine	Psyquil Siquil Vesprin	150-400

1. Phenothiazine derivatives with an aminoalkyl group in the side chain (Table 3)

Alimemazine (Nedeltran, Theralene)

Chemical structure. 10- (3-dimethylamino-2-methylpropyl)-phenothiazine.

Dosage. This compound is generally given by mouth—in the form of tablets, droplets or syrup—but can also be given by intramuscular injection. The oral dose is 50-300 mg per day. Intramuscular administration should not exceed 25-50 mg per injection and 150 mg/24 hours.

Particulars. The sedative effect of this compound prevails over its antipsychotic effect. Since blood pressure and extrapyramidal system are relatively little influenced, this agent is not infrequently used in the treatment of restive demented elderly patients.

Chlorpromazine (Largactil, Thorazine, Megaphen)

Chemical structure. 2-chloro-10-(3-dimethylaminopropyl)-phenothiazine hydrochloride.

Dosage. The therapeutic range of this compound is very wide. The average oral daily dose is 150-600 mg, but amounts up to 1.5-2 g per day are tolerated without undue difficulties.

Chlorpromazine can also be given by intramuscular injection, but this is painful. This compound is but slowly absorbed, moreover, and at the site of injection painful infiltrates soon form, which may be accompanied by fever. It is therefore advisable not to continue parenteral treatment longer than 2-3 days and not to increase the dosage to more than 3-4 × 75 mg daily. Although this "ceiling" is rather low, the calming effect can be substantially potentiated in urgent cases by addition of a barbiturate and/or a sedative antihistamine (chapter XXVII).

Administration of chlorpromazine by continuous drip is possible but not recommended in view of the grave risk of side effects (hypotension!).

Particulars. Chlorpromazine is the prototype of the group of phenothiazine derivatives. Its evolution was outlined in section 3 of chapter VII. It also served as model in the description of the general action profile of neuroleptics, and in this respect it therefore combines the particular with the general.

Laevopromazine (Nozinan, Neurocil)

Chemical structure. 10-(3-dimethylamino-2-methylpropyl)-2-methoxyphenothiazine.

Dosage. Laevopromazine is usually given by mouth (tablets or droplets): 150-300 mg per day. If the daily dose exceeds 400 mg, then side effects rapidly increase in severity and frequency, which shows that the therapeutic range of this agent is not wide.

If parenterally administered, laevopromazine has a pronounced effect on blood pressure. Intramuscular injections are therefore acceptable only if the patient is confined to bed. In that case the daily dose is 100-150 mg, divided over 3-4 fractional doses of 25-50 mg. Intravenous administration is possible in principle but has hardly been used because, in view of the irritant effect of laevopromazine on the vascular wall, a continuous drip is required (50-100 mg in 250-500 ml physiological saline), which is virtually impracticable in restive patients. Intramuscular injections are painful and can cause infiltrates in the muscles. They should not be given for more than a few days.

Particulars. Laevopromazine is undoubtedly an effective and strongly sedative neuroleptic; but it has been claimed to be more. It was introduced as a "broad-spectrum neuroleptic" believed to combine neuroleptic with antidepressant properties and therefore particularly well-suited to the treatment of agitated (vital) depressions. Not all authors are convinced of the antidepressant effect of laevopromazine. At any rate, it is inferior in this respect to tricyclic antidepressants such as imipramine and amitryptiline. It is frequently used in combination with a sedative antidepressant in agitated (vital) depressions.

There have been several reports on agranulocytosis and liver lesions, and it is therefore advisable to monitor blood picture and liver functions.

Promazine (Prazine, Sparine, Protactyl)

Chemical structure. 10- (3-dimethylamino-n-propyl)- phenothiazine hydrochloride.

Dosage. This amounts to about twice that of chlorpromazine. The usual oral daily dose (tablets or suspension) is 300-1000 mg. Parenteral administration is also possible. Since this compound causes no infiltrates, it can be given intramuscularly in larger doses than chlorpromazine, up to a maximum of 200 mg every 4-6 hours. If greatly diluted with physiological saline and slowly injected, promazine can also be given intravenously; however, a dosage of 50 mg per injection and 300 mg per 24 hours should not be exceeded.

Particulars. Promazine lacks the chlorine atom on the phenothiazine core, but otherwise is identical to chlorpromazine. Its neuroleptic as well as its side effects are less marked than those of chlorpromazine. Its hypotensive effect in particular is not pronounced. However, it seems that promazine gives rise to convulsions more frequently than does chlorpromazine, and this would be an exception to the abovementioned rule.

There have been several reports on liver lesions and agranulocytosis. It should also be mentioned that, like chlorpromazine, this compound can give rise to false positive pregnancy tests (melanophore reaction).

Trifluopromazine (Siquil, Vesprin, Psyquil)

Chemical structure. 10-(3-dimethylaminopropyl)-2-(trifluormethyl)-phenothiazine hydrochloride.

Dosage. This compound can be given by mouth (tablets or draught) as well as parenterally (by intravenous or intramuscular injection). When given in equivalent amounts in pharmacological experiments, its effect is slightly stronger than that of chlorpromazine. The daily oral dose is 150-400 mg, and the daily parenteral dose is half as much. Local tissue reactions at the site of injection are rare. The hypotensive effect of trifluopromazine is not pronounced, and intravenous injections can be given without undue risk as long as the compound is greatly diluted in order to prevent phlebitis. Generally, however, intravenous administration of neuroleptics is to be discouraged.

Several phenothiazine derivatives, including trifluopromazine, irritate the oral mucosa after protracted contact. This can pose a problem with the (often demented) patients who keep the tablets in the mouth for a long time. The trifluopromazine emulsion does not irritate the oral mucosa and can therefore be of advantage in these cases.

Particulars. Therapeutically, this compound is regarded as virtually equivalent to chlorpromazine. Its side effects, particularly the hypotensive and the epileptogenic effect, are less pronounced. Dyskinetic changes are rare with the exception of akathisia. Liver lesions and agranulocytosis are very rare.

Table 4. Phenothiazine derivatives with a piperidine ring in the side chain

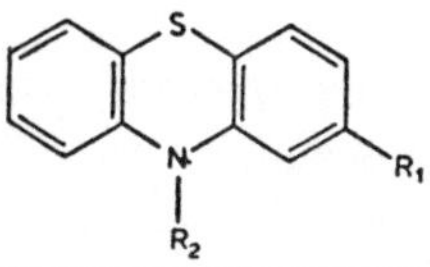

Chemical structure		Generic name	Trade name	Average dose per day in mg by mouth
R_1	R_2			
—	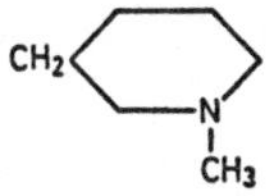	Mepazine	Pacatal Pecazine	100-500
$SOCH_3$	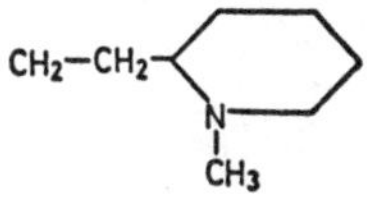	Mesorida- zine	Lidanil Lidanor Serentil	100-400
$COCH_3$	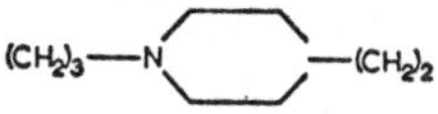	Piperace- tazine	Quide	40-160
CNH	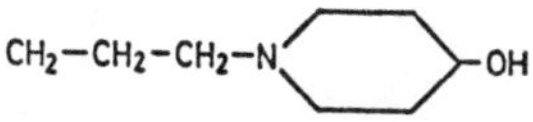	Periciazine Properici- azine	Aolept Neulactil Neuleptil	30-70
SCH_3	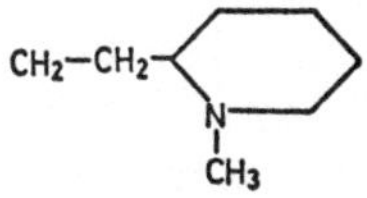	Thioridazine	Mellaril Melleril	150-450

2. Phenothiazine derivatives with a piperidine ring in the side chain (Table 4)

Mepazine (Pacatal, Pecazine)

Chemical structure. 10-(N-methyl-3-piperidylmethyl)- phenothiazine.

Dosage. Mepazine is usually given by mouth, the daily dose being 100-500 mg. Intramuscular injections (75-150 mg per day, in fractional doses) are painful, not infrequently cause local infiltrates, and therefore are not recommended.

Particulars. The anticholinergic effect of this compound is pronounced, and consequently visual complaints, impeded micturition, diminished tear secretion (with the risk of dehydration of corneal epithelium and ulceration), etc., are common. There have been several reports on liver lesions, agranulocytosis and convulsions. Extrapyramidal disorders, however, are rare.

In view of the numerous side effects and the absence of indications that mepazine is therapeutically superior to the other phenothiazine derivatives, this compound is not first choice when neuroleptic medication is to be instituted.

Mesoridazine (Lidanil, Lidanor, Serentil)

Chemical structure. 10-2-(1-methyl-2-piperidyl)-ethyl-2-(methylsulphinyl)-phenothiazine.

Dosage. The oral daily dose is 100-400 mg. The compound can also be given by intramuscular injection: 25-50 mg per injection up to a total of 300 mg/24 hours.

Particulars. This is a sulphoxide derivative of thioridazine. In controlled comparative studies its therapeutic effect does not differ significantly from that of chlorpromazine. Its influence on extrapyramidal system and blood pressure is less pronounced, but ECG changes (increased P-R interval and changes in the T-wave segment) are more marked than with chlorpromazine. Comparative studies with the mother substance thioridazine have not been made. The compound has also been recommended for the treatment of the consequences of alcohol withdrawal, but there are no arguments that in this respect it is superior to benzodiazepines (in adequate doses) and other neuroleptics. There are no indications that this compound has distinct advantages over chlorpromazine and thioridazine.

Piperacetazine (Quide)

Chemical structure. 10-{3-[4-(2-hydroxyethyl)-piperidino] propyl} -phenothiazine-2-yl methyl ketone.

Dosage. The oral daily dose is 40-160 mg.

Particulars. This compound behaves "typically," which is to say that, like the other piperidine phenothiazines, it exerts relatively little influence on motor regulation. It has been recommended in acute types of schizophrenia. There are no indications that this compound has certain advantages over other phenothiazines of the piperidine series.

Periciazine (Aolept, Neulactil, Neuleptil)

Chemical structure. 3-cyano-10-[3-(4-hydroxypiperidino) propyl] -phenothiazine.

Dosage. The oral daily dose (tablets or droplets) is 30-70 mg.

Particulars. Periciazine was introduced as a neuroleptic of specific characteristics, indicated especially in the treatment of behaviour disorders based on demonstrable organic cerebral factors (epilepsy, oligophrenia, head injury, arteriosclerosis, etc.) It was stated that the compound favourably influenced in particular increased aggressiveness, antisocial behaviour and diminished regulation of impulses. Its antipsychotic effect was described as not very pronounced.

I must leave these statements for what they are. There are no strong empirical arguments to support them, nor have they been contradicted. It can only be said that, should the particular suitability of periciazine for the abovementioned indications ever be demonstrated, this would be exceedingly important. So far, after all, we have been fairly powerless precisely against behaviour disorders on the basis of organic cerebral lesions. The conventional neuroleptics can produce some effect in these cases but often only if given in large doses; this means that the therapeutic effect must be bought at the price of inactivity, passivity and extrapyramidal disorders. In the lastmentioned respect, the cards are certainly in favour of periciazine; the affinity of this compound for the extrapyramidal system is small, and it also exerts little influence on activity and initiative. For the time being, however, we can go no further than the statement that periciazine is a strong sedative, which does not significantly interfere with the patient's physical and intellectual activities.

The anti-epileptic *carbamazepine* (Tegretol) has also been described as exerting a regulating influence on behaviour disorders or organic cerebral origin, particularly those in epileptic patients. But on this point, too, there is no certainty. It has been established, however, that apart from its anti-epileptic activity this drug is of importance in the treatment of primary trigeminal neuralgia.

Thioridazine (Melleril, Mellaril)

Chemical structure. 2-methylmercapto-10-[2(N-methyl-2-piperidyl)-ethyl] phenothiazine hydrochloride.

Dosage. The daily oral dose (tablets or draught) is 150-450 mg.

Particulars. The antihistamine, anti-emetic and anticholinergic activity of thioridazine is significantly less marked than that of compounds of the aliphatic series (i.e. compounds with an aminoalkyl group in the side chain). In other respects, too, this agent occupies a special position in pharmacological experiments.

1) Thioridazine has no very pronounced effect on motor activity. As compared with chlorpromazine, a tenfold dose is required to induce in rats a cataleptic state, i.e. a state of extreme motor inhibition.
2) On the other hand, the compound has a pronounced subduing effect on emotions. In rats it inhibits emotional defaecation (i.e. defaecation provoked by anxiety-laden stimuli) much more effectively than, say, chlorpromazine.
3) Neuroleptics inhibit conditioned reflexes, e.g. the conditioned flight reactions. The influence of thioridazine on these reflex mechanisms is relatively feeble.

There is a degree of agreement between the pharmacological and the clinical findings. Thioridazine is an effective agent, but its antipsychotic effect is less marked than that of chlorpromazine. The compound should, in fact, be placed between the ataractics on the one hand and the neuroleptics on the other. It has also been described as having antidepressant properties, but this has not been demonstrated with certainty. Of practical importance is the fact that its side effects are limited. Loss of initiative is rare; blood pressure and extrapyramidal system are hardly influenced. Jaundice has not so far been reported, nor has any serious lesion of the bone marrow. The agent is suitable for the treatment of elderly patients and children.

A remarkable if rare ophthalmological complication is accumulation of brown pigment in the retina. The patient perceives the environment as showing brown discoloration, and complains of diminished visual acuity. The fundus features resemble those of retinitis pigmentosa. This effect can only be produced by large doses (more than 800 mg per day). Whether the daily dose is decisive in this respect or rather the total amount administered is unknown. The changes are reversible if medication is discontinued in time. With large doses of thioridazine (>600 mg per day), regular examination of the ocular fundi is therefore indicated.

3. Phenothiazine derivatives with a piperazine ring in the side chain (Table 5)

Butyrylperazine (Randolectil, Repoise)

Chemical structure. N-[γ-(4′-methylpiperazinyl-1′)-propyl]-3-n-butyrylphenothiazine.

Dosage. The daily oral dose is 15-40 mg. Intramuscular injection is possible: 3 × 5-10 mg per day.

Particulars. German-speaking authors consider this compound to be equivalent to perphenazine and trifluoperazine, but American investigators are more reserved. Conclusion: the significance of butyrylperazine has not been established with certainty and calls for further investigation.

Butyrylperazine exerts but little influence on blood pressure. Extrapyramidal side effects are frequently observed, but disorders of bone marrow and liver functions have not so far been described.

Carphenazine (Proketazine)

Chemical structure. 10-{3-[4-(2-hydroxyethyl)-piperazine-1-yl] propyl}-2-propionylphenothiazine dimaleate.

Dosage. The daily oral dose is 75-300 mg.

Particulars. This compound has been especially recommended for inert patients with chronic psychoses but, like all other phenothiazines, is effective also in acute cases. Data in the literature are not sufficient for comparison with other phenothiazines of the piperazine series in terms of side effects, specifically motor side effects.

Table 5. Phenothiazine derivatives with a piperazine ring in the side chain

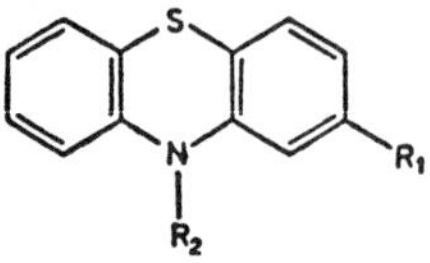

Chemical structure R_1	R_1	Generic name	Trade name	Average dose per day in mg by mouth
$CO-CH_2-CH_2-CH_3$	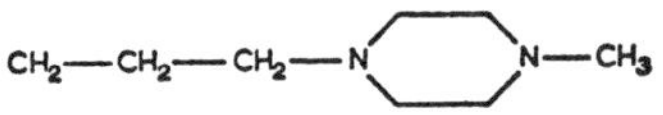	Butyryl-perazine (butaperazine)	Rando-lectil Repoise	15-40
COC_2H_5	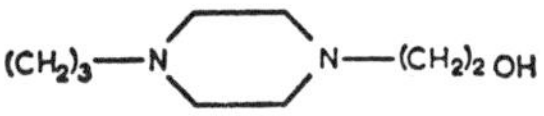	Carphena-zine	Proketazine	75-300
—	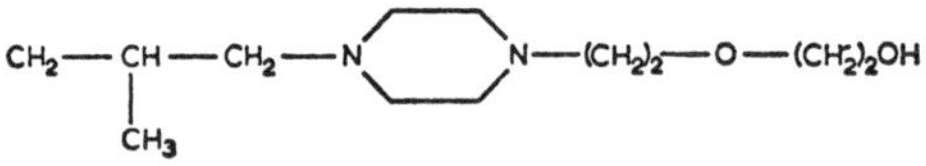	Dixyrazine	Esucos	20-75
CF_3	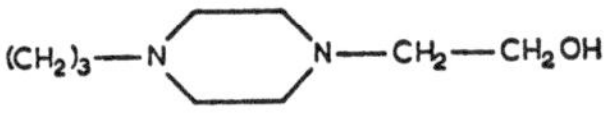	Fluphena-zine	Lyogen Moditen Prolixin	1-10
—	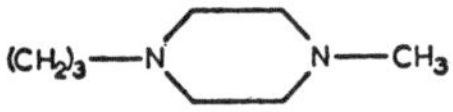	Perazine	Taxilan	100-600
Cl	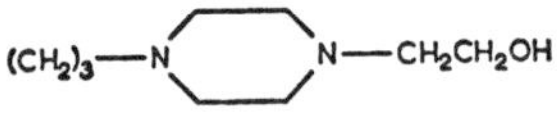	Perphen-azine	Decentan Fentazin Trilafon	6-32
Cl	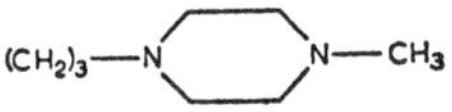	Prochlor-perazine	Compazine Stemetil	30-150
Cl	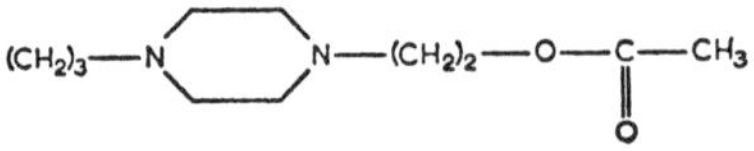	Thiopro-pazate	Dartal Dartalan Vesitan	30-100
$SO_2-N(CH_3)_2$	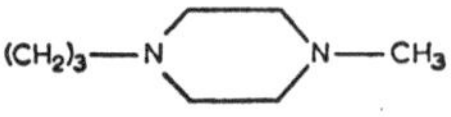	Thiopro-perazine	Majeptil	20-60
CF_3	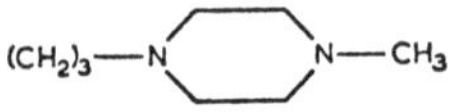	Trifluo-perazine	Jatroneural Stelazine Terfluzine	6-30

Dixyrazine (Esucos)

Chemical structure. 10-[3′-(4″-hydroxyethoxyethyl- 1″-piperazinyl -2′-methylpropyl] phenothiazine.

Dosage. The daily oral or rectal dose of this compound is 20-75 mg.

Particulars. Dixyrazine is a weakling among the phenothiazine derivatives. Neither its sedative nor its antipsychotic effect is very pronounced. Consequently it is not used for neuroleptic purposes but in the symptomatic treatment of neurotic anxiety and anxiety equivalents; in actual fact, therefore, as an ataractic. The compound exerts little influence on blood pressure and motor activity, and its other side effects are also inconsiderable.

Fluphenazine (Moditen, Lyogen, Prolixin)

Chemical structure. 2-trifluormethyl-10-[3-(4-hydroxyethyl- 1-piperazinyl)-propyl] phenothiazine dihydrochloride.

Dosage. The daily oral dose is 1-10 mg. Its effect is probably fairly protracted so that it seems justifiable to give the daily dose at once. This can be of advantage in the treatment of chronic walking patients.

Particulars. This compound has many similarities to trifluoperazine. It is a strong neuroleptic with a relatively pronounced activating component and great affinity for the extrapyramidal system. Motor disorders as a rule do not become manifest until the daily dose exceeds 3 mg. Liver lesions and agranulocytosis have been rarely described.

Perphenazine (Trilafon, Fentazin, Decentan)

Chemical structure. 1-(2-hydroxyethyl)-4[3-(2-chloro-10-phenothiazine)-propyl] piperazine.

Dosage. Perphenazine can be given orally as well as parenterally. The daily oral dose is usually 6-32 mg. For intramuscular injection the "ceiling" is 5 mg per injection and 20 mg/24 hours. If necessary, treatment can be started intravenously after dilution with physiological saline, and if the injection is given very slowly. As already pointed out, however, intravenous administration of neuroleptics is not advisable.

Particulars. Some authors consider perphenazine to be superior to chlorpromazine, particularly in paranoid states. However, this has not been confirmed in a large-scale comparative study by Casey et al. (1964): in schizophrenic patients with a diverse symptomatology, perphenazine (50 mg per day), chlorpromazine (635 mg per day), trifluopromazine (175 mg per day) and prochlorperazine (90 mg per day) were found to be equally effective.

Apart from extrapyramidal disorders (which generally do not occur until the daily dose exceeds 16 mg), this compound is usually tolerated well. Its effect on blood pressure is relatively small. Complaints of dizziness are sporadic, and lesions of liver and bone marrow are exceedingly rare.

Perazine (Taxilan)

Chemical structure. 10-[3-(4-methyl-1-piperazinyl)propyl] phenothiazine.

Dosage. The daily oral dose is 100-600 mg, i.e. about the same as that of chlorpromazine and substantially larger than the doses of the other representatives of the piperazine series. In serious cases this compound can be given by intramuscular injection for a few days: 3-4 × 50 mg per day.

Particulars. German-speaking authors often express considerable appreciation for this compound. They regard it as an effective neuroleptic with a less pronounced influence on motor activity and blood pressure than the other piperazine derivatives of the phenothiazine series, and suitable par excellence for protracted medication. It is believed to cause virtually no stimulation. Experience gained in Anglo-American countries with perazine has been limited, and controlled comparative studies are scanty. The exact position of this compound in the series of piperazine derivatives is therefore not clear. Liver and bone marrow lesions are very rare, but epileptogenic activity is described as pronounced.

Prochlorperazine (Stemetil, Compazine)

Chemical structure. 2-chloro-10-[3-(4′-methylpiperazine-1′-yl) propyl] phenothiazine.

Dosage. Prochlorperazine can be given orally, rectally or intramuscularly. For oral treatment, tablets as well as a syrup are available. The daily oral or rectal dose is 30-150 mg, while the daily parenteral dose is 30-60 mg.

Particulars. It was Broussolle who focused attention on the neuroleptic activity of this compound in 1957. It had previously been used only as an anti-emetic. Prochlorperazine thus became the first of the piperazine derivatives in the phenothiazine series. There are no indications that it has therapeutic advantages over its descendants.

Extrapyramidal symptoms are quite common, especially if the daily dose exceeds 75 mg. There have been several reports on jaundice as well as on agranulocytosis.

Thiopropazate (Dartal, Dartalan, Vesitan)

Chemical structure. 3-chloro-10[3-(4-(2-acetoxyethyl)-1-piperazinyl)propyl] phenothiazine dihydrochloride.

Dosage. The daily oral dose is 30-100 mg.

Particulars. Thiopropazate is the acetic acid ester of perphenazine. There are no indications that it equals the therapeutic potency of the strongest of the piperazine compounds such as perphenazine, trifluoperazine, fluphenazine and thioproperazine. Yet this compound merits attention because, with reserpine and tetrabenazine, it is believed to be useful in the symptomatic treatment of the hyperkinesia of the Huntington patient. Whether in this respect it differs from other phenothiazines has not been established.

The side effects, especially on circulation and motor activity, are not very pronounced; not infrequently, however, one observes signs of parasympathetic hyperactivity (blurred vision, swollen nasal mucosa, xerostomia, etc.) of the type also seen after reserpine medication. There are a few reports on jaundice due to this medication.

Thioproperazine (Majeptil)

Chemical structure. 3-dimethylsulphamyl-10-[3′-(4″-methyl-1″-piperazinyl)propyl] phenothiazine.

Dosage. This compound can be given orally as well as by intramuscular injection. The daily oral dose (tablets or droplets) is 20-60 mg. Different authors give different guidelines for intramuscular administration. Some use a dose equal to the oral dose, while others use half this amount. Yet others consider these doses too large and hold that 1 mg intramuscularly equals 10 mg by mouth.

Particulars. Thioproperazine is among the most effective compounds of the piperazine series. The ratio of sedation to activation is not clear from the literature. Moreover, the practical value of this agent is limited by the risk of serious complications. Motor disorders to begin with: akathisia, dyskinetic syndromes, parkinsonoid syndromes as well as hypokinetic syndromes without hypertonia are not only frequently seen but can also take a fulminating course. In addition, one repeatedly observes a variety of dysregulations of probably diencephalic origin, e.g. hypothermia or hyperthermia, pallor or on the contrary congestion of the face, hyperlacrimation, hypersalivation, hyperhidrosis, hyperactivity of the sebaceous glands, etc.

In rare cases treatment with this compound can lead to vitally dangerous states, characterized by rapid, marked increase in temperature, hypertonia so severe that the patient can hardly move and feed himself, dyspnoea, profuse perspiration and hypersalivation.

To sum up: thioproperazine is an effective neuroleptic, but it should be used with great caution and only under strict clinical supervision.

Trifluoperazine (Terfluzine, Stelazine, Jatroneural)

Chemical structure. 10-[3-(1-methyl-4-piperazinyl)propyl]-2-trifluormethyl-phenothiazine dihydrochloride.

Dosage. This compound can be given orally as well as intramuscularly. The daily oral dose (tablets or draught) is 6-30 mg. The usual intramuscular dose is 3 × 2-3 mg per day; a dose in excess of 10 mg/24 hours is not acceptable with a view to the risk of a cumulative effect.

Particulars. Trifluoperazine is an effective neuroleptic with a relatively strong activating component, due to which it sometimes gives rise to a degree of irritability, harassment and hyperactivity. The compound is therefore particularly well-suited for the treatment of autistic, "anergic" schizophrenics, and for this indication it is superior to chlorpromazine.

With regard to extrapyramidal disorders the therapeutic range is limited (although, as always, there are considerable individual differences in this respect). Doses of less than 8 mg daily produce distinct motor changes in only about 2% of cases. This rate increases to over 50% if the daily dose is increased to 10-20 mg.

Atropine-like side effects occur, but only in response to large doses. A few reports have so far mentioned liver lesions and agranulocytosis.

Table 6. Thioxanthene derivatives

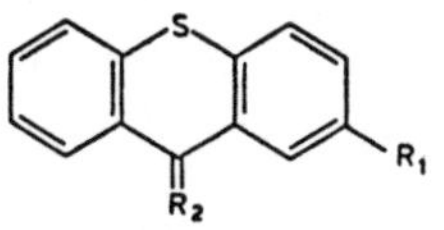

Chemical structure		Generic name	Trade name	Average dose per day in mg by mouth
R_1	R_2			
Cl	$CH-CH_2-CH_2-N(CH_3)_2$	Chlorprothixene	Taractan Truxal	45-400
Cl	$CH-(CH_2)_2-N \quad N-(CH_2)_2-OH$	Clopenthixol	Ciatyl Sordinol	30-150
CF_3	$CH-(CH_2)_2-N \quad N-(CH_2)_2-OH$	Flupenthixol	Fluanxol	6-18
$SO_2-N(CH_3)_2$	$CH-(CH_2)_2-N \quad N-CH_3$	Thiothixene	Navane Orbinamon	20-60

4. Thioxanthene derivatives (Table 6)

The core of the thioxanthene derivatives differs from that of the phenothiazines only in that the central nitrogen atom has been replaced by a carbon atom with double bonds to the side chain (Table 4). The two groups also show many similarities in pharmacological and clinical terms.

Chlorprothixene (Taractan, Truxal)

Chemical structure. 2-chloro-9-(3-dimethylaminopropylidene)-thioxanthene. The central ring carries not a nitrogen atom, as does chlorpromazine, but a carbon atom which double bonds to the side chain. Otherwise the structure is identical to that of chlorpromazine.

Dosage. The daily oral dose is one-half to two-thirds that of chlorpromazine, i.e. about 45-400 mg. In the case of severe agitation, treatment can be started by an intramuscular injection, the usual intramuscular dose being 3-4 × 25 mg per day.

Particulars. Like chlorpromazine, this compound has anti-emetic, histamine-antagonizing, anti-adrenergic and anticholinergic properties. Its anticholinergic activity exceeds that of chlorpromazine.

The compound has a pronounced sedative effect, but its antipsychotic effect is probably inferior to that of chlorpromazine. Chlorprothixene is believed to combine a neuroleptic with a mild antidepressant effect. In fact, for this reason it was marketed as a "broad-spectrum neuroleptic" (like laevomepromazine). However, an antidepressant effect has not been demonstrated with certainty. Yet if one combines an antidepressant with a neuroleptic, one preferably takes a neuroleptic thought to produce a mild antidepressant effect of its own accord.

Chlorprothixene rarely causes severe extrapyramidal symptoms, and exerts little influence also on blood pressure. No reports have so far mentioned liver lesions and agranulocytosis. Mild initial dullness, dizziness and xerostomia are the only side effects more or less regularly observed. The toxicity of this compound is low. Massive overdosage (2-3 g at once) merely proved to produce deep sleep from which the patient could be aroused, to recover without residual symptoms. These two features—few side effects and low toxicity—have caused chlorprothixene to be used also as an ataractic. For the same reasons the compound is useful also in geriatrics.

Clopenthixol (Sordinol, Ciatyl)

Chemical structure. 2-chloro-9-{3-[4-(2-hydroxyethyl)-1-piperazinyl]-propylidene}-thiozanthene dihydrochloride. Apart from replacement of the central nitrogen atom by an unsaturated carbon atom, the structure of this compound is identical to that of perphenazine.

Dosage. Clopenthixol can be given orally as well as parenterally. The daily oral dose is 30-150 mg. The daily intramuscular dose is usually 3-6 × 12.5-25 mg. Infiltrates around the site of injection are unusual. Since it does not irritate the vascular wall, clopenthixol can also be administered, if there is an urgent indication, by slow intravenous injection up to a maximum of 6 × 12.5 mg per day.

Particulars. Clopenthixol has a piperazine group in the side chain and, in terms of clinical effect, closely resembles the piperazine derivatives in the phenothiazine series. The sedative and the antipsychotic components are both strong. Excellent results have been described in particular in states of agitation, but also in hallucinatory syndromes and psychoses accompanied by delusions. Like the phenothiazine derivatives with a piperazine group, clopenthixol has great affinity for the extrapyramidal system. Its hypotensive effect, too, is fairly pronounced, but it exerts little influence on impulses and initiative; an inconvenient degree of passivity is rare. In most cases, in fact, a certain degree of activation occurs and large doses may even lead to irritability, harassment and inner tensions.

Flupenthixol (Fluxanol)

Chemical structure. 2-trifluormethyl-9-{3-[4-(2-hydroxyethyl)-1-piperazinyl]-propylidene-(1) }-thioxanthene. Flupenthixol is a trifluor derivative of clopenthixol.

Dosage. The daily oral dose is 6-18 mg.

Particulars. Flupenthixol is an effective antipsychotic neuroleptic with an activating component. Inert patients with chronic psychoses provide a good indication.

Thiothixene (Navane, Orbinamon)

Chemical structure. N, N-dimethyl-9-[3-(4-methylpiperazine-1-yl) propylidene] thioxanthene-2-sulphonamide. Thiothixene is the analogue of thioproperazine in the phenothiazine series.

Dosage. The daily oral dose is 20-60 mg.

Particulars. This compound is a neuroleptic with a strong antipsychotic effect, but its therapeutic range is limited because larger doses regularly produce motor side effects.

5. Other tricyclic neuroleptics

Clozapine (Leponex)

Chemical structure. 8-chloro-11-(4-methyl-1-piperazinyl)-5-H-dibenz [b,e][1,4]diazepine.

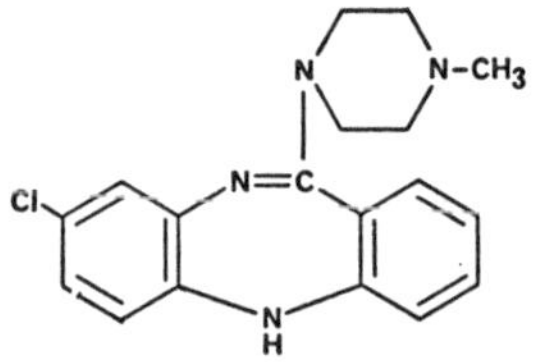

Dosage. The daily oral dose is 150-600 mg. The daily intramuscular dose is 150-300 mg, in 3-4 fractional doses. Although no pharmacokinetic data are available, it is my firm impression that this compound is much more effective when administered parenterally than when given by mouth.

Particulars. Clozapine is a very strong sedative, perhaps the strongest available against psychotic restiveness. Moreover, it rarely produces extrapyramidal symptoms. In some countries it is not commercially available because there is some uncertainty about the agranulocytosis risk. If the compound is used, therefore, regular leucocyte counts are mandatory until the order is revoked. Although it is a superior sedative, this compound probably has a less pronounced antipsychotic effect than that produced by the strongest of the phenothiazines, e.g. perphenazine.

Clozapine is a strong anticholinergic. Hypotension and an increased pulse rate are frequent side effects. Mild, so far unexplained pyrexia sometimes develops during the first week of medication. Fatigue sensations are the rule in the initial phase of treatment. An evening dose of 25-50 mg clozapine can be given to induce sleep. This is not a suitable compound for elderly patients.

Prothipendyl (Dominal)

Chemical structure. 10-(3-dimethylaminopropyl)-10H-pyridol[3,2-b][1,4]benzothiazine.

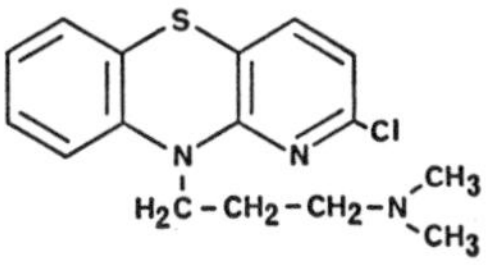

Dosage. The daily oral dose is 200-800 mg. The daily intramuscular dose is 200-400 mg, in 3-4 fractional doses.

Particulars. Prothipendyl is a feeble neuroleptic with few side effects. It can be utilized to induce sleep (40-80 mg one hour before turning in).

6. Butyrophenones (Table 7)

The butyrophenones are chemically related to and derived from the analgesic pethidine. They no longer have an analgesic and anaesthetic effect, however, but behave like typical neuroleptics. The general formula of this group of compounds looks as follows:

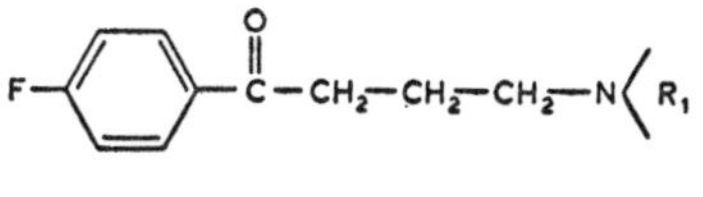

The prototype of the series, haloperidol, was synthesized by Janssen et al. in 1956 and introduced into clinical psychiatry two years later (cf. Janssen, 1967).

Benperidol (Frenactil, Glianimon)

Chemical structure. 4′-fluoro-4-[4-(2-oxo-2,3-dihydro-1-benzimidazolyl)-piperidyl]butyrophenone.

Dosage. The daily oral dose is 1.5-6 mg. The daily intramuscular dose is 0.5-3 mg.

Particulars. Per milligramme, this is the most potent neurolep-

Table 7. Some butyrophenones

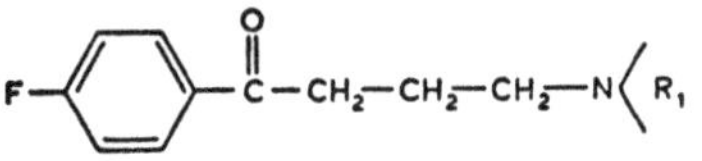

Chemical structure R	Generic name	Trade name	Average dose per day in mg by mouth
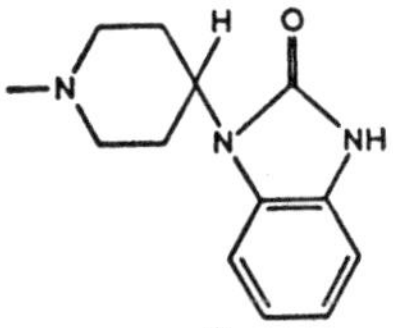	Benperidol	Frenactil Glianimon	1.5–6
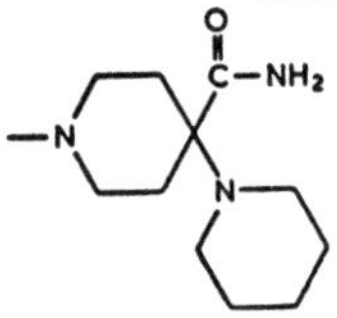	Floropipa-mide	Dipiperon	300-500
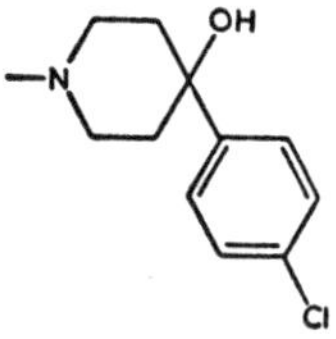	Haloperidol	Haldol Serenase Serenace	3-20
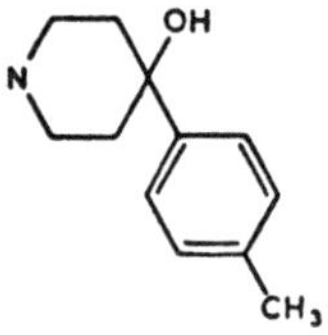	Methyl-peridol	Luvatren Luvatrena	20-40
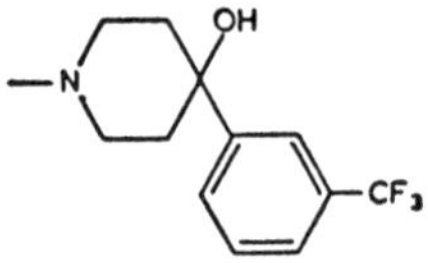	Triflu-peridol	Triperidol	0.5-6

tic so far known. There are no indications that this compound has advantages over haloperidol in the treatment of psychoses. It has been used in the treatment of sexual disorders at a daily dosage of 0.5-1.5 mg (chapter XXIV). With these relatively small doses, the risk of extrapyramidal side effects is inconsiderable.

Droperidol (Dehydrobenzperidol, Inapsine, Innovar)

Chemical structure. 1-[3-(p-fluorobenzoyl)-propyl]-1,2,3,6-tetrahydro-4-pyridyl]-2-benzimidazolinone. Except for a double bond in the piperidine ring, the structure is identical to that of benperidol.

Dosage. The daily oral dose is 2.5-60 mg. The parenteral (intramuscular or intravenous) dose is 10-40 mg per day.

Particulars. Droperidol is a quick- but short-acting butyrophenone, virtually without anticholinergic activity. It is used as premedication in anaesthesia, but is also of importance in the treatment of motor agitation. In the latter cases it is given intramuscularly (intravenously in emergencies) at a rate of 5-10 mg per injection, to be repeated after 15-30 minutes if necessary, up to a parenteral maximum of 40 mg/24 hours. Extrapyramidal symptoms are rare after short medication. Hypotension is a risk in particular after intravenous administration. No comparative studies with haloperidol are available.

Haloperidol (Serenase, Serenace, Haldol)

Chemical structure. 4′-fluoro-4-(4″-chlorophenyl)-4′-hydroxypiperidine-butyrophenone.

Dosage. Haloperidol can be given orally (tablets or droplets) as well as parenterally. The daily oral dose is 3-20 mg. The daily intramuscular dose is 3-15 mg in fractional doses. Intravenous injections (1-2.5 mg per injection) are to be considered only as initial "booster therapy" in the case of very marked agitation.

Particulars. Haloperidol is a very strong sedative in psychotic or maniacal agitation. As an antipsychotic, it is slightly inferior to the strongest among the phenothiazine derivatives. With clozapine, haloperidol ranks as the agent of choice in the treatment of the aggressive psychotic patient with motor unrest. Which of the two is most effective has not been established. Haloperidol has the disadvantage of a high affinity for the extrapyramidal system. In large doses, it has to be combined with an anti-parkinson agent. Clozapine has only a minimal effect on motor activity but has the disadvantage of a more marked hypotensive effect than haloperidol. This is why haloperidol can be very useful in the treatment of agitated elderly patients, whereas clozapine is better avoided in such cases.

The epileptogenic activity of haloperidol is less pronounced than that of the phenothiazines. The compound is used as an anti-emetic in internal medicine, and in neurology in the treatment of the Gilles de la Tourette syndrome.

Trifluperidol (Triperidol)

Chemical structure. 4′-fluoro-4-[4′-hydroxy-4′-(3″trifluoromethyl)-phenyl]piperidinobutyrophenone.

Dosage. The daily oral dose (droplets) is 0.5-6 mg. The dose per intramuscular injection is 0.5-2.5 mg up to a maximum of 5 mg per day (1 droplet contains 0.05 mg active principle).

Particulars. The therapeutic position of this compound is uncertain. As a sedative, it is probably inferior to haloperidol. The drive level is increased rather than decreased and the agent is therefore suitable in principle for the treatment of inert and autistic patients. The literature warrants no conclusion concerning the antipsychotic potency of this compound.

Like haloperidol, it strongly influences the extrapyramidal system but has little effect on blood pressure. So far there have been no reports on liver lesions and changes in the blood picture.

The group of the butyrophenones comprises several other agents, of which we mention *floropipamide* (Dipiperon), *fluanisone* (Haloanison) and *methylperidol* (Luvatren). So far there have been no indications that these agents have any particular advantages over the original haloperidol. A detailed discussion is therefore omitted.

7. Diphenylbutylpiperidines (Table 8)

Compounds of this group are chemically related to the butyrophenones. The group consists of three agents: pimozide,

Table 8. Some diphenylbutylpiperidines

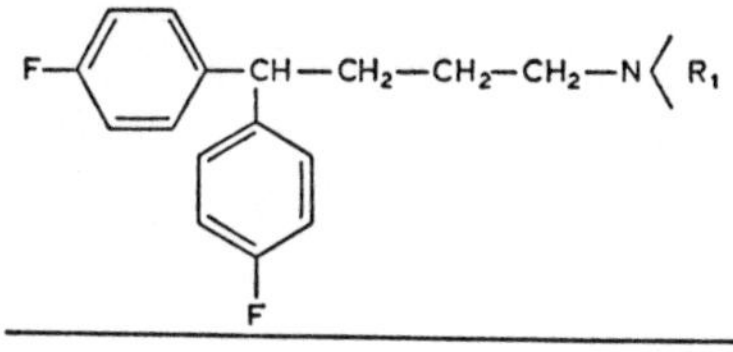

Chemical structure R_1	Generic name	Trade name	Average dose
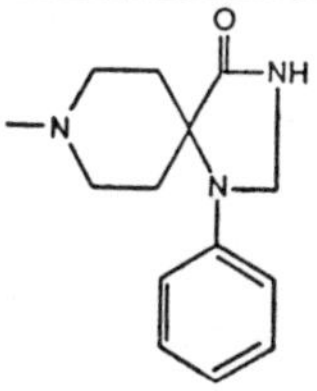	Fluspirilene	Imap	2-6 mg i.m./ week
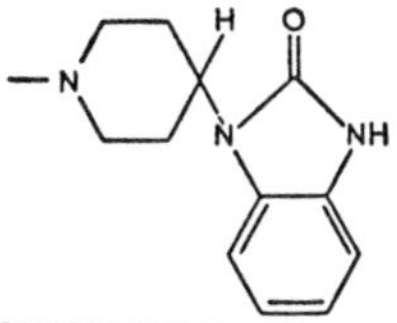	Pimozide	Orap	2-6 mg orally/ day

penfluridol and fluspirilene. They are characterized by relatively protracted activity. Somewhat arbitrarily, I discuss pimozide with a duration of action of 24 hours, here. The other two compounds, with a duration of action of about a week, are discussed in the section of long-acting neuroleptics.

Pimozide (Orap)

Chemical structure. 1-{1-[4,4-bis(4-fluorophyl)-butyl]-4-piperidyl} -2-benzimidazolinone.

Dosage. The daily oral dose is 2-6 mg. The agent need be given only once every 24 hours.

Particulars. This compound is recommended especially for maintenance therapy of chronic, apathic psychotic patients. Its extrapyramidal side effects have been described as mild, but untoward inner restiveness is not uncommon in the initial phase of medication. Pimozide has not been sufficiently compared with other types of neuroleptic to warrant definite conclusions concerning its value. Biochemically the compound is interesting because it is the most selective DA antagonist among the neuroleptics.

8. Indole derivatives

Only one indole neuroleptic is commercially available: oxypertine. A few others, including *molindone*, are still under investigation.

Oxypertine (Forit, Integrin, Opertil)

Chemical structure. 5,6-dimethoxy-2-methyl-3-[2-(4-phenyl-1-piperazinyl)ethyl]indole.

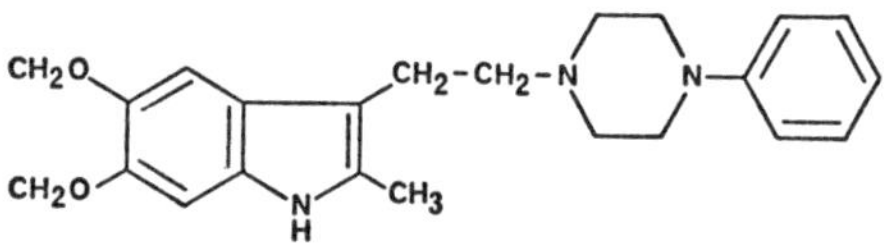

Dosage. The daily oral dose is 100-300 mg. The daily oral dose often indicated in the literature (150 mg average) is too small. In many cases no results are obtained until larger doses are given.

Particulars. Oxypertine is not a strong antipsychotic but has a pronounced activating effect, while the antipsychotic effect is still sufficient to prevent activation of delusions and hallucinations. However, anxiety or a degree of inner unrest may be provoked. The agent is indicated for the treatment of inert patients with chronic psychoses. It exerts little influence on blood pressure, and its effect on the extrapyramidal system is likewise relatively small.

In biochemical terms, oxypertine forms a separate group with reserpine and tetrabenazine: the neuroleptics of the store-depleting type. Their mode of action is discussed in chapters IV and XI.

9. Rauwolfia alkaloids

The group of the Rauwolfia alkaloids is chemically unrelated to the above discussed neuroleptics. It was the most effective compound of this group—reserpine—that heralded the era of the neuroleptics along with chlorpromazine. The other Rauwolfia alkaloids have hardly been used in psychiatry.

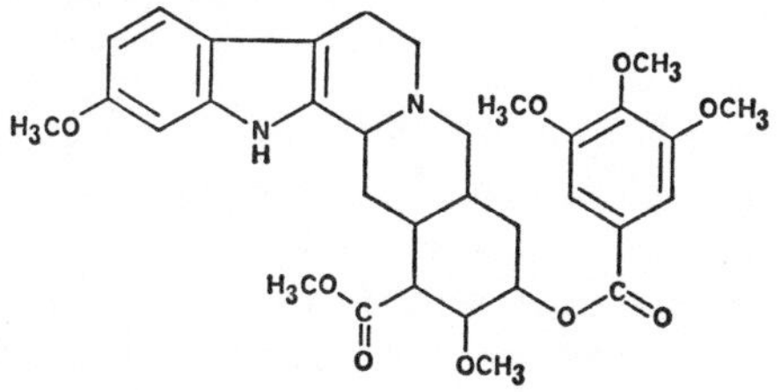

Reserpine (Serpasil)

Chemical structure. 3,4,5-trimethoxybenzoylmethyl reserpate.

Dosage. The daily oral dose is 3-12 mg. The daily intramuscular dose is 1-3 mg per injection, to a maximum of 12 mg/24 hours.

Particulars. As a neuroleptic, reserpine retains only historical significance. To begin with, it is not a good neuroleptic: its sedative potency is considerable but its antipsychotic effect is feeble. Moreover, the use of this agent carries certain risks when large doses are given: hypotension, depression, nausea, diarrhoea, in rare cases even haematemesis due to increased motility of the stomach and increased acidity of peptic juice. Cholinergic effects such as bradycardia, miosis, ptosis, hypersalivation, swelling of the nasal mucosa and conjunctival vasodilatation can be very inconvenient. Finally, the agent also has a pronounced affinity for the extrapyramidal system.

10. Benzoquinolizine derivatives

The first and most important representative of this group is tetrabenazine (Nitoman). Other benzoquinolizine derivatives have been used in animals experiments but not in clinical psychiatry. These compounds are chemically unrelated to the other categories of neuroleptics.

Tetrabenazine (Nitoman)

Chemical structure. 2-keto-3-isobutyl-9,10-dimethoxyhexahydrobenzoquinolizine.

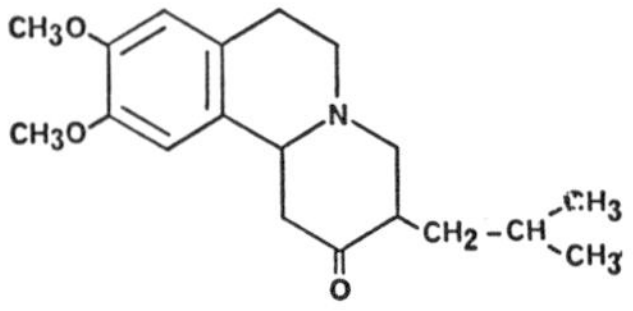

Dosage. The daily oral dose is 75-200 mg. In serious cases treatment can be introduced by intramuscular injection, to a maximum of 50 mg per injection and 150 mg/24 hours. The effect develops rapidly, unlike that of reserpine.

Particulars. Tetrabenazine is a neuroleptic that has always lived in the shadow of other agents. In the past it was used sporadically, and nowadays hardly if at all. Why this is so remains unexplained. It has not been demonstrated that it is inferior to the more conventional neuroleptics and, apart from extrapyramidal symptoms, the agent produces few side effects. In terms of biochemical activity it is related to reserpine and oxypertine in that, like these compounds, it depletes the central monoamine stores.

11. Other neuroleptics

Sulpirid (Dogmatil)

Chemical structure. N-[1-ethyl-2-pyrrolidinyl)-methyl]-2-methoxybenzamide-5-sulphonamide.

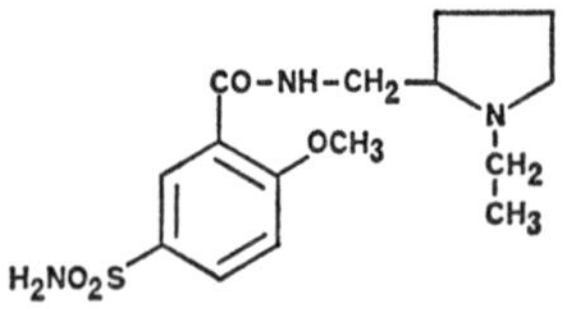

Dosage. The usual daily oral dose is 300-600 mg.

Particulars. The position of this compound, only recently introduced, is not yet clear. There are claims that it combines neuroleptic with antidepressant properties, but these statements are not well-documented. The preliminary impression from the clinical literature is that sulpirid is a neuroleptic of average potency, with a component of motor activation and relatively few motor and cardiovascular side effects. In view of its activating properties, it has been advised that the last dose be given no later than 3 p.m.

12. Long-acting neuroleptics

Neuroleptics of which a single administration produces an effect which lasts one or several weeks, are indicated in:

1) Chronic recurrent psychoses.

2) Psychoses which have developed mainly in response to marked emotional pressure (psychogenic psychoses), when it is believed that hospitalization can be avoided by rapid sociotherapeutic and psychotherapeutic intervention if the patient can be made accessible to this approach. The latter requires: a) neuroleptics, and b) the certainty that the patient does in fact take them. This certainty exists only if the medication is personally administered, which is virtually impossible if several doses have to be given each day. But it can be ascertained with the aid of long-acting neuroleptics.

Medication with long-acting neuroleptics also has its disadvantages.

1) It is difficult to ensure a high ratio between desired and undesired effects, because the doses required can be less accurately determined than with short-acting neuroleptics.

2) Perfectly even blood levels cannot be attained. The blood concentration shows a peak during the first few days after administration, and during this period there is consequently an accumulation of side effects, particularly extrapyramidal disorders, hypotension and fatigue sensations. This is why elderly patients should not be given long-acting neuroleptics.

3) The question of compatibility with other compounds is even more urgent with long-acting compounds than with "ordinary" agents. In this respect the neuroleptics stand out rela-

tively favourably. They can be combined with most other compounds without difficulty. The principal exception to this rule is alcohol, because several of its effects are potentiated by neuroleptics. There are no general rules for the practical problems arising from this fact. Benefit and risk must be balanced from case to case, and in each individual case from time to time. The effect of barbiturates is likewise potentiated. The risk of an emergency operation, should this be required, is not or hardly increased by a long-acting neuroleptic, provided the anaesthetist is aware of its involvement. It seems advisable to give the walking patient some sort of document which specifies the long-acting drug given, and to instruct his family accordingly.

4) On several occasions I have observed severe depression of the "vital" type during the first few months of medication with long-acting neuroleptics. I have rarely observed such syndromes during medication with short-acting neuroleptics. This can develop also in patients who have no history of depression. Other authors have reported similar observations. There is no certainty that these cases in fact involve pharmacogenic depressions (they could be a feature of the natural history of the disease), but one is nevertheless well-advised to bear this possibility in mind.

The disadvantages of long-acting neuroleptics, however, are outweighed by their advantages. I have discussed this on page 102.

There are long-acting phenothiazines, thioxanthenes and diphenylbutylpiperidines, of which I list the following principal representatives.

1) *Fluphenazine enanthate* (Anatensol enanthate, Moditen enanthate) is a phenothiazine derivative of which the average intramuscular dose is 25 mg/2 weeks. More recommendable is:

   Fluphenazine decanoate (Anatensol decanoate, Modecate), which acts slightly longer (3-4 weeks) and produces fewer extrapyramidal side effects. The intramuscular dose averages 25 mg/3-4 weeks.

2) *Pipothiazine undecylenate* (Piportil Medium) and *pipothiazine palmitate* (Piportil Longum) are phenothiazine derivatives which act during 2 and 4 weeks, respectively. The average dose per administration is 100 mg. There have been no comparative studies with long-acting fluphenazines. According to the manufacturer, motor complications are infrequent.

3) *Flupenthixol decanoate* (Fluxanol depot, Depixol) is a long-acting thioxanthene derivative. The average intramuscular dose is 20 mg/2 weeks. With this compound, too, severe motor side effects are not uncommon.

The abovementioned compounds are all esters of the corresponding neuroleptics, dissolved in oil, which are administered by intramuscular injection. Their extended effect is based on two factors: 1) slow release of the ester from the oil depot; 2) hydrolysis of the ester, releasing the free (active) base.

4) *Fluspirilene* (Imap) is a diphenylbutylpiperidine derivative for intramuscular injection, which in the muscle forms a microcrystalline depot from which the active principle is gradually released (Table 8). The average dose is 4 mg/week. It exerts relatively little influence on motor activity and blood pressure.

5) *Penfluridol* (Semap) is likewise a diphenylbutylpiperidine derivative, and the only long-acting neuroleptic given *by mouth:* 40-60 mg/week. Its extended effect is explained by the fact that it slowly enters the brain and as slowly leaves it, without being locally degraded.

The advantage of an injection is that the drug is certain to reach the appropriate site, and that the "magic load" of a syringe exceeds that of a tablet. On the other hand, the oral route is very practical for the "field worker" (family doctor, social psychiatrist). Penfluridol exerts little influence on motor activity and blood pressure.

The dosages indicated are all averages; they should be adapted to individual requirements by varying the dose administered and/or the frequency of administration.

BIBLIOGRAPHY

Bobon, J. and J. Collard (1972). Present treatment of manic states. *Acta. psychiat. belg.* 72, 617.

Broussolle, P., J. Perrin and P. Maurel, et al. (1957). La prochlorperazine en psychiatrie; expérience tirée de 240 cures. *Presse méd.*, 65, 1628.

Casey, J. F., J. J. Lasky, C. J. Klett and L. F. Hollister (1964). Treatment of schizophrenic reactions with phenothiazine derivatives. A comparative study of chlorpromazine, triflupromazine, mepazine, prochlorperazine, perphenazine and phenobarbital. *Amer. J. Psychiat.* 117, 97.

Cole, J. O. and J. M. Davis (1975). Antipsychotic agents. In: *Comprehensive Textbook of Psychiatry*. (Eds.) A. M. Freedman, H. I. Kaplan and B. J. Sadock. Baltimore: Williams and Wilkins.

DiMascio, A. and R. F. Shader (Eds.) (1972). *Butyrophenones in Psychiatry*. New York: Raven Press.

Elizur, A. and S. Davidson (1975). The evaluation of the anti-autistic activity of sulpiride. *Current Ther. Res*. 18, 578.

Forrest, I. S., C. J. Carr and E. Usdin (Eds.) (1974). *Thioxthixene and the Thioxanthenes*. New York: Raven Press.

Gallant, D. M. and M. P. Bishop (1972). Quide vs. Mellaril in chronic schizophrenic patients. *Cur. Ther. Res*., 14, 10.

Janssen, P. A. J. (1967). Haloperidol and related butyrophenones. In: *Psychopharmacological Agents*. (Ed.) M. Gordon. New York, London: Academic Press. 2, 199.

Klein, D. F. and J. Davis. (1969). *Diagnosis and Drug Treatment of Psychiatric Disorders*. Baltimore: Williams and Wilkins.

Kline, N. S. (1954). Use of rauwolfia serpentina in neuropsychiatric conditions. *Ann. New York. Acad. Sci*. 59, 107.

Leeuwen, A. M. H. van, J. Molders, P. Sterkmans, P. Mielands, C. Martens, Ch. Toussaint, A. M. Hovent, M. F. Desseilles, H. Koch, A. Devroye and M. Parent Droperidol in acutely agitated patients. A double-blind placebo-controlled study. *J. Nerv. Ment. Dis.,* 1977, 164, 280.

Lingjaerde, O. (1963). Tetrabenazine (Nitoman) in the treatment of psychoses. *Acta Psychiat. Scand*. Suppl. 170.

Neff, K. E., D. Denney and P. H. Blachly (1972). Control of severe agitation with droperidol. *Dis. Nerv. Syst*. 33, 597.

Pöldinger, W. and P. Schmidlin (1972). *Index psychopharmacorum*. Bern, Stuttgart, Wien: Huber.

Pragg, H. M. van, T. Schut, L. C. W. Dols and R. van Schilfgaarden (1971). Controlled trial of penfluridol in acute psychosis. *Brit. Med. J*. 4, 710.

Praag, H. M. van, and L. C. W. Dols (1973). Fluphenazine enanthate and fluphenazine decanoate: A comparison of their duration of action and motor side effects. *Amer. J. Psychiat*. 130, 801.

Praag, H. M. van, L. C. W. Dols and T. Schut (1975). Biochemical versus psychopathological action profile of neuroleptics: A comparative study of chlorpromazine and oxypertine in acute psychotic disorders. *Compr. Psychiat*. 16, 255.

Praag, H. M. van, J. Korf and L. C. W. Dols (1976). Clozapine versus perphenazine. The value of the biochemical mode of action of neuroleptics in predicting their therapeutic activity. *Brit. J. Psychiat.,* 129, 547.

Rifkin, A., F. Quitkin, J. Kane and D. F. Klein (1976). Long-term use of antipsychotic drugs. In: *Progress in Psychiatric Drug Treatment*. (Vol. 2) (Eds.) D. F. Klein and R. Gittelman-Klein. New York: Brunner/Mazel.

Swazey, J. (1974). *Chlorpromazine: The History of the Psychiatric Discovery*. Cambridge, Mass.: MIT Press.

XI

Biological Aspects of Psychoses and Their Treatment

1. Research into biological determinants of (schizophrenic) psychoses

For many years, far into the sixties, research into biological determinants of psychoses, more especially of schizophrenic psychoses, had suffered from a lack of more or less well-founded and testable working hypotheses. Efforts were confined to a fairly unsystematic search for abnormal metabolites in a variety of body fluids. Strange people, strange substances—not a very effective research strategy. It has recently come to be understood, however, that neuroleptics can serve as pacemakers of biological psychosis research, much as antidepressants have been pacemakers of biological depression research. I shall now briefly discuss the train of thoughts which has led to this conclusion.

2. Neuroleptics and central catecholamine metabolism

All known neuroleptics influence the central catecholamine (CA) metabolism in two different ways: by receptor block or by interference with CA storage.

a. Neuroleptics of the receptor-blocking type

The one group, that of the so-called neuroleptics of the receptor-blocking type, comprises the phenothiazines, butyrophenones, and the chemically related groups of the diphenylbutylpiperidines and thioxanthenes. Administration of such a compound to a test animal is followed by an increase in the cerebral concentration of catecholamines (CA) metabolites, while the concentration of the CA themselves remains unchanged. This is suggestive of increased CA degradation in combination with increased CA synthesis which compensated the CA loss; thus, it indicates an increased CA turnover. The correctness of this hypothesis has been verified with the aid of isotope kinetics and by the method of synthesis inhibition. In isotope kinetics, a radioactive CA precursor is administered, and the rate of incorporation of radioactivity in CA is measured. A synthesis inhibitor is used to inhibit CA production, whereupon the rate of disappearance of CA is measured. The serotonin (5-hydroxytryptamine, 5-HT) turnover proved not to be influenced by these compounds.

In functional terms, an increase in turnover can have two completely different implications: increased transmission activity in CA-ergic synapses or, alternatively, block of transmission in CA-ergic synapses. Increased transmission activity leads to an increased need for transmitter substance and so to an increased CA synthesis. Transmission block leads to an increased impulse frequency in the presynaptic element and, probably via this way, to increased CA synthesis. It is logical in this respect to think of a compensatory mechanism aimed at breaking the block (Fig. 14).

With the abovementioned neuroleptics, the increase in turnover is probably secondary to block of transmission. This theory is supported by the following arguments.

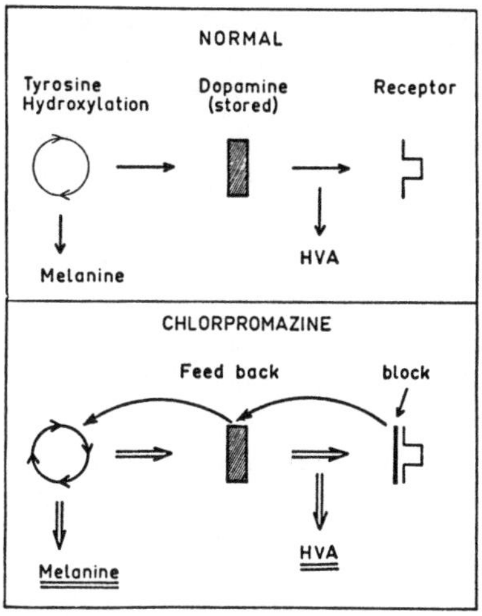

Figure 14. CA-sensitive receptors are localized in the presynaptic and in the postsynaptic membrane of a CA-ergic synapse. Activation of both types of receptor, it is assumed, leads to reduction of CA synthesis via negative feedback. CA synthesis increases when these inhibitory mechanisms are blocked.

1) On the level of behaviour, neuroleptics antagonize manifestations of CA-ergic hyperactivity, e.g. the motor hyperactivity provoked by amphetamines. Via several different mechanisms (MAO inhibition, re-uptake inhibition, release of CA into the synaptic cleft), amphetamines increase the amount of CA available at the CA receptors. This effect is believed to underlie the motor activity they produce.

2) Neuroleptics cause reduction of motor activity. Motor hypoactivity is a constant phenomenon when CA-ergic activity is suppressed, e.g. by inhibition of CA synthesis or via destruction of CA-ergic neuronal systems. This is why hypokinesia is a characteristic feature of Parkinson's disease, with its typical defects in the nigro-striatal DA system.

3) Neuroleptics inhibit adenylcyclase, an enzyme involved in the production of cyclic AMP. This substance is required for activation of postsynaptic CA receptors, and reduced production indicates, or leads to, reduced transmission activity.

In a CA-ergic synapse, receptors are probably localized at two sites: not only in the postsynaptic but also in the presynaptic membrane. The former cause a state of stimulation of the postsynaptic element. The task of the presynaptic receptors is believed to be regulation of the rate of CA synthesis on the basis of the amount of CA contained in the synaptic cleft. It is assumed that both types of receptor are blocked by neuroleptics. Block of the postsynaptic receptors inhibits transmission, while block of the presynaptic receptors is believed to contribute to the increased turnover of the transmitter via elimination of the feedback inhibition.

Another important point is that the extent to which neuroleptics of this type block dopamine (DA) and noradrenaline (NA) receptors differs from one compound to the other; a classification of neuroleptics on the basis of this ratio is quite at odds with their classification according to chemical structure.

Finally, there are indications that neuroleptics of this type inhibit release of DA into the synaptic cleft, which normally occurs after stimulation of the axon. This mechanism, like that of receptor block, should lead to reduction of transmission activity.

b. Neuroleptics of the store-depleting type

Another type of neuroleptic interferes with the uptake of CA into the storage (synaptic) vesicles, causing their accumulation in the cytoplasm, where they are degraded by monoamine oxidase (MAO) so that their concentration decreases. It is assumed that degradation takes place before the amine can reach the synaptic cleft. Consequently no stimulation of postsynaptic CA receptors occurs. The decrease in concentration leads to inhibition of transmission.

Neuroleptics of this category include reserpine, which depletes the DA, NA and serotonin (5-HT) stores, and the indole derivative oxypertine, which shows some predilection for NA stores.

c. Conclusions

Neuroleptics show marked individual differences in chemical structure, but seem similar in their net effect on central CA metabolism. Neuroleptics of the phenothiazine and the butyrophenone series are believed to block presynaptic and postsynaptic CA receptors, and possibly also block release of DA into the synaptic cleft after nerve stimulation. The ratio between DA receptor and NA receptor-blocking potency differs from one neuroleptic to the next. Reserpine and oxypertine interfere with the storage of CA in intraneuronal stores, as a result of which CA degradation increases and the concentration available for transmission decreases.

Neuroleptics reduce transmission in DA-ergic and NA-ergic neurons, but in different proportions and via different mechanisms. This function seems to be a group characteristic.

3. Research strategy

Neuroleptics are substances which differ in chemical structure, but they have two features in common. In *biochemical* terms: they reduce transmission in CA-ergic systems, either by inhibition of postsynaptic receptors or by reduction of the amount of transmitter available. In *psychopathological* terms: they reduce motor unrest, anxiety and psychotic disorders of thinking and experiencing.

These data logically raise a number of closely interrelated questions:

1) Do neuroleptics reduce transmission also in human central CA-ergic neurons?

2) If so, is there a relation between this effect and a) the therapeutic and b) the extrapyramidal (side) effects of neuroleptics?

3) Is the ratio between the DA receptor-blocking and the NA receptor-blocking potency predictive of the precise therapeutic action profile of a neuroleptic? I note that their chemical structure is of little use in this respect.

4) Is the activity in central CA-ergic neurons increased in (schizophrenic) psychoses?

These questions together indicate a research strategy in biological research into psychotic disorders. At least I have used them as such. The principal results of the relevant research will be briefly discussed in the following sections. In this context the NA metabolism has only sporadically been studied, and the following considerations therefore refer chiefly to the DA metabolism.

4. Do neuroleptics reduce human central CA-ergic transmission?

This question can be divided into two parts: 1) Are there indications that neuroleptics of the phenothiazine and the butyrophenone type increase human central CA turnover and, if so, 2) is this phenomenon associated, as it is in test animals, with reduced activity in postsynaptic CA receptors?

a. Neuroleptics and central CA turnover

Influence on DA turnover. There are two methods by which an impression can be gained of the DA and NA metabolism in the human CNS: determination of the concentrations in the CSF of their principal degradation products, i.e. homovanillic acid (HVA) and 3-methoxy-4-hydroxyphenyl glycol (MHPG); and determination of the accumulation of HVA in the CSF after blocking its transport from the CNS to the blood stream with the aid of probenecid. The probenecid technique has been briefly discussed in chapter IV. It cannot be used in studies of the central NA metabolism because MHPG transport is probenecid-insensitive.

Central DA is mainly localized in three systems: the nigro-striatal, the mesolimbic/mesocortical and the tubero-infundibular DA system. The concentration of HVA in the CSF reflects chiefly DA degradation in the nigro-striatal system. Since the spinal cord contains hardly any DA-ergic neurons or DA-ergic nerve endings, the spinal contribution to the HVA concentration in lumbar CSF is negligible. MHPG in lumbar CSF, however, is of mixed spinal and cerebral origin.

The neuroleptics studied in this context—a few phenothiazines and the butyrophenone haloperidol—all cause an increase in the baseline HVA concentration in CSF as well as in probenecid-induced HVA accumulation (Fig. 15). The increase is dose-dependent, i.e. more marked as a larger dose of the neuroleptic is given. These changes are indicative of an increased DA turnover in the CNS.

Oxypertine, a neuroleptic of the store-depleting type which in animal experiments exerts little influence on DA stores, does not influence the HVA concentration in CSF.

Influence on NA turnover. Much less is known about the effect of

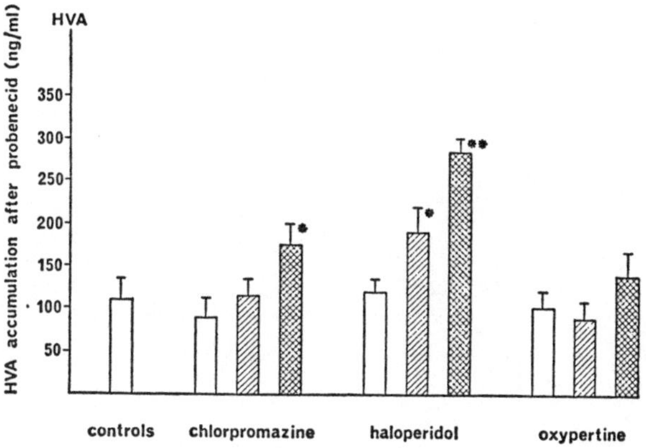

Figure 15. Influence of various types of neuroleptics on the probenecid-induced HVA response in CSF.

This study included 33 patients (aged 18-64) with acute psychoses. They were treated with chlorpromazine (150-225 or 300-450 mg per day), haloperidol (3-4.5 or 9-12 mg per day) or oxypertine (50-100 or 150-200 mg per day). The second probenecid test was carried out at the end of the second week of medication.
Clear columns: before medication.
Hatched columns: during medication with small doses.
Cross-hatched columns: during medication with large doses.
$^*p<0.05$ $^{**}p<0.01$ (Student's t-test)

neuroleptics on MHPG concentration in CSF. Clozapine and oxypertine cause an increase, but chlorpromazine does not. This does not necessarily mean that it exerts no influence on central NA metabolism, for the baseline concentration of a monoamine (MA) metabolite is a less faithful reflection of central MA degradation than its accumulation after probenecid administration.

Influence on 5-HT turnover. None of the neuroleptics studied influenced post-probenecid accumulation of the main 5-HT metabolite: 5-hydroxyindoleacetic acid (5-HIAA) (Fig. 16), and this suggests that they left 5-HT turnover intact.

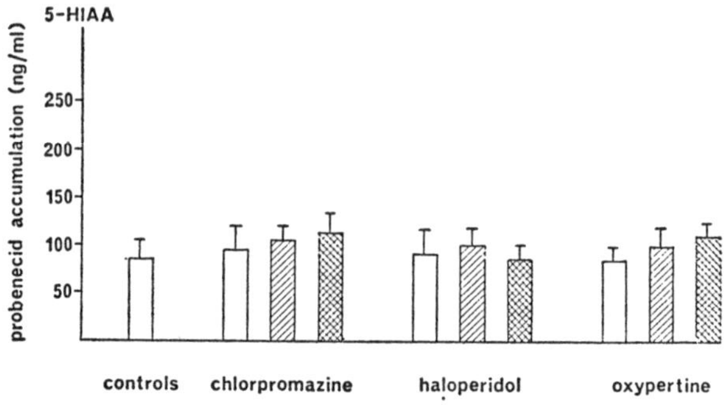

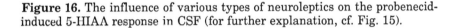

Figure 16. The influence of various types of neuroleptics on the probenecid-induced 5-HIAA response in CSF (for further explanation, cf. Fig. 15).

b. Neuroleptics and activity of postsynaptic DA receptors

The prolactin concentration in blood (and CSF) can be accepted as an indicator of the activity in postsynaptic DA receptors, at least those in the tubero-infundibular DA system. We have no such indicator for postsynaptic NA receptors. Prolactin is a hormone produced exclusively in the anterior pituitary, and its production and release are regulated by the prolactin-inhibiting factor (PIF). PIF is a peptide produced in the hypothalamus, and its production is influenced by DA-ergic neurons of the tubero-infundibular DA system. An increase in DA-ergic activity causes an increase in PIF production, causing decreased production and release of prolactin and consequently a decrease of its concentration in blood and CSF. The reverse occurs if DA-ergic activity diminishes: the PIF production decreases, and the prolactin concentration in blood and CSF increases. If a substance reduces the activity of postsynaptic DA receptors, therefore, an increase of the prolactin concentration in blood and CSF can be expected. This effect is indeed observed in response to neuroleptics of the phenothiazine series (Fig. 17), and this is a strong argument that transmission in central DA-ergic neurons diminishes.

c. *Duration of the effect of neuroleptics on DA-ergic transmission*

The effect of neuroleptics on probenecid-induced HVA accumulation gradually diminishes in the course of a few weeks. Accumulation is normalized after about 3 weeks. This does not mean that the block of the postsynaptic DA receptors is abolished, for the prolactin effect persists unchanged (Fig. 17). The compensatory increase in DA turnover apparently abates after a few weeks. This may explain the fact that the optimal therapeutic effect of neuroleptic medication often does not occur immediately but only after a few weeks. As long as DA production is increased, after all, the receptor block can be abolished entirely or in part, for this block is of a competitive type, which means that it can be overcome by an excess of substrate. Conceivably, transmission inhibition does not become maximal until receptor block is accompanied by normalized DA synthesis. An argument in support of this hypothesis is that the therapeutic effect of neuroleptics is potentiated by combination with α-methyl-p-tyrosine—an inhibitor of DA and NA synthesis.

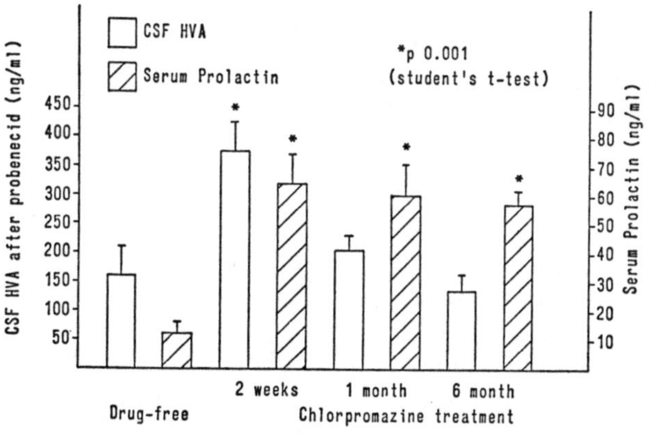

Figure 17. The long-term influence of chlorpromazine on the probenecid-induced HVA response in CSF and on the serum prolactin concentration.

In this group of 20 patients (aged 19-57), treated exclusively with chlorpromazine (300-450 mg per day), the initially markedly increased probenecid-induced accumulation of HVA in CSF returned to its original value after about a month. The increased prolactin concentration, however, persisted unchanged.

d. Conclusion

Neuroleptics of the phenothiazine and butyrophenone type increase the central DA turnover, and in this respect haloperidol is the most effective. This effect is dose-dependent. The increase in central DA turnover is accompanied by an increase of the prolactin concentration in blood and CSF. This indicates that the effect on turnover is based on inhibited transmission in DA-ergic neurons, *not* on increased DA-ergic activity. The DA effect is a transient one, but the prolactin effect is not. It is possible that inhibition of transmission does not become maximal until DA turnover is normalized. This might explain the fact that the therapeutic effect of neuroleptics often gradually increases, to reach a maximum only after a few weeks. The 5-HT turnover is not influenced by neuroleptics.

These findings are in agreement with expectations based on results obtained in animal experiments. MHPG in CSF has not yet been systematically studied in this context. The few data so far available do not warrant any general conclusion.

5. Is there a relation between decreased CA-ergic transmission and the clinical effects of neuroleptics?

a. Therapeutic effects

There are several arguments to support the plausibility of a relation between the therapeutic effect of neuroleptics and their influence on central CA.

To begin with, promethazine (Phenergan), a phenothiazine derivative with no antipsychotic potency, exerts no influence on the probenecid-induced HVA accumulation in CSF. As already demonstrated in animal experiments, therefore, the stimulant effect on DA turnover seems to be a property of phenothiazines with antipsychotic potency.

The second argument derives from a personal study of 32 patients suffering from acute psychoses of varying symptomatology and aetiology, who were treated with chlorpromazine, haloperidol or perphenazine and in whom the therapeutic effect of this medication was compared with the degree of intensification of the HVA response to probenecid during medication (van Praag and Korf 1976). Every day the neuroleptic dosage was adapted to requirements by a psychiatrist not involved in behaviour rating. Patient and evaluator were unaware of the type of neuroleptic given, its dosage and the results of the probenecid test.

A positive correlation was found between the degree of improvement during the second week of medication and the percent increase in HVA response as compared with the pretherapeutic value (Fig. 18). In other words: the clinical improvement was as much more pronounced as the HVA response showed a more marked increase. This correlation proved not to be determined only by the sedative action component of the neuroleptics, for it persisted when results were evaluated not on the basis of total scores but on the basis of improvement in the two prototypical psychotic symptoms, delusion and hallucination, in combination with anxiety (Fig. 19). Sedvall et al. (1977) likewise reported a positive correlation between the increase in the baseline concentration of HVA in CSF and the therapeutic effect of neuroleptics.

Finally, an argument of a different order: If therapeutic efficacy of a neuroleptic and CA-ergic block are linked, then it can be expected that the profile of the clinical (side) effects of a neuroleptic is influenced by the ratio between DA receptor block and NA receptor block. There are indications that such an influence indeed exists—a statement based on no more than the results of two experiments (van Praag et al. 1975, 1977). The conclusions of these experiments should therefore be regarded as tentative. With regard to a neuroleptic, it seems justifiable to maintain that: 1) its inertia-inducing potency increases with its DA receptor-blocking potency; 2) its antipsychotic activity diminishes with its DA receptor-blocking potency; 3) its sedative activity increases with its NA receptor-blocking potency.

These findings indicate that the manner in which a neuroleptic influences central CA is predictive of the pattern of its clinical effects; and as such they support the hypothesis that therapeutic efficacy of neuroleptics and suppression of central CA-ergic activity are interrelated.

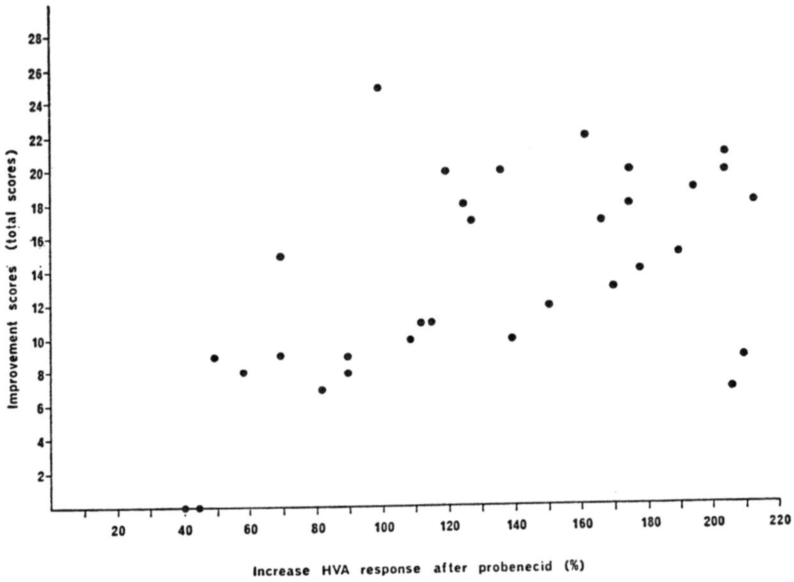

Figure 18. Relation between the increased HVA response to probenecid and the overall clinical improvement at the end of the second week of neuroleptic medication.

Of the 32 patients with various types of acute psychosis, 12 were given chlorpromazine, while 10 received haloperidol and 10 were given perphenazine. Dosage was flexible, and was optimized daily by a psychiatrist who did not score and was unaware of the biochemical findings.

X-axis: percent increase in HVA response during the second week of medication as compared with the original level.

Y-axis: difference between pretherapeutic total score and total score at the end of the second week of medication, using a 10-item 5-point rating scale.

The correlation is significant: $p<0.05$ (Bravais-Pearson correlation coefficient).

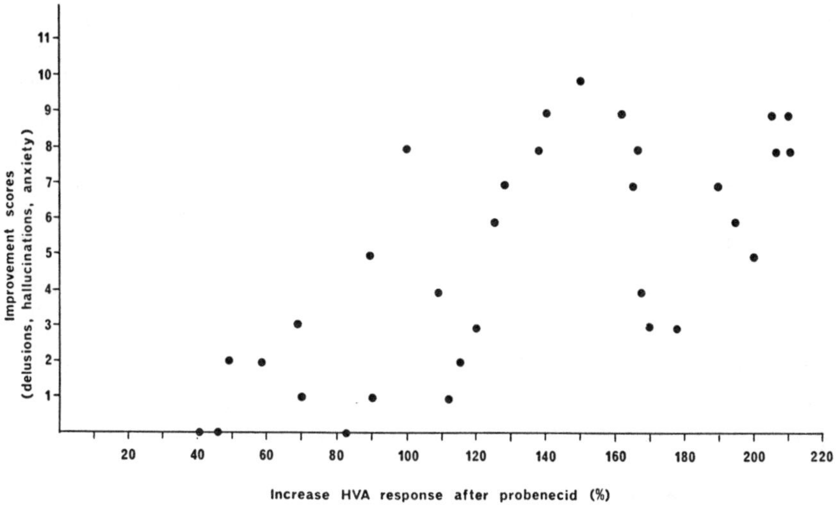

Figure 19. Relation between the increased HVA response to probenecid and improvement of the symptoms delusion, hallucination and anxiety at the end of the second week of neuroleptic medication. For further explanation, cf. Fig. 18.

b. Motor side effects

Since the pathogenesis of Parkinson's disease can be described at least in part in terms of central DA deficiency, it seems logical to assume a causal relation between neuroleptic parkinsonism and block of (nigro-striatal) DA receptors. This assumption would be given a firmer foundation if it were found that: 1) l-DOPA was therapeutically active also in neuroleptic parkinsonism, and 2) a correlation was demonstrable between HVA concentration in CSF and the development of neuroleptic parkinsonism.

Data relevant to the first criterion are scanty. l-DOPA has been little used in neuroleptic parkinsonism because it can aggravate psychotic symptoms (vide infra). The few data available, however, suggest that l-DOPA abates symptoms of hypokinesia and rigidity provoked by neuroleptics.

There is a relation between HVA concentration in CSF and

neuroleptic parkinsonism (van Praag and Korf 1976). During the second week of medication with neuroleptics of various types, the HVA response to probenecid in patients who had developed hypokinetic-rigid symptoms proved to exceed that in patients without motor pathology (Fig. 20). This possibly indicates that DA receptor block is more pronounced in patients of the former category.

In addition it was established that, in patients with hypokinetic-rigid symptoms *during* medication, the *pretherapeutic* HVA response to probenecid was less marked than that in patients without these symptoms (Fig. 21). The interpretation of this finding was that the risk of neuroleptic parkinsonism increases by as much as the pretherapeutic DA turnover is lower. This was believed to afford an explanation of the interindividual differences in susceptibility to the motor side effects of neuroleptics.

In view of all these findings, it seems plausible that the development of hypokinetic-rigid symptoms during neuroleptic medication is related to changes in DA metabolism. Many neuroleptics are not only DA antagonists but also antagonize acetylcholine in varying degrees. Snyder et al. (1974) assumed that it was the anticholinergic potency that determined the degree of extrapyramidal activity of a neuroleptic in the human organism: the stronger its anticholinergic effect, the fewer extrapyramidal symptoms. The above described findings are not consistent with this assumption. They suggest that the degree of DA antagonism is indeed one of the factors which determine the occurrence or non-occurrence of extrapyramidal (at any rate hypokinetic-rigid) symptoms.

Hyperkinesias and dyskinesias induced by neuroleptics have not been studied in this context. Chase (1972) assumed that the occurrence of hypo- or hyper(dys)kinetic symptoms is determined by the balance between receptor block and increased DA turnover. If the former predominates, then hypokinetic-rigid symptoms should result. If the increase in DA turnover is sufficiently marked to break the receptor block (overshooting its target, so to speak), then hyper(dys)kinetic symptoms should result. In principle, this hypothesis could be tested in human individuals, for we have a (gross) standard for the central DA turnover (CSF HVA after probenecid) as well as a standard for postsynaptic activity in DA neurons (serum prolactin).

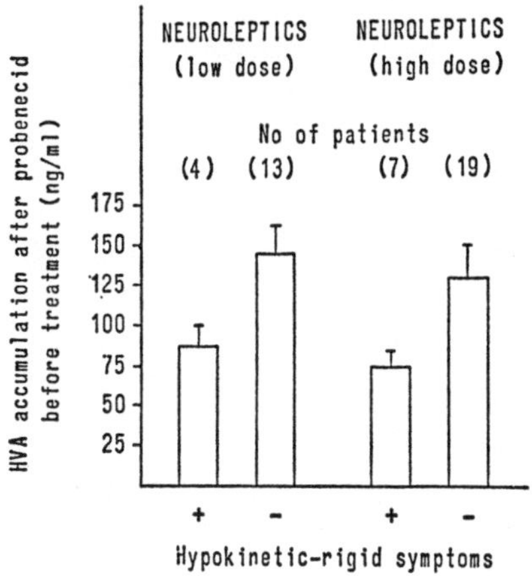

Figure 20. Increased HVA response to probenecid in patients who, during medication with chlorpromazine, haloperidol or perphenazine, developed no (−), mild (+), moderate (++) or marked (+++) hypokinetic-rigid symptoms. The HVA response was more pronounced in the 12 patients who did than in the 20 who did not develop parkinsonoid symptoms ($p<0.05$, Student's t-test).

c. Conclusions

The increase in CA turnover (read: decrease in CA-ergic transmission) induced by neuroleptics seems to be a prerequisite for the development of their therapeutic effects. It is consistent with this conclusion that the ratio between DA receptor block and NA receptor block has proved to be a better predictor of their clinical (side) effects than their chemical structure.

Neuroleptic parkinsonism is probably also related to central DA-ergic hypoactivity, although this conclusion would have been more convincing if the therapeutic efficacy of l-DOPA could have been more intensively studied in these cases. The pathogenesis of neuroleptic hyper(dys)kinesia has remained obscure.

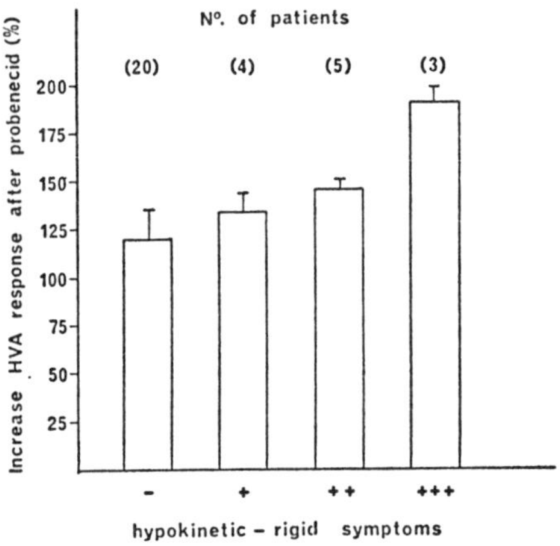

Figure 21. Relation between probenecid-induced HVA accumulation in CSF *before*, and development of hypokinetic-rigid symptoms *during* medication with neuroleptics of the receptor-blocking type.

In patients who developed parkinsonoid symptoms the HVA response before medication was less pronounced than that in those in who did not develop these symptoms. The patients were divided into a low-dosage and a high-dosage group in order to eliminate the possibility that low HVA responders, accidentally, were given mostly large doses of neuroleptics and thus ran an increased risk of extrapyramidal side effects.

The significance of NA effects of neuroleptics for their clinical (side) effects has not yet been adquately studied.

6. CA metabolism in acute schizophrenic psychoses

If it is true that 1) suppression of CA-ergic transmission in the brain is a common characteristic of neuroleptics, and 2) this potency is related to their therapeutic efficacy, then it is justifiable to raise the question whether hyperactivity of CA-ergic systems exists in psychoses which show a favourable response to these compounds. The so-called dopamine (DA) hypothesis is a particularization of this general argumentation. This hypothesis postulates a causal relation between DA-ergic hyperactivity and the development of schizophrenic psychoses.

Two indirect arguments can be advanced in support of a relation between CA, more specifically DA, and psychoses. The first argument is that of *amphetamine-induced psychosis*. This is a syndrome provoked by large doses of amphetamines, as a rule given parenterally; it shows close similarity to paranoid types of schizophrenia. Moreover, amphetamines aggravate schizophrenic psychoses. In biochemical terms, these compounds potentiate neuronal activity in the central DA-ergic systems by various mechanisms (cf. 2a). There is another compound used in the treatment of human individuals with a similar potency: l-DOPA. And this compound, too, can provoke psychoses. This so-called *DOPA-induced psychosis* supplies us with the second, likewise indirect, argument in support of the DA hypothesis. This second argument, however, is not a strong one: DOPA-induced psychoses vary widely in symptomatology, and rarely resemble amphetamine-induced psychosis or "true" schizophrenia.

So far there have been no direct indications of a disorder of central CA metabolism in psychoses. MHPG concentrations in CSF are normal. Postprobenecid HVA accumulation can be increased, but there are reasons to assume that this phenomenon is related to motor agitation, and not so much to prototypical psychotic symptoms such as delusion, hallucination, incoherence or disorientation (Fig. 22). Moreover, the serum prolactin concentration has always been found normal in schizophrenic psychoses of widely diverse symptomatology (Fig. 23).

A possible explanation of the negativity of these findings lies in the fact that the HVA concentration in CSF mainly reflects DA metabolism in the nigro-striatal DA system, whereas serum prolactine is a function of DA activity in the tubero-infundibular DA system. There are no methods to obtain information on the human limbic DA system, and yet it is possibly precisely this system that is involved in the pathogenesis of psychotic symptoms. MHPG in lumbar CSF is only partly of cerebral origin; moreover, there are no inhibitors of MHPG transport. Consequently it may well be that cerebral changes in NA metabolism cannot be traced in lumbar CSF.

Finally, it should of course be borne in mind that the mechanism of action of a therapeutically active compound does not necessarily coincide with or come close to the substrate of the disease symptoms

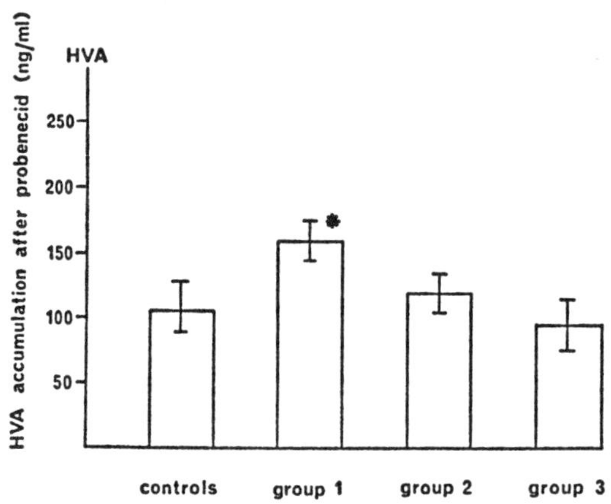

Figure 22. Probenecid-induced HVA accumulation in CSF in 33 untreated psychotic patients with manifest delusions and/or hallucinations at the time of admission.
Group 1: marked motor unrest and anxiety.
Group 2: marked anxiety but no or no pronounced motor unrest.
Group 3: motor unrest and anxiety either absent or not pronounced.
*$p<0.05$ (Student's t-test).

which it is used to control. Example: anticholinergic agents are effective anti-parkinson compounds. Yet it is not the cholinergic but the DA-ergic system that plays the principal role in the pathogenesis of many cases of Parkinson's disease.

7. Conclusions

Animal experiments have demonstrated that, regardless of their chemical structure and via different mechanisms, all known neuroleptics probably inhibit transmission in central CA-ergic systems. In terms of clinical psychiatry, this raises a number of questions: 1) Does this apply to human individuals as well? 2) If so, is this mechanism of importance for the clinical (side)effects of neuroleptics? 3) Do patients with (schizophrenic) psychoses show evidence of central CA-ergic hyperactivity.

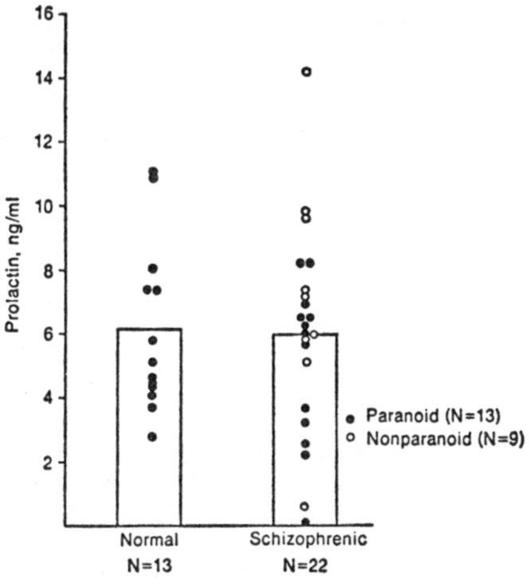

Figure 23. Serum prolactin levels in untreated patients with various types of schizophrenia at the time of admission, and in a control group. There are no differences between the different groups (after Meltzer et al. 1974).

The first two questions can be answered in the affirmative, at least so far as the DA system is concerned. In this system, inhibition of transmission occurs and the therapeutic effects of neuroleptics as well as their ability to provoke hypokinetic-rigid symptoms seem to be related to this fact. In this respect the NA metabolism has not yet been adequately studied. The ratio between the DA receptor-blocking and the NA receptor-blocking potency of a given neuroleptic appears to be predictive of its therapeutic activity. This, too, is an argument in favour of a relation between therapeutic effects and CA effects. The relation between CA metabolism and neuroleptic hyper(dys)kinesia has not yet been studied.

The hypothesis that DA-ergic hyperactivity is an important pathogenetic mechanism in schizophrenic psychoses is based solely on indirect arguments; direct studies of DA metabolism have so far failed to yield evidence to support this hypothesis. This is probably related to the fact that the DA system most important in this context (the limbic DA system) has not been accessible to investigation in human individuals. Finally, it is of course possible that DA play no role of significance in the pathogenesis of (schizophrenic) psychoses, even though the therapeutic efficacy of neuroleptics is related to their influence on DA systems.

BIBLIOGRAPHY

ANDÉN, N. E., S. G. BUTCHER, H. CORRODI, K. FUXE AND U. UNGERSTEDT (1970). Receptor activity and turnover of dopamine and noradrenaline after neuroleptics. *J. Pharmacol.* 11, 303-314.

BOWERS, M. B. JR. (1974). Central dopamine turnover in schizophrenic syndromes. *Arch. gen. Psychiat.* 31, 50-54.

CARLSSON, A., T. PERSSON, B-E. ROOS AND J. WÅLINDER (1972). Potentiation of phenothiazines by α-methyl-tyrosine in treatment of chronic schizophrenia. *J. Neural. Transm. 33*, 83-90.

CHASE, T. N. (1972). Drug-induced extrapyramidal disorders. In: *Neurotransmitters* (Ed.) I. J. Kopin. Baltimore: Williams and Wilkins. 448-471.

FREEDMAN, D. X. (Ed.) (1975). *Biology of the Major Psychoses: A Comparative Analysis*. New York: Raven Press.

HASSLER, R., I. J. BAK AND J. S. KIM (1970). Unterschiedliche Entleerung der Speicherorte für Noradrenalin, Dopamin und Serotonin als Wirkungsprinzip des Oxypertins. *Nervenartz.*, 41, 105-118.

IVERSEN, L. L. (1975). Dopamine receptors in the brain. *Science* 118, 1084-1089.

MATTHIJSSE, S. (1973). Antipsychotic drug actions: a clue to the neuropathology of schizophrenia? *Feder. Proc.* 32, 200-205.

MELTZER, H., E. J. SACHAR AND A. G. FRANTZ (1974). Serum prolactin levels in unmedicated schizophrenic patients. *Arch. gen. Psychiat.* 31, 564-569.

MUNKVAD, I., R. FOG AND A. RANDRUP (1975). Amphetamine psychosis: A useful model of schizophrenia? In: *On the Origin of Schizophrenic Psychoses*. (Ed.) H. M. van Praag, Amsterdam: De Erven Bohn B. V.

NYBÄCK, H. AND G. SEDVALL (1970). Further studies on the accumulation and disappearance of catecholamines formed from ^{14}C in mouse brain. Effect of some phenothiazine analogues. *Eur. J. Pharmacol.* 10, 193-205.

POST, R. M., E. FINK, W. T. CARPENTER AND F. K. GOODWIN (1975). Cerebrospinal fluid amine metabolites in acute schizophrenia. *Arch. Gen. Psychiat.* 32, 1063-1069.

POST, R. M. AND F. K. GOODWIN (1975). Time-dependent effect of phenothiazines in dopamine turnover in psychiatric patients. *Science* 190, 488-489.

PRAAG, H. M. VAN (1967). The possible significance of cerebral dopamine for neurology and psychiatry. *Psychiat. Neurol. Neurochir.* 70, 361-379.

PRAAG, H. M. VAN (1977). *Depression and Schizophrenia. A Contribution on Their Chemical Pathology.* New York: Spectrum Publications.

PRAAG, H. M. VAN, L. C. W. DOLS AND T. SCHUT (1975). Biochemical versus psychopathological action profile of neuroleptics: A comparative study of chlorpromazine and oxypertine in acute psychotic disorders. *Compr. Psychiat.* 16, 255-263.

PRAAG, H. M. VAN AND J. KORF (1975). Neuroleptics, catecholamines and psychotic disorders. A study of their interrelation. *Amer. J. Psychiat.* 132, 593-597.

PRAAG, H. M. VAN AND J. KORF (1976). Importance of the dopamine metabolism for the clinical effects and side effects of neuroleptics. *Amer. J. Psychiat.* 133, 1171-1177.

PRAAG, H. M. VAN, J. KORF AND L. C. W. DOLS (1976). Clozapine versus perphenazine or the value of the biochemical mode of action of neuroleptics in predicting their therapeutic activity. *Brit. J. Psychiat.* 129:547-555.

PRAAG, H. M. VAN (1977). The significance of dopamine for the mode of action of neuroleptics and the pathogenesis of schizophrenia. *Brit. J. Psychiat.* 130:463-474.

SEDVALL, G., G. ALFREDSON, L. BJERKENSTEDT, P. ENEROTH, B. FYRÖ, C. HÄRNRYD AND B. WODE-HELGODT (1977). In: *The Impact of Biology on Modern Psychiatry.* (Eds.) E. S. Gershon, R. H. Belmaker, S. S. Kety and M. Rosenbaum. New York, London: Plenum Press.

SEEMAN, P. AND T. LEE (1975). Antipsychotic drugs: direct correlation between clinical potency and presynaptic action on dopamine neurons. *Science* 188, 1217-1219.

SNYDER, S. H. (1973). Amphetamine psychosis: a "model" schizophrenia mediated by catecholamines. *Amer. J. Psychiat.* 130, 61-66.

SNYDER, S. H., S. P. BANERJEE, H. I. YAMAMURA AND D. GREENBERG (1974). Drugs, neurotransmitters and schizophrenia. *Science* 184, 1243-1253.

Symposium on catecholamines and their enzymes in the neuropathology of schizophrenia (1974). *J. Psychiat. Res.* 11, 1-361.

WILSON, R. G., J. R. HAMILTON, W. D. BOYD, A. P. M. FORREST, E. N. COLE, A. R. BOYNS AND K. GRIFFITHS (1975). The effect of long-term phenothiazine therapy on plasma prolactin. *Brit. J. Psychiat.* 127, 71-74.

PART THREE

Pharmacotherapy of Disorders of Mood Regulation

As we look at this whole field, the most challenging, and the least conquered and understood, is that set of phenomena which we associate with the mind. Here is the great challenge to the physician and to the scientist. To the physician because it is particularly in this respect that one individual differs from another, and because the meeting and mutual understanding of minds constitute the essence of the doctor-patient relationship; to the scientist because here is presented an elementary problem of scientific method—namely, that of classifying the facts in such a way that allows numerical values to be assigned to them, and formulation of these in terms of a simple hypothesis. This challenge has been offered before to the scientific method, and I cannot believe that it will, this time, go unanswered.

J. Pickering
British Medical Journal
26 December 1964.

XII

Diagnosis of Depressions

1. Depression and antidepressants

Antidepressants—otherwise also known as thymoleptics*—are compounds which primarily improve the mood in certain types of depression. The word "primarily" distinguishes the antidepressants from the neuroleptics and ataractics—compounds which can likewise exert a favourable influence on the mood, but indirectly, via reduction of the intensity of various pathological and alarming experiences. Although the effect of antidepressants is not confined to affective life, it is this activity that gives them their identity.

The above definition encompasses a second restriction: it is stated that antidepressants are effective not in all but only in *certain* types of depression. This implies that it would be wrong to prescribe these agents indiscriminately in all states of depressive dys-

*Delay (1965) pointed out that the term thymoleptic is not a felicitous term because it denotes suppression of affective life, whereas in fact this type of compound activates. The term "thymoanaleptic" would have been more appropriate, but this has never been widely accepted.

phoria. Determination of their indications requires careful differentiation of the various types of depression. A discussion of the range of indications for antidepressants should therefore be preceded by considerations on the diagnosis of depressions. In the context of this book, these considerations cannot be comprehensive. They will be confined to aspects which, in my opinion, are relevant to the pharmacotherapy of depressions.

2. Imperfections in depression diagnosis

Depressions are usually designated after the most prominent aetiological factor. One refers to, say, endogenous depression, involutional depression, psychogenic depression, neurotic depression, arteriosclerotic depression, etc. In the classification of depressions, therefore, use is made of a single criterion: aetiology. This method of classification can give rise to misunderstanding because it seems to warrant one of the following two conclusions: 1) In spite of their diverse aetiology, depressions are highly similar in symptomatological terms; or 2) there are different depressive syndromes, but each type is characterized by a well-defined aetiology, and can be identified by mentioning the aetiology.

Neither conclusion is correct. Depressions are not a homogeneous category, and individual depressive patients show substantial differences both in symptomatology and in subjective experiences. Nor is there a predictable relation between aetiology and the type of disease symptoms produced in depressions. Let us consider the random example of involutional depression. This can have the features of a largely vital depression, but anxiously agitated and/or paranoid syndromes are likewise encountered. In other cases we find a predominantly hysterical symptomatology, and a hysterical personality structure is not a prerequisite for this finding. Finally, a patient suffering from involutional depression can show a syndrome of deep despondency which is evoked by the problems of this phase of life and, as such, is entirely understandable.

By way of discursion I may add that the absence of specific relations between aetiology and syndrome is no reason for immediate rejection of the principle of specificity in psychiatry. I consider it quite possible that research into the pathogenesis of depressions (chapter V) may re-establish this principle—that on a cerebral level there will certainly prove to be specific relations between psychological dysfunctions and the complex of cerebral functional disorders which generates them.

The paired concepts "unipolar" and "bipolar" depression have in the past few years been accepted in depression diagnosis (section 9 below). These concepts, too, are incomplete because they give information on the course of the depression but not on its symptomatology and aetiology.

The diagnosis of depressions, to put it briefly, is not consistently three-dimensional. This is a serious shortcoming for, if an adequate therapeutic plan is to be made, one needs expertise on symptoms as well as on aetiology and course. This is why I intend to focus some attention on these diagnostic dimensions. For the unwary reader (without psychiatric training), it is to be noted in advance that the diagnostic terminology is unfortunately not yet normalized. I shall primarily discuss the concepts which I personally use, but will attempt to "translate" them into the terms conventionally used in the literature, and particularly in the Anglo-American literature.

3. Mood disturbances in depressions

As early as 1920, Kurt Schneider was acutely aware of the symptomatological diversity of depressions. On the basis of Scheler's (1928) division of affective life into four "layers," he compared melancholia with psychogenically determined depression. The psychogenic depression, Schneider maintained, involves the sphere of the psychological feelings in the sense indicated by Scheler, i.e. the feelings which can be motivated. Melancholia, however, involves the "layer" of the vital feelings, i.e. the conglomerate of feelings of content and discontent that cannot be precisely localized and are experienced in the somatic sphere. Schneider characterized melancholia as "eine primäre Depression in der Schicht der Vitalgefühle" (a primary depression in the layer of vital feelings).

Accepting Schneider's principle of classification, we can now roughly distinguish *two basic types of depression*. The one involves the sphere of psychological feelings, and in this type the substance of the dysphoria coincides, so to speak, with what has prompted it. The patient perceives a comprehensible relation between the one and the other. He says: "I am downhearted because. . . ," and then gives expression to what is bothering him. The existence of this depression is experienced as meaningful. With reference to depressions of this category I use the term *personal*. Why? Why not simply retain the "psychogenic depression" concept? Because the word psychogenic explicitly alludes to an aetiology, not to a syndromal form, "psychogenic depression" means no more than a depression which is conditioned mainly by factors of a psychological nature. The syndromal form remains uncertain. However, psychological factors can give rise to depressions of the comprehensible kind, but equally well to vital depressions (section 8 below). There are psychogenically (or neurotically) conditioned personal depressions, but there are also psychogenically (or neurotically) conditioned vital depressions.

The other basic type of depression involves the sphere of the vital feelings, and I therefore refer to these depressions as *vital* depressions. The affective anomaly in these cases shows the following features:

1) It is of an unmotivated character. The word unmotivated should in this context be understood to mean: absence of a sense of comprehensibility. The dysphoria is experienced as meaningless (apart from a possible interpretation in the metaphysical sense). The patient says: "I do not know how I came to be this way; it has come over me." If we characterize the category of personal depressions as "geistnah" (psyche-oriented), then the term "leibnah" (body-oriented) is appropriate for the category of vital depressions.

   It should be explicitly noted that by "unmotivated" I do not mean that precipitating factors of a psychotraumatic nature are necessarily always absent. In some cases they are indeed absent; the period preceding manifestation of the depression is psychopathologically quite "vacuous." The patient indicates that the origin of his complaints is a mystery to him. In other cases, however, the patient does mention a reason for his complaints in the first instance. Further investigation in these cases shows, however, that this "reason" is no longer experienced as an adequate explanation of the existing condition. The depression proves to have become detached from its original motivation. In other words: the continuity, i.e. the comprehensible relation between the dysphoria and what has prompted it, is lost. The depression could be described, not very elegantly, as having been vitalized. In such cases the patient experiences as painful the very fact that he can no longer be really sad about the original psychotraumatic event.

2) Particularly in the milder instances of vital depression, sad feelings are not predominant. The patient often does not give the outsider an impression of marked sadness. Some impress as resigned, and others as rather irritable and caustic. The patient himself also regards the term despondent as inadequate to characterize his condition. He is not so much downhearted as spiritless, and full of a sense of displeasure and discontent. Without knowing why, he lacks zest in living. His condition might be described as a persistent hangover or, to use Schneider's words, as a depressio sine depressione. Westerman (1922) used the term "körperliche Traurigkeit" (somatic sadness) in this context in order to indicate that these feelings are usually experienced as "leibnah" (body-oriented). One should beware in these cases of the fact that, although despondency is not prominent, taedium vitae can be very pronounced.

It is only in a later stage that the striking, massive, intractable melancholy develops with which vital depression is not infrequently (but erroneously)identified.

4. Vital depressive symptoms outside the affective sphere

Vital depressions manifest themselves not exclusively in affective life, but also in other disorders, the most important of which will be briefly discussed. This discussion will be confined to the early symptoms, i.e. manifestations seen in incipient or mild vital depression.

Psychomotor disorders

In principle, these disorders carry a minus sign. Initially there is no question of objective manifestations of the motor retardation which characterizes the fully developed vital depression. In the initial phase, retardation manifests itself only in subjective experiencing. The patient notices that his work is not what it used to be. His tempo diminishes. He has a sense of being held back, and can no longer cope with his duties. Nothing goes easily and smoothly anymore; every activity requires a conscious effort (retarded vital depression).

In some cases, particularly in patients of more advanced age, there may be more or less pronounced agitation *as well* (agitated vital depression). The patient feels tense and anxious, and may show visible signs of motor unrest. I emphasized the words "as well"; in these cases retardation and agitation are not polar features. The agitation is superimposed on the retardation, so to speak, and this is experienced in this way by the patient himself. An increased level of tension can also, or even mainly, express itself in somatic functional disorders, e.g. palpitations, tremors and atypical precordial pain.

Cognitive disorders

The insufficient impetus also manifests itself in cognition. The patient notices that it takes longer for things to penetrate. He experiences difficulties in fathoming a particular correlation. His thoughts "will not come." There is a certain paucity of inventiveness, of ideas. The patient himself often speaks of disturbed concentration. Not infrequently there is also a degree of irresoluteness; decision making poses great problems. It should be emphasized that these manifestations occur long before there is any unequivocal retardation of the flow of thoughts. Manifest bradyphrenia is a late phenomenon.

Disturbed time sense

The time sense is involved in the general retardation. The patient states that time just does not seem to pass; that the days last so long. Straus (1928), who was the first to mention this phenomenon, described it as a lagging behind of the "ego-time" in relation to the "world-time"—two time dimensions which normally coincide.

Hypoaesthesia

The early symptoms also include a category of manifestations which the patient often describes as indifference. He loses his interest in work, family and hobbies. Nothing touches him anymore. In this way the patient himself experiences what could be interpreted as reduced emotional susceptibility to exogenous and endogenous affective stimuli. The stimuli are perceived undisturbed, but their emotional load is removed. As a result, the patient feels cut off from himself as well as from the world around him, which he experiences as—literally—cold and colourless. He can no longer experience pleasure and, often in a somewhat later stage, is equally unable to experience sadness. He feels "empty inside." The reduced emotional susceptibility as such is often experienced very vividly. This is a peculiar paradox which Schulte (1961) described as "erlebte Leblosigkeit" (experienced lifelessness).

In its extreme form, this experiential impoverishment leads to the so-called feeling of unfeelingness which characterizes the syndrome of *melancholia anaesthetica*.

Somatic disorders

Beside psychopathological symptoms, somatic complaints also develop. Some of these are objectively verifiable (insomnia, constipation, etc.), but others are not (disagreeable sensations in the upper abdomen, fatigue, etc.). Not infrequently, these complaints are assimilated in a hypochondriacal way; they become the focus of attention and the patient gradually becomes unable to detach himself from them. In this way, somatic symptoms can come to be so predominant in the syndrome as to disguise the origin almost completely *(masked vital depression)*. In some cases this leads to diagnostic errors. The perturbation produced by these complaints is mistaken for their origin; or the complaints are primarily interpreted in an organic sense, and this can greatly delay the patient's visit to a psychiatrist, much to his disadvantage.

The somatic disorders which can develop in the course of a vital depression are numerous. A nearly constant triad is: *reduced appetite, disturbed sleep* and *fatigue*; this combination is found even in mild cases. The amount of food taken can still be normal, but it no longer tastes well. As regards the disturbed sleep, complaints about premature awakening are more common than those about difficulties in getting to sleep. In rare cases, sleep requirements are increased (hypersomnia). Rest hardly alleviates the sense of fatigue (which in any case is most pronounced in the morning hours and therefore is, in fact, independent of performance). Contrary to the conventional view, constipation has proved to be a symptom which is often absent in vital depression, and especially in the milder forms.

Another important fact is that *disturbances in sexual functions* can develop in the context of a vital depression, specifically, amenorrhoea, reduced libido, and disturbed potency. These symptoms often show an excellent response to antidepressants, which simply means that they abate as the depression abates. If their origin is not recognized, or is mistakenly considered to be neurotic, then a psychotherapeutic approach could be erroneously taken.

The above enumeration is not complete, and in fact comprises only the most important symptoms. A detailed survey of somatic manifestations can be found in the monographs of Kraines (1957) and Kiev (1974). It remains for me only to make mention of a misconception. Many publications in the literature describe vital depressions as "dry" depressions; this refers to the alleged unusual dryness of the skin of these patients. In its generality, this statement is erroneous. The humidity of the skin of a vitally depressed patient depends on the degree of agitation. Agitated vital depressions, even if mild, are often anything but "dry."

Spontaneous diurnal fluctuation

This is the most typical, virtually pathognomonic feature of the vital depressive symptom complex. Retardation and dysphoria are most marked in the morning hours, and gradually diminish in intensity in the course of the day. Improvement starts at the end of the morning or towards the beginning of the afternoon. The time of improvement is as much later as the vital depression is deeper, and in these cases the diurnal fluctuation is often less pronounced. Finally, fluctuations in intensity can disappear completely.

In some vital depressions there is no diurnal fluctuation; it is absent throughout all phases of the disease. Whether these cases represent a special subtype is unknown.

Seasonal influences, depressions occurring mainly in autumn and spring, are classical but by no means present in all cases.

5. Vital depression

The series of symptoms discussed in section 4, in combination with a depression in the sphere of vital feelings, is described by me as vital depressive syndrome or, more succinctly, vital depression. The term vital depression is strictly *syndromal* and has *no* aetiological and prognostic implications.

The vital depression equates to the syndrome described in Anglo-American literature as *endogenous depression.* I prefer the former designation for three reasons: a) the concept "endogenous" is not syndromal but aetiological, for it alludes to involvement of hereditary factors and is therefore unsuitable as a designation of a syndrome; b) a vital depression is an aetiologically non-specific syndrome; endogenous factors may be involved, but the same applies to factors of a different nature; c) endogenous factors are not exclusively linked with the vital depression; Shields (1976) found indications that they can be equally significant in personal depression.

The syndrome of vital depression does not always manifest itself in its complete form. These incomplete depressions are described not as vital depressions but as depressions with vital features. The risk entailed here is that one is satisfied with so few "features" that the concentration of the vital depression concept approaches zero value. I describe a condition as a depression with vital features if *at least* the following symptoms are in evidence: decreased mood level, hypoaesthesia and, of the somatic series, disturbed sleep and reduced appetite.

In very severe vital depressions there can be delusions with typical contents: hypochondriacal (the patient's body literally deteriorates), poverty (material existence deteriorates), and sin (existential deterioration). I describe a deep vital depression with delusions as *melancholia.*

Some authors maintain that depressions which involve the sphere of psychological feelings (i.e. personal depressions) generally take a mild course, whereas vital depressions invariably take a serious course. I consider this view to be incorrect. Personal and vital depressions are qualitatively different categories, and each can take either a mild or a more serious course. Vital depressions with a mild course are quite common; yet experience shows that this diagnosis is only too often missed. This results from the fact that vital depressions are sometimes erroneously identified with the features of a massively despondent, seriously inhibited patient. This is to be regretted, because it is precisely these milder forms of vital depression that often show an excellent response to antidepressant medication.

It is to be noted that the word "mild" is used here in a strictly formal psychopathological sense. The suffering of the vitally depressed patient is always serious, whatever the depth of the depression may be in clinical terms.

6. Personal depressive symptoms outside the affective sphere

In personal depressions, disorders outside the affective sphere are less common, and their pattern is less constant, than in vital depressions. I shall describe the syndrome of personal depression by comparing it with that of vital depression.

Psychomotor disorders

These are much less pronounced than those of vital depression. Retardation of any significance is rare. Unrest, anxiety feelings, and somatic anxiety equivalents (chapter XIX) are much more common. Cognitive processes can be impeded because the patient is preoccupied with his problems, but there is no real blocking of the flow of thoughts (as if each thought has to be produced by a great effort). There is no irresoluteness, and the time sense remains normal.

Hypoaesthesia

Hypoaesthesia is absent; there may be depersonalization, but these are different phenomena. In both depersonalization and hypoaesthesia, perception is undisturbed. In the case of hypoaesthesia, perception no longer elicits any feeling, or only to a reduced extent; in the case of depersonalization, perception is associated with an unusual feeling.

Somatic disorders

These are frequently observed, but largely concern symptoms of vegetative dysregulation such as palpitations, atypical anginous pains, disagreeable sensations at various sites of the body, etc. Sleep is often disturbed, i.e. getting to sleep is more often difficult than continuing sleep. Complaints about appetite and sexual functions are uncommon.

Spontaneous diurnal fluctuation

There are no consistent variations in the intensity of symptoms in the course of the day. Occasionally there may be a so-called reversed diurnal fluctuation: unlike the patient with a vital depression, these patients feel worst in the evening. It is often psychogenic factors that seem responsible for this, e.g. coming home to the marital partner, or worry about the night with its insomnia and/or anxious dreams.

7. Personal depression

The symptoms described in section 6, together with a depression which involves the "layer" of psychological feelings, are described by me as personal depressive syndrome or, briefly, personal depression. The features of the personal depression are less sharply defined than those of the vital depression. This is because there is a gradual transition between personal depression and the vast field of the psychosomatic illnesses, anxiety-neuroses, neurotic personality disorders, etc. As long as the latter field has not been more accurately charted, an outline of the personal depression cannot be more precise.

The boundary between personal and vital depression is likewise ill-defined, as apparent from the fact that it was necessary to introduce a concept such as "depression with vital features." In other words: the vital and the personal depression are prototypes, and mixed forms are quite common. Is it possible and useful further to differentiate these mixed forms? We do not know. Further investigation will have to settle this point.

The syndrome of personal depression is described in Anglo-American literature as psychogenic, neurotic or reactive depression. For several reasons I do not consider this terminology to be felicitous: 1) because it is illogical to describe a syndrome in terms which have an aetiological significance; 2) because genetic and environmental as well as psychological factors can play a role in the pathogenesis of this type of depression; 3) because psychological factors need not inevitably lead to a personal depression. They can equally well be responsible for a vital depression. These are sufficient reasons, therefore, for the consistent use of appropriate terms to characterize aetiology and syndrome, e.g. by referring to a chiefly neurotically determined personal depression, or to a personal depression largely conditioned by environmental factors.

As already mentioned in section 5, I consider it a misconception to assume that vital and personal depressions differ only quantitatively; that the vital depression is merely a severe variant of the personal depression. They are qualitatively different syndromes, each of which can take either a mild or a more severe course. The development of typical depressive delusions (hypchondriacal, poverty and sin delusions) is characteristic of the severe vital depression. They do not occur in personal depressions.

8. Aetiological aspects of the vital and the personal depression

In the aetiological context, an estimate is made of the extent to which endogenous (genetic), exogenous (acquired somatic), psychogenic (intrapsychical), or sociogenic (relational) factors contribute to the development of a given syndrome.

In the individual case, the sole clue to involvement of an endogenous factor is a tainted family history; and the taint should not be found exclusively in linear descent because in that case pseudo-heredity (transmission via a learning process) cannot be excluded. Exogenous factors are investigated on the basis of the history and findings obtained by physical examination.

A psychogenic "charge" becomes plausible if there are positive indications of an unresolved psychological conflict situation and a personality structure with weak spots which indicate why the conflict remained unresolved. Sociogenic stress factors have their origin in the patient's life environment. Their pathogenetic activity, however, is always a result of the interaction between the psychotraumatic factors and the personality structure. The majority of human individuals can cope with most frustrations. A minority decompensates. Consequently there must be demonstrable features in their personality structure which explain their "susceptibility." Examples of depression-susceptible personalities are: the passive personality, highly dependent on the judgement of others and with a great need for gratification; and also the compulsive individual, who experiences every interference with the rigid pattern of his life as a threat or an injury.

The *vital depression* is an aetiologically non-specific syndrome which can be provoked by endogenous as well as by exogenous (acquired), psychogenic and social factors. In some cases provoking factors are not discernible at all (idiopathic form). The vital depression has long been identified erroneously with its idiopathic or endogenous form; with the patient who is overwhelmed by despondency, without understanding why. Vital depressions, however, can also develop in response to (combinations of) intrapsychical tensions and social pressure. In this respect there are two possibilities:

1) Psychogenic (and social) factors provoke a depression which from the start shows the symptomatological features of a vital depression; or:

2) The psychogenically (and/or socially) conditioned depression is initially experienced in the personal sphere but, sooner or later, gradually assumes the character of a vital depression. This development is sometimes described, somewhat ambiguously, as the *vitalization* of a personal depression. This complication is one of several possible causes of stagnation of a psychotherapeutic approach. Since it is often possible to correct it fairly quickly with the aid of antidepressants, it is of great importance that this complication be identified as such as soon as possible.

Vital depressions can also develop in response to somatic illness. In this respect cerebral arteriosclerosis is a valid example. A similar development is repeatedly seen after infectious diseases. Particularly, viral infections such as influenza, infectious hepatitis and infectious mononucleosis are notorious in this respect. The non-psychiatrist says: convalescence often requires a long time in these diseases. In psychiatric terms, many of these cases involve a vital depression.

In the actual case, combinations of these factors are often involved. For example: an individual living under stress, with a depression-tainted family history, develops a vital depression after suffering from a somatic disease.

Psychological and environmental factors always play a role in the pathogenesis of *personal depressions*. There are strong indications, however, that a genetic factor can be of importance in this type of depression as well.

9. Classification according to course

In terms of course (or prognosis), two types of vital depression are distinguished: unipolar and bipolar depressions. A *unipolar depression* is defined as a recurrent vital depression without (hypo)manic phases; a *bipolar depression* is a recurrent vital depression in which (hypo)manic phases also occur in the course of life. In other respects, too, unipolar and bipolar depressions differ. The mode of hereditary transmission differs (genetic factors are by no means in all cases demonstrable). Also different are the age of onset of the first phase, the duration of asymptomatic intervals, and the premorbid personality structure.

The terms unipolar and bipolar have no aetiological implications. Classical examples are cases in which the depressive phases occur for no apparent reason and in which the family history is depression-tainted—the classical endogenous aetiology. However, cases in which exogenous and/or psychosocial factors provoke (or cause?) the phases are certainly no exception, particularly so far as the initial phases are concerned. Not infrequently, later phases develop more and more "spontaneously."

The term *manic-depressive psychosis* can be regarded as a collective name for unipolar and bipolar depressions. I dislike using the term because: 1) some patients (the majority) never develop (hypo)-manic phases, and 2) some patients (the majority) never become psychotic either during depressive or during (hypo)manic phases.

If left untreated, the psychogenic (neurotic) personal depressions also tend to become recurrent. This is not surprising. As long as the patient's personality structure and his situation in life remain unchanged, he remains subject to the threat of ever-repeated minor or major conflicts which can lead to a depression. The natural history of personal depressions, unlike that of vital depressions, has hardly been studied systematically so far.

I personally use the term unipolar depression exlusively with reference to the recurrent vital depression, not to the recurrent personal depression. In the literature, it is by no means always clear whether or not this definition is adhered to, and in such cases the term unipolar (which is after all one-dimensional) can be confusing.

Once it develops, the vital depression takes its independent course subject to its own rules, regardless of causative factors. An excellent example of this is the reserpine-induced depression. Discontinuation of reserpine often fails to lead to recovery. This requires antidepressant medication. As judged by the older literature (before the introduction of specific therapy), the vital depression is also a self-limiting disease, which can last from a few days to many years, but tends to disappear spontaneously in the end. This prompts the question: Is it justifiable to distinguish between exogenous and psychogenic depressions? Is every vital depression perhaps essentially of endogenous origin, with psychogenic and exogenous factors playing only a subordinate role as precipitating factors? It is difficult to answer this question. Since electroshock therapy and antidepressants have become available, it is no longer justifiable to study the natural history of vital depressions. Perhaps modern biochemical genetic research (marker research) can supply some information. A discussion of its results, however, is not within the scope of this book.

10. Other diagnostic classifications

In Anglo-American literature a distinction is made between *primary* and *secondary affective disorders*. This distinction is based on premorbid factors. The primary depression develops in individuals with a more or less normal personality structure and a psychiatric history which is "clean," apart from possible depressive or manic episodes. A depression is described as secondary if the patient has a history of psychiatric disorders other than depression and mania, as well as an imperfect personality structure.

The "primary depression" concept in actual fact covers the classical vital depression with a unipolar or bipolar course in non-neurotic individuals; the secondary depression seems to approximate the neurotic depression, but insufficient information is given on the symptomatology. I am not very happy with this pair of concepts. The terms are not multi-dimensional, disregard the possibility that vital depressions (with a unipolar or bipolar course) can develop in neurotic individuals, and disregard the fact that there are no indications that mainly neurotically and mainly non-neurotically determined vital depressions should fundamentally differ in therapeutic or prognostic terms.

Winokur et al. (1969), on the basis of an extensive family study, distinguished two subtypes within the unipolar group: *depression spectrum disease*, and *pure depressive disease*. The prototype of the former group is the woman whose first depressive phase develops before age 40, and in whose family depression is more common in women than in men—a "depression deficit" which is filled out in the men by alcoholism and sociopathy. The prototype of the latter group is the man whose first depressive phase develops after age 40 and in whose family depressions show no male or female predominance, while alcoholism and sociopathy are not overrepresented.

Finally we find the term *hysterodepression*. This is an ambiguous term, sometimes used to indicate the presence of certain symptoms (e.g. unauthenticity and theatricality) and at other times used to characterize an aetiological mechanism (e.g. hysterical neurosis). The two criteria do not coincide. Hysterodepressive symptoms can develop in a not evidently hysterical personality (e.g. in association with organic cerebral lesions, but also if the personality is shaken by exogenous conditions such as war, disasters of nature, marital infidelity, etc.). Inversely, a depression in hysterical neurosis need not necessarily show a hysterical "colouring." Since it is an ambiguous concept, hysterodepression should be divided into two categories. That of a personal depression with hysterical manifestations, sometimes but not always caused by hysterical-neurotic mechanisms, and that of a personal depression without pronounced hysterical symptoms but nevertheless caused by hysterical mechanisms.

11. Conclusions

This chapter marshals arguments in favour of a three-dimensional classification of depressions according to: symptomatology, aetiology and course. This is necessary because: 1) the type of syndrome gives insufficient information on its aetiology; 2) a particular aetiology does not necessarily produce a particular syndrome; 3) the course of a depression cannot be reliably predicted on the basis of either its aetiology or the features of its syndrome. A three-dimensional approach is of practical importance in that it facilitates therapeutic planning. Schematically and by way of example: the decision whether a depression is mainly vital or mainly personal determines whether or not antidepressants will be given; the decision concerning the "weight" of the psychosocial factors determines whether some form of focused psychotherapy will be instituted; and the decision whether a depression is unipolar or bipolar determines whether or not lithium prophylaxis is to be instituted.

For research purposes, a three-dimensional approach is quite indispensable.

BIBLIOGRAPHY

ANGST, J. (1966). *Zur Ätiologie und Nosologie endogener depressiver Psychosen: eine genetische, soziologische und klinische Studie*. Berlin: Springer.

BECKER, J. (1974). *Depression: Theory and Research*. New York, Toronto, London, Sydney: John Wiley.

BURROWS, E. (1977). *Handbook of Studies on Depression*. Amsterdam: Elsevier, Excerpta Medica.

DELAY, J. (1965). Psychotropic drugs and experimental psychiatry. *J. Neuropsychiat.* 1, 104.

FEIGHNER, J. P. et al. (1972). Diagnostic criteria for use in psychiatric research. *Arch. gen. Psychiat.* 26, 57.

FLACH, F.F. AND S. C. DRAGHI (1975). *The Nature and Treatment of Depression*. New York: Wiley.

FRIEDMAN, R. J. AND M. M. KATZ (1974). *The Psychology of Depression: Contemporary Theory and Research*. Washington, D.C.: V. H. Winston & Sons.

KENDELL, R. E. (1968). *The Classification of Depressive Illnesses*. London: Oxford Univ. Press.

KIEV, A. (1974). *Somatic Manifestations of Depressive Disorders*. Int. Congress Series No. 332, Amsterdam, New York: Excerpta Medica.

KRAINES, S. H. (1957). *Mental Depressions and Their Treatment*. New York: Macmillan.

PERRIS, C. (1966). A study of bipolar (manic-depressive) and unipolar recurrent depressive psychoses. *Acta Psychiat. Scand.* 42, suppl. 194, 1.

PRAAG, H. M. VAN (1962). *A Critical Investigation of the Importance of Monoamineoxidase Inhibition in the Treatment of Depressions*. Thesis, Utrecht.

PRAAG, H. M. VAN, A. M. ULEMAN AND J. C. SPITZ (1965). The vital syndrome interview. A structured standard interview for the recognition and registration of the vital depressive symptom complex. *Psychiat. Neurol. Neurochir.* 68, 329.

ROBINS, E., R. A. MUNOZ, S. MARTIN AND K. A. GENTRY (1972). In: *Disorders of Mood*. Ed. by J. Zubin and F. A. Freyhan, Baltimore: John Hopkins Press, pp. 33.

SCHELER, M. (1928). *Die Stellung des Menschen im Kosmos*. Darmstadt: Fischer.

SCHNEIDER, K. (1920). Die Schichtung des emotionalen Lebens und der Aufbau der

Depressionszustände. *Z. ges. Neurol. Psychiat.* 59, 281.
SCHULTE, W. (1961). Nichtraurigseinkönnen im Kern Melancholischen Erlebens. *Nervenarzt* 32, 314.
SELIGMAN, M. E. P. (1976). Depression and learned helplessness. In: *Research in Neurosis.* Ed. H. M. van Praag, Amsterdam: Bohn/Scheltema/Holkema.
SHIELDS, J. (1976). Genetic factors in neurosis. In: *Research in Neurosis.* Ed. H. M. van Praag, Amsterdam: Bohn/Scheltema/Holkema.
STRAUS, E. (1928). Das Zeiterlebnis in der endogenen Depression und in der psychopathischen Verstimmung. *Mschr. Psychiat. Neurol.* 68, 640.
WESTERMAN, N. (1922). Über die vitale Depression. *Z. ges. Neurol. Psychiat.* 77, 391.
WINOKUR, G., P. J. CLAYTON AND T. REICH (1969). *Manic Depressive Illness.* St. Louis: C. V. Mosby.

XIII

Antidepressants I: General Part

1. Classification

Focused therapy of depressions with the aid of biological methods dates back to 1938, when electroshock therapy (EST) was introduced. Methods used until then could produce some transient alleviation of certain symptoms, e.g. reduction of anxiety and tension by opiates, and reduction of fatigue sensations by amphetamines. The affective disorder as such, however, was only marginally influenced, and the course of the syndrome not at all. If successful, EST restores the patient to his premorbid level within a few weeks (6-10 sessions). The same applies to antidepressants, with the restriction that medication should be continued for some considerable time in order to prevent relapse (section 7 below). EST arrests a (vital) depressive phase, whereas with antidepressants it is bridged, so to speak.

In actual practice, three groups of antidepressants are now in

In this chapter all antidepressants are referred to by their generic names. The principal trade names are listed in the tables of chapter XV.

Figure 24. Basic structure of the tricyclic antidepressants. *Left*: iminodibenzyl-nucleus; *Right*: dibenzocloheptene-nucleus.

use: tricyclic compounds, tetracyclic compounds, and monoamine oxidase (MAO) inhibitors. The former two derive their names from their chemical structures: a core of three condensed rings (Fig. 24) and a basic structure of four coupled rings, respectively. The lastmentioned group derives its name from the ability of these substances to inhibit the enzyme monoamine oxidase (MAO). This enzyme is involved in the degradation of monoamines: substances which in the brain act as neurotransmitters (chapter IV).

According to the structure of the side-chain at R, tricyclic antidepressants can be divided into two groups.

1) Compounds with a terminal aminodimethyl group: $(CH_3)_2$

2) Compounds with a terminal aminomonomethyl group: $-N\left\langle {}^{H}_{CH_3} \right.$

The best-known compounds of the first group are imipramine and amitriptyline. The second group includes the demethylation products of imipramine and amitriptyline: desipramine and nortriptyline, respectively.

MAO inhibitors can be divided into those with and those without a hydrazine group (R_1-NH-NH-R_2). The tetracyclic group has so far comprised only two compounds: maprotiline and mianserine.

Pharmacologically, the current antidepressants differ from the neuroleptics in that: a) they antagonize the effects of reserpine and tetrabenazine (e.g. catalepsy, hypotonia and ptosis) instead of potentiating them, as the neuroleptics do; b) they potentiate the various effects of catecholamines (e.g. hypertension and contraction of the nictitating membrane) instead of antagonizing them, as the neuroleptics do.

The three groups of antidepressants mentioned were discovered by coincidence rather than as a result of research which focused on possibilities to exert a particular influence on particular metabolic processes in the brain. Today, this latter research strategy is being used. For example, deliberate efforts are made to identify substances which selectively increase the amount of noradrenaline (NA) or serotonin (5-hydroxytryptamine; 5-HT) available at the central post-synaptic receptors. Indications that certain types of depression can be associated with disorders of central NA and/or 5-HT metabolism have catalysed these efforts (chapter XVI). Studies of the clinical efficacy of compounds of this type have only recently started and will not be further discussed here.

2. History

At the time of their discovery, antidepressants represented a new therapeutic principle. The two prototypes—the tricyclic compound imipramine and the first MAO inhibitor, iproniazid—are chemically unrelated. Rather remarkably, the two were discovered almost simultaneously but quite independently, and purely by coincidence.

In view of its relatedness to chlorpromazine, imipramine was offered for clinical trials as a possible neuroleptic. After a series of careful observations, Kuhn (1957) reached the conclusion that imipramine was not a chlorpromazine-like compound but a substance which showed a new action pattern: antidepressant action.

The origin of the MAO inhibitors lies in a field far remote from psychiatry. In the early fifties, two new tuberculostatic agents were being studied: isonicotinic acid hydrazide (INH; isoniazid; Nidaton), and its isopropyl derivative (iproniazid; Marsilid). Both proved to be effective in various forms of tuberculosis. In addition it was found that one of them (iproniazid) made some patients much more active and cheerful than could be attributed to the improvement of the tuberculous process. This led to iproniazid studies in psychiatric clinics and to the discovery of its antidepressant properties. Kline was the first to report on this fact at a meeting of the American Psychiatric Association on 6th April 1957.

In historical terms, maprotiline is a derivative from the tricyclic series. The other tetracyclic antidepressant (mianserine) is of quite different origin. It was evolved in a program which focused on new serotonin antagonists. Its antidepressant action was discovered accidentally.

3. Range of action of antidepressants, more specifically of tricyclic antidepressants

Antidepressants are compounds which primarily have a mood-improving effect in certain types of depression. This definition poses three questions: 1) What does "primarily" mean in this context? 2) How do we know that substances with an antidepressant effect do at all exist? 3) Which are the "certain types of depression" that are particularly suitable for antidepressant medication? These three questions will be discussed in succession.

Mediate and immediate influences on mood

Apart from the antidepressants, there are other groups of psychotropic drugs which can influence mood. An example is the group of the neuroleptics, of which chlorpromazine is a prototype. When a psychotic patient (e.g. one suffering from delusions or hallucinations) is given chlorpromazine, the intensity with which he experiences these phenomena is often reduced. Since the substance of delusions and hallucinations is far more likely to be menacing and depressing than cheerful, reduction of their intensity is usually accompanied by improvement of the patient's mood. Chlorpromazine thus influences the mood, but this effect is secondary to another effect: the antipsychotic. This is why chlorpromazine is not counted among the antidepressants. The latter compounds exert a direct influence on the central mood-regulating mechanisms, and it is to this that the adverb "primarily" in the definition refers.

Overall efficacy of tricyclic antidepressants

Imipramine and amitriptyline are the oldest antidepressants, with which the greatest clinical experience has been amassed. Their efficacy in depressions has been well documented in various controlled studies. The documentation on the other tricyclic compounds is less abundant, but leaves little doubt about their therapeutic efficacy. It is impossible to review the entire available literature in this context. I confine myself to a sample of studies made with a few reputable agents (Lehmann 1966). In 42 studies which encompassed a total of 2705 depressive patients, imipramine was found to cause unmistakable improvement in an average of 66.7% of patients. About one-third of the patients showed a favourable response to a placebo. With amitriptyline (16 studies, 872 patients), the rate of improvement averaged 65%, the corresponding rates with desmethylimipramine (11 studies, 355 patients) and with nortriptyline (7 studies, 250 patients) being 72.5% and 78.8%, respectively. All these data concern placebo-controlled studies. The range of the rates of improvement, however, is wide (for imipramine and amitriptyline 19-100 and 15-81, respectively). This is probably due to the fact that the results were not arranged according to syndromal type but simply summated for all types of depression.

Morris and Beck (1974) analysed 93 double-blind placebo-controlled studies on tricyclic antidepressants (Table 9), in some 66% of which the antidepressant was superior to the placebo. The percentage of studies in which the placebo equalled the antidepressant is undeniably large, but probably also exaggerated because these analyses likewise did not account for the syndromal type.

Specificity

Apart from the question of the efficacy of antidepressants, that of their specificity arises. Are antidepressants more effective than other psychotropic drugs in depressions? They very probably are. I cannot fully commit myself because relevant research data are scanty. This type of research is difficult because it makes severe demands on accuracy and technique of assessment. Many depressions are associated with feelings of anxiety and tension. Neuroleptics are strong sedatives and can reduce the severity of these feelings, which secondarily benefits the mood. On the other hand, several antidepressants have sedative properties (section 4 below). There is therefore substantial overlap between antidepressant and neuroleptic effects. This is why results obtained with the two types of psychotropic drugs were found to be equivalent as long as syndromal classifica-

Table 9. Controlled studies comparing tricyclics with placebo (93 treatment group comparisons in 85 studies) (Morris and Beck, 1974)

	Inpatients		Outpatients		Mixed Group		Total All Groups	
Drug Studied	Superior to Placebo*	Not Superior	Superior to Placebo	Not Superior	Superior to Placebo	Not Superior	Superior to Placebo	Not Superior
Imipramine	23	15	6	4	1	1	30	20
Desipramine	3	2	1	0	0	0	4	2
Amitriptyline	7	4	7	2	0	0	14	6
Nortriptyline	4	3	1	0	0	0	5	3
Protriptyline	1	0	2	0	0	0	3	0
Doxepin	1	0	0	0	0	0	1	0
Amitriptyline + perphenazine	1	1	3	0	0	0	4	1
Totals	40	25	20	6	1	1	61	32

*Superior in each column indicates statistical significance at least at 0.05 level.

tion of the depressions was omitted. When they were thus classified, and the psychopathological profiles before and after medication carefully compared, the antidepressants invariably proved to be superior, at least in the group of vital depressions.

Indications of choice

Many authors hold that the vital depressive syndrome is the indication of choice for the current antidepressants, and that the results in personal depressions are significantly less favourable. Yet there is no agreement on this point. Some authors refute this difference. Our own data, however, decidedly argue in favour of the former contention. I have analysed the data on 412 depressive patients whom I treated with tricyclic antidepressants between 1958 and 1977 (drugs used in 85% of the cases: amitriptyline, imipramine and chlorimipramine). The best results were obtained in the group of vital, and the least good results in that of personal depressions. The depressions with vital "features" (minimally: the typical mood quality of vital depression, hypoaesthesia, anorexia and disorders of sleep) occupied an intermediate position (Table 10). The aetiology of the vital depression exerted no distinct influence on the therapeutic effect (Table 11).

Table 10. Efficacy of tricyclic antidepressants (mainly imipramine, amitriptyline and chlorimipramine) in 412 hospitalized patients with depressions.
The concepts "vital depression" and "personal depression" are discussed in chapter XII. Depressions with vital "features" are depressions with elements of the vital depressive syndrome, minimally: decreased mood level, hypoaesthesia, anorexia and disorders of sleep.

		Recovery or marked improvement		No or only slight improvement	
Syndrome	Number	number	%	number	%
Vital depression	174	127	73	47	27
Depression with vital features	126	61	48	65	52
Personal depression	112	31	28	81	72

Table 11. Efficacy of tricyclic antidepressants (mainly imipramine amitriptyline and chlorimipramine) in 174 patients with vital depressions, in relation to the predominant aetiological factor.

Aetiology	Number	Recovery or marked improvement		No or only slight improvement	
		number	%	number	%
Mainly hereditary	82	64	78	18	22
Mainly psychosocial	61	44	72	17	28
Mainly exogenous (acquired somatic factors)	31	19	61	12	39

I can think of two possible causes of the abovementioned controversy.

1) Some antidepressants have sedative properties (section 4 below) and have some therapeutic effect on depressions associated with manifest anxiety. If analysis of the profile of therapeutic actions is omitted, then this therapeutic effect can be mistaken to be a really antidepressant effect.

2) The three-dimensional classification system discussed in the preceding chapter is not commonly used. Many authors are unfortunately still using a one-dimensional system, e.g. classification based on aetiology alone (psychogenic/endogenous) or on the clinical course alone (unipolar/bipolar). This is asking for confusion. The category of psychogenic (neurotic, reactive) depressions can comprise patients with vital depressive as well as others with personal depressive symptoms; the category of unipolar depressions can encompass patients with recurrent vital as well as others with recurrent personal depressions, and so forth. The difference in response to antidepressants between vital and personal depressions can easily become vague as a result of the use of this one-dimensional system.

Antidepressants are effective in some 70% of the typical vital depressions. However, they exert no influence on the aetiology of the depression. If psychogenic or sociogenic factors play an important role, then systematic psychotherapy is indicated besides pharmacotherapy in order to improve the patient's psychological stability and adjustment to his environment.

In many vital depressions it is an error to confine therapy to antidepressant medication; but it is no less an error to give a vitally depressed patient exclusively psycho(socio)therapy. In the depressive phase, he is in any case hardly accessible to it, and in this way precious months, or even years, might be wasted quite unnecessarily.

In the typical personal depressions there is but a small chance that antidepressants will be effective. In other words: there are as yet no agents capable of enhancing the mood level in this type of depression (a possible exception being phenelzine, the action of which is discussed in section 13 below). These cases primarily require a psycho(socio)therapeutic approach. If in a given phase of therapy rapid reduction of anxiety and tension is required, then an ataractic (e.g. a benzodiazepine derivative) is the agent of choice. It should be explained to the patient that the purpose of this medication is not to achieve a cure but to give some temporary support in a difficult phase. It is important that the temporary character of the medication be emphasized as soon as it is started; it is best described as a "course"—otherwise it may be difficult to persuade the patient that the medication should be discontinued.

The vital and personal depressive syndromes are prototypes. Mixed forms are quite common. Should these be treated with antidepressants? I believe they should, on the basis of data listed in Table 11; it is to be understood, however, that the chance of success is smaller than in the prototypical vital depression. To this statement I add two practical guidelines. The first is that the use of antidepressants is as much more justifiable as a given depressive syndrome shows more features of a vital depression. The second is that the duration of the period of evaluation should be limited: One may wait 4-6 weeks, but no longer. If in the course of this period a favourable turn has failed to occur, then the strategy should be revised (section 7 below). The chance that the agent may after all produce a pharmacological effect has then become minimal. In brief, therapeutic expectations should be curbed. This applies to typical vital depressions, but even more to the more dubious indications.

Effects in normal test subjects

These have hardly been systematically studied. Apart from some very scanty experimental psychological data, only general impressions after a single dose are available. Tricyclic compounds are believed mainly to sedate when administered to normal individuals. But this is certainly not the only possible effect. We observed disinhibition after clomipramine administration. The effects of more protracted medication have never been studied.

4. Inter-agent differences in effect

In chemical terms, tricyclic antidepressants are iminodibenzyl or dibenzocycloheptene derivatives (Fig. 24). They are qualitatively similar in their mood-improving effect in (vital) depressions. They are likewise virtually equivalent in terms of intensity of this effect. But they differ in their influence on motor activity, drive level and anxiety. In these terms, three groups are distinguished and this classification has some practical value even though the boundaries are far from well-defined.

To begin with there are tricyclic compounds which, apart from their influence on mood, have a marked *sedative effect*. These are: 1) amitriptyline; 2) trimeprimine; 3) doxepine.

Secondly there are tricyclic antidepressants which do not sedate but in fact *activate* motor function and drive. It should be understood that this statement is based not so much on hard experimental facts as on clinical experience. Not much focused research has been done in this context. It is beyond doubt, however, that anxiety and tension can be aggravated by these compounds. If this occurs, then it is advisable to combine the agent with a neuroleptic (e.g. chlorpromazine) or an ataractic (e.g. diazepam). The more activating antidepressants include: 1) nortriptyline (i.e. demethylated amitriptyline); 2) protriptyline; 3) desipramine (i.e. demethylated imipramine). These are all compounds with one methyl group in the side-chain.

Thirdly there are compounds of an *intermediary* group, which exert relatively little influence on motor activity and drive level. If they do produce an effect of this type, then it is more likely to be activating than inhibitory. The degree of anxiety, too, is hardly influenced and virtually never increased. These compounds, therefore, have a wide range of action but their effect is less focused than that of the antidepressants of the other two categories. In agitated vital depressions they can be combined without difficulty with a neuroleptic or ataractic. The intermediary group includes: 1) imipramine; 2) clomipramine; 3) dibenzepine.

It can be stated in summary that antidepressants are indicated in vital depressions and that the choice of agent is determined by the patient's degree of motor activity and anxiety. Activating antidepressants are indicated in largely retarded vital depressions, and sedative antidepressants in agitated vital depressions; agents of the intermediary group can be tried in both cases.

5. Dosage

Mode of administration

Tricyclic antidepressants are usually given orally in three daily doses. Several compounds such as imipramine and amitriptyline can also be administered by (deep) intramuscular injection. Sometimes (but in actual fact only rarely) this mode of administration can have its advantages (if the patient is not cooperating or markedly inhibited, which makes it difficult for him to swallow). The risk of hypotensive reactions is higher than after oral administration, however, and the patient should therefore be confined to bed for at least an hour after the injection—a rule which is particularly stringent for elderly patients. Clomipramine can also be administered by intravenous drip. There is no convincing evidence that parenteral administration of an antidepressant potentiates its effect or hastens its occurrence.

Amitriptyline is now available also in long-acting form (Lentizol; Sarotex Retard), which makes it possible to administer a 24-hour dose at once. It remains to be established, however, that a more or less constant blood level for 24 hours can thus be ensured. Some authors advise that the total daily dose of non-long-acting tricyclic compounds be also given at once, immediately before sleep. Side effects should then be less marked, or rather they should occur during sleep and could not interfere with the therapeutic efficacy. However, no comparative pharmacokinetic studies have been made, and I would rather wait for their results before recommending this procedure. Anyhow, this treatment regime seems not advisable in cardiac patients (section 9 below).

Dosage scheme

In chapter XV the mean and maximum therapeutic doses for each antidepressant are listed. I recommend the following procedure. The initial dose is increased to the mean therapeutic dose in 3-4 days. If the patient fails to respond to this after 3-4 weeks, then the doses are (gradually) increased to the maximum, provided: 1) the blood pressure is regularly determined (especially in elderly patients), and 2) the cardiac history is "clean." The meaning of these two restrictions will become clear in section 9.

If after 2-4 weeks on the maximum dose the patient still shows no response, then medication should be discontinued because the chance that a pharmacological effect will subsequently occur is minimal. In such cases another attempt may be made with a different antidepressant of the tricyclic or the tetracyclic series; insensitivity to one agent need not necessarily imply insensitivity to the entire series. If a second attempt is likewise unsuccessful, then the patient should be hospitalized for medication with a MAO inhibitor or for EST.

Once an optimal therapeutic effect is attained, the minimum effective dose is determined by very gradual reduction of dosage.

6. Pharmacokinetic aspects

Antidepressant-refractory vital depressions

The group of the vital depressions provides the indication of choice for tricyclic antidepressants. Within this diagnostic category, however, some 30-35% of patients show no or no adequate response. In principle, this could have several causes.

1) The aetiology of the vital depression is more important for the efficacy of tricyclic antidepressants than we now suspect.

2) The group of vital depressions, although relatively homogeneous in psychopathological terms, is heterogeneous in terms of pathogenesis. In other words: vital depressive syndromes can be based on disparate cerebral processes, and the biochemical action profile of a tricyclic antidepressant therefore influences its range of therapeutic action. This possibility is discused in some detail in chapter XVI.

3) Finally the pharmacokinetic factor: It is possible that individual differences exist in the way in which the organism "handles" tricyclic antidepressants. It is with this possibility that this section concerns itself.

Differences in pharmacokinetics

There can be no doubt that such differences do exist. After a given dosage of a tricyclic antidepressant, the steady-state concentration differs widely in different individuals; for example, the difference is 40-fold for nortriptyline (150 mg/day) and desipramine (75 mg/day). Since there are only slight differences between these compounds in intestinal absorption, binding to plasma proteins and renal excretion, the wide range of the steady-state concentrations is probably based on individual differences in their degradation rate.

Generally speaking, differences in the degradation rate of a drug can be determined genetically or by environmental factors. Of the latter, exposure to another drug is probably the most important. Both factors have proved also to influence the metabolism of tricyclic antidepressants. Alexanderson et al. (1969) administered a standard dose of nortriptyline during 8 days to a group of non-identical and a group of identical twins, and found virtually identical steady-state concentrations per pair in the latter group, whereas those in the former group differed widely. This difference can only be explained genetically. However, exogenous factors can also play a role. For example, the steady-state concentration in plasma after a given dose of nortriptyline is reduced by barbiturates, but increased by certain neuroleptics, e.g. chlorpromazine.

Blood level and therapeutic effect

Another question (and one to which there is no certain answer) is whether the plasma level of a tricyclic antidepressant faithfully reflects its concentration at its site of action. There are some indirect arguments which indicate that it probably does. I need not discuss these (in this respect, cf. Asberg 1976), however, because there is only one conclusive argument: a correlation between plasma level and therapeutic effect. Views on such a correlation have so far been controversial. A typical example is found in studies with nortriptyline, which have so far produced three different results: 1) no correlation between plasma level and therapeutic efficacy; 2) a positive (rectilinear) correlation; 3) a so-called curvilinear correlation, which is to say that both low and very high plasma nortriptyline levels were associated with little therapeutic effect, whereas an optimal effect was obtained at an intermediate level.

Several different factors may have contributed to the marked disparity of the results: 1) Differences in criteria of selection: some authors studied "depressions" in general, while others selected vital ("endogenous") depressions. 2) Differences in methods of determination. 3) The possibility of a curvilinear correlation may have been overlooked so that the correlation between concentration and effect within a certain range of concentrations remained unrecognized. Recent findings (Åsberg 1976) indicate the likelihood of a curvilinear correlation between plasma concentration and therapeutic effect for amitriptyline and maprotiline as well. 4) It may well be that metabolites of tricyclic antidepressants are therapeutically more important than the mother substances. The degradation of these compounds has not yet been accurately studied, let alone detailed information obtained on the pharmacological properties of the various metabolites. 5) So far, total plasma concentrations have always been measured, even though it is known that tricyclic antidepressants can bind themselves to plasma proteins. It is therefore possible that not the total concentration but the free fraction correlates with the clinical (side) effects. 6) Finally it is, of course, possible that no correlation exists between plasma concentration and concentrations at strategic sites in the brain.

Tentative conclusions

At this time it is impossible to make any statement concerning the value which determination of plasma concentrations of tricyclic antidepressants may assume in actual practice. However, research so far justifies two conclusions. The dosage of a tricyclic antidepressant does not reliably predict the effective concentration that will be attained. Therefore, the dosages listed in chapter XV are no more than a very rough guideline; it is urgently necessary to determine dosages individually! The second conclusion is that additional drugs can influence the therapeutic efficacy of an antidepressant. This indicates the necessity of exercising restraint in combining drugs.

7. Duration of treatment with tricyclic antidepressants

Latency

No immediate effect should be expected of a tricyclic antidepressant. If a therapeutic effect occurs, then it does so only after 10-24 days. Why this is so we do not know (the same has been observed with the other group of antidepressants: MAO inhibitors). In view of this latency, outpatients who have threatened suicide should be frequently examined during the first few weeks, the more so because the improvement of mood can be preceded by reduction of motor retardation and apathy; during such a "dissociation phase" the suicide risk is increased. Another consequence is that the effect of the medication cannot be evaluated until after about a month. Desisting earlier because no effect has yet been observed in as much of an error as persisting too long in cases showing no effect, hoping for what would have to be a pharmacological miracle.

Desipramine and nortriptyline were expected to produce a therapeutic effect more rapidly. The mother substances (imipramine and amitriptyline) are demethylated in the organism, and the demethylation products (desipramine and nortriptyline) proved to be therapeutically active. It was then postulated that not so much imipramine and amitriptyline as their demethylation products were active, and consequently the latter could be expected to be more quickly effective than the mother substances. This postulate has not been empirically confirmed: The various tricyclic compounds have very similar latencies.

Discontinuation of medication

Antidepressants alleviate or eliminate the symptoms of depression but do not arrest it. With this fact in mind, how long should antidepressant medication be continued? This question can be answered only in general terms. A vital depression is a self-limiting disease, but the duration of the disease period ranges from a few days to several years, the peak of the curve being observed at about six months. Assuming that a patient is not likely to seek medical advice until one to two months after the onset of symptoms, it would seem to be advisable to continue medication (if successful) for at least four months. It can then be gradually reduced at frequent follow-ups, and finally discontinued if the condition does not deteriorate. In the case of a relapse, medication is resumed at the old (minimum effective) dosage. The procedure described is then repeated one to two months later.

Prophylactic use of tricyclic antidepressants

The question whether it is of any use to prescribe tricyclic antidepressants prophylactically in unipolar and bipolar depressions will be discussed in chapter XVII.

8. Combination with other drugs

There are two depressive symptoms which make it necessary to prescribe additional drugs along with antidepressants: insomnia and anxiety. So far as we know, there are no objections to combination with conventional hypnotic agents. In order to reduce anxiety, tricyclic antidepressants can be combined with ataractics (e.g. diazepam, 3 × 5-10 mg daily) or neuroleptics (e.g. chlorpromazine, 3 × 50-100 mg daily). It is to be borne in mind, however, that according to Gram and Overø (1972) the metabolism of tricyclic antidepressants is inhibited by certain neuroleptics. This would imply that, administered in combination, a substance such as chlorpromazine not only has its own effects but also potentiates the clinical (side) effects of the antidepressant.

There are several commercial preparations which combine an antidepressant with a neuroleptic or ataractic, e.g. *Mutabon* (a combination of amitriptyline and perphenazine), *Limbatril* and *Limbritol* (which combine amitriptyline with chlordiazepoxide). Personally I prefer to give these drugs separately, because the sedative substance can then be carefully "titrated."

There is no objection to combining tricyclic compounds with lithium. On the contrary, if a depressive phase develops during lithium prophylaxis, then an antidepressant should be prescribed and lithium medication continued.

Tricyclic compounds potentiate the effects of atropine and amphetamine derivatives, and some effects of alcohol. Alcohol is to be avoided during antidepressant medication (even a small amount precludes driving). This is even more necessary when the antidepressant is used in combination with a neuroleptic or ataractic. The peripheral and central actions of adrenaline and noradrenaline are likewise potentiated. This is of practical importance when local anaesthetics are given in combination with catecholamines as vasoconstrictors.

Another important interaction is that with the antihypertensive agents of the guanidine-type, such as guanethidine and bethanidine—compounds taken up into the noradrenergic neurons, there to inhibit the release of noradrenaline. Tricyclic compounds hamper the uptake into the noradrenergic neurons, and consequently the antihypertensive effect diminishes.

Until recently it was an accepted rule of thumb that tricyclic antidepressants should not be combined with MAO inhibitors because this could lead to vitally dangerous complications, e.g. hypertensive crises. Meanwhile, some investigators have used this combination successfully and without difficulty in therapy-resistant patients. The combination so far most widely tested is that of amitriptyline (25-100 mg daily) with isocarboxazid (10-20 mg daily) or phenelzine (45 mg daily) as MAO inhibitor. I consider the use of this combination justifiable only in a clinical setting, under close supervision, after other methods of treatment have failed.

There are indications that the therapeutic effect of imipramine is enhanced and accelerated by combining it with the thyroid hormone tri-iodothyronine (T_3, 25 μg daily). The mechanism of this potentiation is still obscure. Nothing is known about combinations of T_3 with other antidepressants.

There are also studies which indicate that the serotonin precursors tryptophan (5-9 g daily) and 5-hydroxytryptophan (200 mg daily, combined with a peripheral decarboxylase inhibitor) are capable of enhancing the therapeutic effect of clomipramine. The theoretical implications of these observations are discussed in detail in chapter XVI.

The number of observations on the three lastmentioned combinations is still too small to warrant their recommendation for use in practice.

9. Side effects and toxic effects of tricyclic antidpressants

Side effects

This discussion focuses mainly on the two compounds in longest use and best known: imipramine and amitriptyline. However, it seems plausible that these observations apply also to the entire tricyclic series.

Frequently observed are *atropine-like side effects* such as xerostomia, constipation, palpitations, accelerated pulse, diminished accommodation (which may lead to blurred vision), and impeded micturition. This is why these compounds should be used with caution in patients suffering from glaucoma and hypertrophy of the prostate. Pointed questions should be asked in advance concerning a feeble flow of urine or after-drip, and concerning intermittent blurred vision associated with periocular pain or pain in the eye and seeing rainbow-like rings around light sources. It is also to be borne in mind that atropine-like side effects are potentiated when antidepressants are combined with substances that likewise act anticholinergically, e.g. phenothiazines (chlorpromazine) and the conventional anti-parkinson drugs. Paradoxically, hyperhidrosis is not uncommon, particularly with imipramine. The mechanism underlying this phenomenon is still unknown.

During the first few days to at most weeks of medication, many patients complain of *fatigue, drowsiness and a sensation of lightness in the head.* Most patients soon become habituated to this.

Practically, the most important side effect of tricyclic compounds is *orthostatic hypotension*. Elderly patients in particular are prone to this, especially during the first weeks of medication. The phenomenon as a rule disappears spontaneously within 4-6 weeks—the vascular system evidently adapts itself—and it can be minimized, moreover, by ensuring that the dosage is very slowly increased. The ECG often shows flattening, sometimes reversal of the T-wave—a phenomenon which may also occur, surprisingly, in response to lithium. As a rule it develops 1-2 weeks after starting medication, and disappears after its discontinuation.

Muller et al. (1961) compared the hypotensive effect of imipramine in 41 patients without and 50 with pre-existent cardiovascular disease. No complications of significance occurred in the former group. In the latter group, four patients developed cardiac decompensation and two had myocardial infarction during a hypotensive period. Other authors have reported similar developments. Nevertheless it is impossible to reach a definite conclusion concerning the role of imipramine in the aetiology of cardiovascular disorders, because we do not know how common (or uncommon) these disorders are in a matched group of depressive patients not treated with imipramine. Bearing this in mind, and considering the fact that vital depression is a serious, disabling disease with a high mortality, I regard it as a mistake simply to deprive cardiac patients of needed antidepressants. However, benefit and risk should be regularly weighed throughout the medication, preferably in consultation with an internist. In any case, the blood pressure should be regularly measured (recumbent and upright) in cardiac patients receiving tricyclic antidepressants. Any pronounced orthostatic decrease is an indication to reduce or even discontinue medication.

Photosensitization and other cutaneous *allergic manifestations* occur sporadically; eosinophilia is slightly less uncommon. Jaundice (of the cholangiolitic type, like that after chlorpromazine) is a rare complication, and so is agranulocytosis. The lastmentioned complication develops exclusively between the second and eighth week of medication. In brief: allergic manifestations are very uncommon.

The *extrapyramidal symptoms* so frequently observed with phenothiazine derivatives and other neuroleptics, are rarely seen in patients given tricyclic antidepressants. Some 10% of these patients develop a fine tremor of the hands, and sometimes of the tongue. Like the phenothiazine derivatives, tricyclic compounds (particularly in large doses) can provoke grand mal *seizures* even in patients with no history of epilepsy.

Finally, the *psychological side effects*. To begin with, manic symptoms can develop especially, but not exclusively, in patients with a history of manic phases receiving tricyclic compounds in large doses. Elderly patients occasionally develop a delirious syndrome with a lowered level of consciousness and hallucinations, possibly (in part) as a result of diminished cerebral circulation on the basis of hypotension. Specifically, the activating compounds in the tricyclic series may provoke or intensify anxiety and tension, and cause an untoward increase in motor activity (agitation). Some authors, finally, have indicated that imipramine and amitriptyline can disturb sleep during the first few weeks. However, it is uncertain whether this is a true side effect or rather a component of the depressive syndrome per se.

Psychological dependence on tricyclic compounds does not develop any more than on neuroleptics. After abrupt discontinuation of high-dosage treatment, however, withdrawal symptoms may occur, e.g. malaise, nausea, diarrhoea, coryza and myalgia. Habituation to the atropine-like side effects and the hypotensive effect develops, but not to the therapeutic effects.

Acute *overdosage* of tricyclic antidepressants chiefly causes symptoms from the central nervous system and the cardiovascular system. Dependent on the dosage, the patient may either show a lowered level of consciousness with delirious symptoms, or enter a comatose state. Hypertonia and hyperreflexia occur, and 20% of patients show varying types of convulsions. Extrapyramidal symptoms, either parkinson-like or of a more hyperkinetic type, may occur. On the other hand, there may be disorders originating from the level of the brain stem, e.g. hyperpyrexia.

Cardiac damage is a grave risk. Tricyclic compounds in large doses are a cytotoxin to the myocardium. Arrhythmias and conduction disturbances may develop. The force of contraction diminishes. The blood pressure can fall, the patient entering shock. On the other hand, an increase in blood pressure is also possible. This is probably a central effect.

There is no specific therapy. Heart and circulation demand expert attention and severely intoxicated patient should be transferred to an intensive care unit. Convulsions are dealt with in the conventional manner.

10. Contraindications to tricyclic antidepressants

A history of agranulocytosis and severe disorders of liver and kidney function are to be regarded as absolute contraindications.

Relative contraindications are glaucoma, hypertrophy of the prostate and cardiovascular disorders (e.g. a history of myocardial infarction, severe hypertension, cardiac decompensation, arteriosclerosis). Under these circumstances tricyclic antidepressants may be prescribed only after consultation with the relevant specialists, and if the patient can be carefully monitored.

Caution is indicated also in dealing with epileptic patients and diabetics. Tricyclic compounds lower the convulsion threshold and have a slight antidiabetic effect; in some cases it may therefore be necessary to adjust the dosage of anti-epileptic and anti-diabetic agents, respectively.

There are no indications that tricyclic antidepressants can adversely affect a foetus or neonate. Nevertheless I consider it advisable not to prescribe these drugs during the first half of pregnancy and during lactation.

11. Tetracyclic antidepressants

Maprotiline is the oldest known representative of this group. Its range of therapeutic action does not seem to differ much from that of the tricyclic antidepressants, but research so far has been strictly confined to psychopathological aspects. However, there are indications that vital depressive syndromes, although tending towards homogeneity in psychopathological terms, are heterogenous in biochemical terms (chapter XVI). It would therefore seem advisable also to consider biochemical criteria in studies of the therapeutic efficacy of maprotiline, the more so because this compound is biochemically selective: it inhibits the uptake of noradrenaline into neurons, but exerts no influence on that of serotonin. It is therefore conceivable that, within the vital depression group, there are categories of patients with a particular sensitivity to this compound. In terms of its influence on tenseness and motor activity, maprotiline should be regarded as one of the sedative antidepressants.

Mianserine has only recently been introduced. It is not known with certainty whether its range of indications coincides with or differs from that of the tricyclic and tetracyclic antidepressants. In terms of animal pharmacology it differs from them in that it has no anticholinergic properties and does not antagonize the effects of reserpine and tetrabenazine. There are biochemical differences as well: mianserine does not inhibit the (re)uptake of monoamines into the neuron, and is not a MAO inhibitor either. Yet it is not without any influence on central monoamines: it increases the turnover of catecholamines. In terms of its influence on tenseness and motor activity, it is believed to activate rather than sedate.

12. Monoamine oxidase (MAO) inhibitors: opinions and biases

The MAO inhibitors have been less thoroughly studied in clinical psychiatry than the tricyclic antidepressants. There are several reasons for this. Patients being treated with iproniazid, the first MAO inhibitor, showed an alarmingly high incidence of damage to the liver parenchyma; and shortly after its introduction the compound was withdrawn. This has discredited the entire group of MAO inhibitors. Moreover, MAO inhibitors are not so readily manageable in practice: They must not be combined with certain drugs and foods (section 14). Finally, some MAO inhibitors proved to be therapeutically less effective than the conventional tricyclic compounds.

Without wishing to minimize the disadvantages, I nevertheless believe that justice has not been done to the MAO inhibitors and that they have been sidetracked too easily. To support this opinion I present the following arguments.

1. The jaundice epidemic in iproniazid-treated patients coincided with an epidemic of viral hepatitis. Reports on liver damage in association with the other MAO inhibitors have been exceedingly rare. The conclusion that the group of MAO inhibitors should be regarded as potential hepatic toxins is consequently a rash one, to say the least.

2. It is an error to regard the MAO inhibitors as a homogeneous group. They are not homogeneous in terms of chemical structure (section 1 above), and possibly not in terms of biochemical action either, since it has been established that the enzyme MAO is not a homogeneous enzyme but rather a series of related enzymes with a different affinity for different monoamines. There are indications that MAO inhibitors inhibit different components of the MAO complex in a different degree. This possibly explains why the notorious "cheese reaction" (hypertensive crises after eating cheese containing tyramine during medication with a MAO inhibitor) was repeatedly observed with some, but never with other MAO inhibitors.

3. Generalizations about the clinical efficacy of MAO inhibitors are likewise erroneous. Some compounds (for example,

isocarboxazid) are therapeutically inferior. Others are the equals of imipramine (for example, iproniazid, with which I have gained considerable experience, and tranylcypromine, which has been tested in several double-blind comparative studies).

4. Finally, even the qualification "inferior" as used above must not be applied hastily. In none of the studies from which this qualification arose was the degree of MAO inhibition measured. Recent studies with phenelzine have demonstrated that, in order to produce a therapeutic effect, at least 80% of the MAO in blood platelets should be inhibited. The dosage required to achieve this level of inhibition is related to the rate at which phenelzine is inactivated; and this rate varies individually. It is therefore not impossible that the poor reputation of some MAO inhibitors is in fact based on underdosage.

13. Range of indication of MAO inhibitors

The range of indication of the two MAO inhibitors considered of old to be most effective—iproniazid (long since withdrawn as a commercial drug) and tranylcypromine—does not differ from that of the tricyclic antidepressants. The best results are obtained in vital depressions, and especially in those with motor retardation. These MAO inhibitors, therefore, are activating antidepressants. Comparative studies have shown that their efficacy is not inferior to that of imipramine.

Attention has re-focused on "the" MAO inhibitors in recent years. They have been reported to be indicated (also) in the group of personal depressions, and more specifically in those in which anxiety, phobic fears, somatic anxiety "equivalents," irritability and fatigue are predominant. I have apostrophized "the" because only phenelzine has been demonstrated to be effective in the range of indication given. Other preparations have not been studied in this context. For an optimal effect, at least 80% of the MAO in blood platelets should be inhibited. In most patients, at least 60 mg phenelzine per day is required to achieve this. If no response has developed after a month, then the daily dosage should be increased to 75-90 mg because the patient may be a "rapid acetylator," who unusually quickly inactivates (acetylates) phenelzine.

These observations are very interesting. Phenelzine is the first antidepressant available for clinical practice which is effective in the group of personal depressions (we ourselves have studied a group of compounds with a similar range of indication—chloramphetamines—but they have not been made commercially available). An urgent question now is whether all MAO inhibitors have this efficacy or whether it is confined to phenelzine, and, if so, why.

For the duration of treatment with MAO inhibitors, the same guidelines are valid as for tricyclic antidepressants (section 7 above). MAO inhibitors are not combinable with a large number of other compounds. For this reason it is expedient to limit their use to clinical patients.

14. Combinations of MAO inhibitors with other drugs

MAO inhibitors must not be combined with several drugs and food constituents, but we do not know whether this is equally stringent for all preparations. The following substances are of importance in this respect.

1) Sympathicomimetic amines. Owing to inhibition of their degradation, their effects are enhanced, be they central or peripheral (e.g. increased blood pressure). This applies to the catecholamines themselves as well as to the indirectly acting sympathicomimetics such as amphetamines and ephedrine (e.g. in nasal sprays).

2) Foods which contain a large amount of tyramine (fermented cheese, red wine, liver, broad beans, herring). Inhibition of tyramine degradation can lead to severe hypertensive crises.

3) In a few patients under treatment with MAO inhibitors, the analgesic pethidine (Dolantine) has led to symptoms of violent cerebral irritation with hypertonia, lowered level of consciousness and convulsions. The mechanism underlying this idiosyncratic reaction is still unknown.

4) Combinations of MAO inhibitors with antihypertensive agents are undesirable. To begin with, the former themselves exert an antihypertensive influence. Secondly, untoward reactions may occur, e.g. with methyldopa (Aldomet). This amino-acid is decarboxylated in the organism to active amines, the degradation of which is probably inhibited by MAO inhibitors. Increased blood pressure can result.

5) MAO inhibitors increase the glucose tolerance, and this is of practical importance in diabetic patients.

6) The risks of combining MAO inhibitors with tricyclic antidepressants have been discussed in section 8.

A combination alleged to be *beneficial* is that of a MAO inhibitor with large doses of the serotonin precursor 1-tryptophan (5-9 g daily). This enhances the therapeutic efficacy of the MAO inhibitor. This combination merits consideration in persistently refractory cases. Its theoretical justification is discussed in chapter XVI.

15. Side effects and toxic effects of MAO inhibitors

Side effects

Orthostatic hypotension is one of the most common and most inconvenient side effects of MAO inhibitors. Once it develops, this effect usually persists as long as medication continues; this is in contrast with the hypotension seen in response to neuroleptics and tricyclic antidepressants, which as a rule gradually disappears after a few weeks. The phenomenon is dose-dependent, and its intensity and incidence increase as the dose is increased more rapidly and more markedly. Elderly patients with hypertension are high-risk patients. It can be stated in general that MAO inhibitors must not be prescribed to patients over 65.

As regards *prophylaxis*, the following points are of importance: 1) the increase in dosage should be made very gradually; 2) the minimum effective dose should be scrupulously adhered to; 3) the blood pressure should be determined regularly, once or twice weekly. If a decrease in blood pressure occurs, it is usually gradual, and regular determinations can thus prevent disastrous consequences. Once the patient is stabilized on a maintenance dose, less frequent determinations of blood pressure are sufficient.

Since there are no hypertensive drugs which can be given in long-term medication without risk, the *treatment* of this complication remains confined to either not further increasing or reducing the dosage. Discontinuation of medication, if necessary, can be effected abruptly; withdrawal symptoms rarely occur. Should the severity of the hypotension necessitate vasoconstrictor medication, then it is to be borne in mind that the enzyme MAO is involved in the degradation of catecholamines. Consequently, MAO inhibitors potentiate (part of) their effects, and vasoconstrictors of this type should therefore be given in cautious doses.

Damage to the liver parenchyma has been repeatedly observed in the course of iproniazid medication (however, cf. section 12). So far as we know, MAO inhibitors now commercially available leave the liver intact. A few cases of jaundice have been reported, but the correlation with the medication in these cases was dubious. To be sure, it is nevertheless advisable to examine liver function before medication is started, and to continue liver function tests in patients with a hepatic history. MAO inhibitors are contraindicated in cases with manifest disturbances in liver function.

Vegetative symptoms are quite common. I mention constipation and impeded micturition, the latter mostly in male patients: the flow of urine becomes feeble and the patient has the sensation of urinating against a resistance. Both symptoms are dose-dependent and abate as medication is reduced. The micturition symptoms, although rarely so severe as to require treatment, respond well to parasympathicomimetics such as carbachol (Doryl). Impotence and/or anorgasm, frequently observed during iproniazid medication, are rare with the more recent MAO inhibitors. Few complaints are likewise heard about xerostomia and blurred vision (deficient accommodation).

Muscle twitches in the limbs, particularly during and just before sleep, and hyperreflexia are among the most frequent *side effects involving the central nervous system*.

Paraesthesia of the fingers and toes may be observed, but is rare. The original theory that these paraesthesias are based on a pyridoxine (vitamin B_6)-antagonizing activity of MAO inhibitors and might be prevented by administration of this vitamin has not been corroborated.

Unlike the tricyclic antidepressants, these drugs have an anticonvulsive rather than an epileptogenic effect, at least in animal experiments. Sleep disorders may develop, but only if the antidepressant is administered just before bedtime.

An unexplained complication of medication with MAO inhibitors is *oedema* of the lower limbs, unilateral or bilateral. The phenomenon is dose-dependent but, once it develops, it usually does not disappear completely until after medication is discontinued.

Changes in the white blood picture and allergic dematoses are virtually not observed in response to MAO inhibitors now available.

The principal *psychological side effects* are mental restiveness and motor hyperactivity. These symptoms of agitation can be very well controlled with neuroleptics or classical sedatives.

In (melancholic) patients with delusions, the morbid thought contents may be accentuated by MAO inhibitors so that symptoms are aggravated. Occasionally there may be a maniacal turn. In rare cases, and especially in elderly patients, delirious symptoms may develop. As pointed out, however, patients in this category should not be given MAO inhibitors.

With a view to the many *risky combinations* (cf. section 8), it is customary not to prescribe other drugs during medication with MAO inhibitors, and to give patients careful instructions about foods to be avoided or, even better, to hospitalize them for clinical treatment.

Hypertensive crises (section 8) have been successfully controlled by means of phentolamine (Regitine): up to 5 mg by slow intravenous drip.

Symptoms of overdosage

Acute overdosage of MAO inhibitors leads to a lowered level of consciousness, but rarely to complete loss of consciousness. In addition, the patient is often restive, and a syndrome of a delirious type may develop. The greatest risk in these intoxications is abrupt hypotension, as a result of which the patient may enter deep shock. Seizures are exceedingly rare.

Treatment of these intoxications is symptomatic. After gastric lavage (if necessary), attention and necessary corrective measures focus in particular on the circulation, lung ventilation, and fluid and electrolyte balance. Since MAO inhibitors interfere with the degradation of pressor amines, hypertensive agents of the noradrenaline type should be given very cautiously and under strict supervision (this of course in order to prevent overdosage).

16. Antidepressants and electroshock therapy

Electroshock therapy (EST), i.e. provocation of an epileptic seizure by means of an electric current, was introduced in 1938 by Cerletti and Bini and, until the introduction of antidepressants, was the method of choice in the treatment of vital depressions, and more specifically of melancholia. Melancholia is a severe vital depression in which the patient has delusions (of inferiority, poverty and sin, hypochondriacal delusions, etc.). Convulsions can also be chemically provoked. Before the EST era, pentetrazole (Metrazol) was used for this purpose, but this has become obsolete. An agent more recently introduced is hexafluorodiethyl ether (Indoklon), which is inhaled or injected. This method has never been used on a large scale, and it is unknown whether it has advantages over EST.

Before an EST session, the patient is usually anaesthetized with the aid of a short-acting intravenous barbiturate (in order to make treatment more acceptable), and succinylcholine or another muscle relaxant is given (in order to prevent fractures and luxations).

Another modification, but not one generally used, is unilateral EST which makes use of a single electrode placed over the non-dominant hemisphere. This is believed greatly to reduce the principal side effects of EST (transient amnesia and memorizing defects), while leaving the therapeutic efficacy unaffected.

There can be no doubt about the efficacy of EST in the treatment of vital depressions. In nine studies covering a total of 2314 patients mainly suffering from vital depressions, the improvement rate averaged 87% (80-97%) after an average of 9 (6-17) shocks (Hordern et al. 1965). The effect of EST is superior to that of no treatment, placebo and brief barbiturate anaesthesia ("placebo-EST").

How do EST and tricyclic antidepressants compare? Not much research has been devoted to this question, and such little as was done chiefly concerned imipramine. Some authors consider the two methods to be equivalent, but the majority regard EST as superior in the sense that it produces a higher improvement rate than imipramine (80-95% versus 60-70%). The therapeutic effect does not occur more quickly. The superiority of EST is particularly evident in the severe vital depressions with delusions (melancholia). Not a single study has claimed superiority of imipramine over EST. Imipramine does not potentiate the effect of EST. Some 50% of patients who fail to respond to imipramine or amitriptyline show improvement after EST.

EST surpasses the tricyclic antidepressants in therapeutic efficacy. That these compounds should nevertheless be regarded as a major asset in the treatment of vital depressions is due to the fact that they can be easily used in a non-clinical setting, and hardly inconvenience (or terrify) the patient. On the other hand, EST is by no means obsolete, even though its range of indication has substantially diminished.

Another category of depressions in which EST is often still indispensable is that of the involutional depressions. They are symptomatically characterized by greater diversity: Hysterical and paranoid features occur alongside the features of vital depression, and motor disinhibition may be very marked. In these cases antidepressants are often inadequate, but EST has produced satisfactory-to-good results in many cases.

17. Somatic contraindications to antidepressant medication

Manifest disorders of liver function are an absolute contraindication to both groups of antidepressants. In view of their numerous atropine-like side effects, neither MAO inhibitors nor tricyclic compounds should be prescribed for patients showing glaucoma or a tendency to urinary retention. The latter compounds should be used with great prudence in epileptic patients.

The hypotensive effect of all antidepressants so far introduced necessitates great caution, particularly in elderly patients with poor cardiac function and/or hypertension. In these patients, a rapid decrease in blood pressure can easily lead to cardiac and cerebral complications. In this respect MAO inhibitors are even more risky than tricyclic compounds. It therefore seems a wise policy to refrain from prescribing MAO inhibitors in the treatment of patients over 65.

18. Non-psychiatric applications of antidepressants

The only antidepressant so far accepted as a hypotensive agent is pargyline—a MAO inhibitor whose antidepressant activity does not seem to be very pronounced.

Imipramine is being successfully used in the treatment of nocturnal enuresis. Reduction of depth of sleep and relaxation of the bladder musculature may be of importance in this context. The initial dose is 10 mg, to be taken before bedtime. If necessary, the dose can be increased to 20 mg daily for patients aged 1-7, and to 50 mg daily for those aged 8-14. Imipramine is also being used in narcolepsy (3 × 50-75 mg daily).

BIBLIOGRAPHY

ÅSBERG, M. (1976). Treatment of depression with tricyclic drugs—pharmacokinetic and pharmacodynamic aspects. *Pharmakopsychiat.* 9, 18.

ALEXANDERSON, B., D. A. P. EVANS, F. SJÖQVIST (1969). Steady state plasma levels of nortriptyline in twins. Influence of genetic factors and drug therapy. *Brit. Med. J.* 4, 764.

BIEL, J. H. AND B. BOPP (1974). *Antidepressant Drugs. Psychopharmacological Agent, Vol. III.* New York, San Francisco, London: Academic Press.

BRAITHWAITE, R. A., R. GOULDING, G. THEANO, J. BAILEY, A. COPPEN (1972). Plasma concentration of amitriptyline and clinical response. *Lancet* I, 1297.

BURROWS, G. D., B. DAVIES, B. A. SCOGGINS (1972). Plasma concentrations of nortriptyline and clinical response in depressive illness. *Lancet* II, 619.

COPPEN, A., D. M. SHAW AND J. P. FARRELL (1963). Potentiation of the antidepressive effect of a monoamine oxidase inhibitor by tryptophan. *Lancet* I, 79.

FINK, M., S. KETY, J. MCCAUGH AND T. A. WILLIAMS (1974). *Psychobiology of Convulsive Therapy.* Washington, D.C.: Winston & Sons.

GRAM, L. F. AND K. F. OVERØ (1972). Drug interaction: inhibitory effect of neuroleptics on metabolism of tricyclic antidepressants in man. *Brit. Med. J.*, 1, 463.

GRAM, L. F., N. REISBY, I. IBSEN, A. NAGY, S. J. DENCKER, P. BECH, G. O. PETERSEN AND J. CHRISTIANSEN (1975). Plasma levels and antidepressive effect of imipramine. *Clin. Pharmacol. Therap.* 19, 318.

HORDERN, A., C. G. BURT AND N. F. HOLT (1965). *Depressive States. A Pharmacotherapeutic Study.* Springfield, Ill.: Charles C Thomas.

HUSSAIN, M. Z. AND Z. A. CHAUDHRY, (1973). Single versus divided daily dose of trimipramine in the treatment of depressive Illness. *Amer. J. Psychiat.* 130, 1142.

JOHNSTONE, E. C. (1976). The relationship between acetylator status and inhibition of monoamine oxidase, excretion of free drug antidepressant response in depressed patients on phenelzine. *Psychopharmacologia* 46, 289.

KLERMAN, G. L. (1972). Drug therapy of clinical depressions—current status and implications for research on neuropharmacology of the affective disorders. *J. Psychiat. Res.* 9, 253.

KRAGH-SØRENSEN, R., C. E. HANSEN, P. C. BAASTRUP, E. F. HVIDBERG (1976). Relationship between antidepressant effect and plasma level of nortriptyline. Clinical studies. *Pharmakopsychiat.* 9, 27.

KUHN, R. (1957). Über die Behandlung depressiver Zustande mit einem iminobenzyl derivat (G 22355). *Schweiz. Med. Wschr.* 87, 1135.

LEHMANN, H. E. (1966). Depression: categories, mechanism and phenomena. In: *Pharmacotherapy of Depression.* Eds.: J. O. Cole and J. R. Wittenborn. Springfield, Ill.: Charles C Thomas.

MAÎTRE, L., P. C. WALDMEIER, P. M. GREENGRASS, J. JAEKEL, S. SEDLACEK AND A.

Delini-Stula (1975). Maprotiline—Its position as an antidepressant in the light of recent neuropharmacological and neurobiochemical findings. *J. Int. Med. Res.* 3, supplement (2) 2.

Monoamine oxidase and its inhibition (1976). City Foundation Symposium 39 (new series). Amsterdam, Oxford, New York: Elsevier, Excerpta Medica, North-Holland.

Montgomery, S. (1975). The relationship between plasma concentrations of amitriptyline and therapeutic response. Paper read to the British Academy of Psychopharmacology July 1, London.

Morris, J. B. and A. T. Beck (1974). The efficacy of antidepressant drugs—A review of research (1958 to 1972). *Arch. gen. Psychiat.* 30, 667.

Muller, O. F., N. Goddman and S. Bellet (1961). The hypotensive effect of imipramine hydroethoride in patients with cardiovascular disease. *Clin. Pharmacol. Ther.* 2, 300.

Murphy, J. E. (1975). A comparative clinical trial of org. GB 94 and imipramine in the treatment of depression in general practice. *J. Int. Med. Res.* 3, 251.

Paykel, E. S. (1972). Depressive typologies and response to amitriptyline. *Brit. J. Psychiat.* 120, 147.

Praag, H. M. van and B. Leijnse (1965). Depression, glucose tolerance, peripheral glucose uptake and their alterations under the influence of antidepressive drugs of the hydrazine type. *Psychopharmacologia* 8, 67.

Praag, H. M. van, J. Korf and L. C. W. Dols (1976). Clozapine versus perphenazine or the value of the biochemical mode of action of neuroleptics in predicting their therapeutic activity. *Brit. J. Psychiat.*, 129, 547.

Raskin, A. and T. H. Cook (1976). The endogenous-neurotic distinction as a predictor of response to antidepressant drugs. *Psychol. Med.* 6, 59.

Ravaris, C. L., A. Nies, D. S. Robinson, J. O. Ives, K. R. Lamborn and L. Korson (1976). A multiple-dose, controlled study of phenelzine in depression-anxiety states. *Arch. Gen. Psychiat.* 33, 347.

Stewart, M. M. (1976). MAOIs and food. Fact and fiction. *Adverse Drug Reaction Bulletin.* No. 58, 200.

Turek, I.S. and T. F. Hanlon (1977). The effectiveness of electroconvulsive therapy. *J. Nerv. Ment. Dis.*, 164, 419.

Tyrer, P. (1976). Towards rational therapy with monoamine oxidase inhibitors. *Brit. J. Psychiat.* 128, 354.

Vogel, H. P., D. Bente, J. Feder, H. Helmchen, B. Müller-Oerlinghausen, N. Bohacek, M. Mihovilovic, A. Brändli, J. Fleischhauer and W. Walcher (1976). Mianserine versus amitriptyline. A double blind trial evaluated by the AMP system. *Int. Pharmacopsychiat.* 11, 25.

Whyte, S. F., A. J. Macdonald, G. J. Naylor and J. P. Moody (1976). Plasma concentrations of protriptyline and clinical effects in depressed women. *Brit. J. Psychiat.* 128, 384.

XIV

Antidepressants II: Practical Guidelines for Antidepressant Medication

The principal data from chapter XIII are presented in summary in the following subsections.

1) The group of vital depressions form the range of indications par excellence for the tricyclic and tetracyclic antidepressants. These compounds are equivalent in their mood-improving effects. The patient's psychomotor status is the decisive factor in the choice of antidepressant. Vital depressions with predominance of retardation are suitable for activating antidepressants, specifically the monomethyl compounds of the tricyclic series. Whenever retardation is superposed by a degree of agitation, sedative antidepressants are indicated. In the case of severe agitation, neuroleptics or ataractics can be combined with antidepressants. Combination with neuroleptics, however, calls for more intensive monitoring of blood pressure. Psychotherapy is indicated in cases in which psychosocial factors have contributed to the development of a vital depression.

Vital depressions complicated by delusions (melancholia) often show an inadequate or even an adverse response to antidepressants. Electroshock therapy is often required in these cases.

Whether antidepressants of this type can be used in the treatment of personal depressions remains uncertain. The only certainty is that this type of depression requires some form of systematic psychotherapy.

2) MAO inhibitors are also effective in vital depressions. Of the compounds now available, only tranylcypromine has proved to be equivalent to imipramine; in terms of influence on motor function, it activates. In view of its possible side effects, this compound should be considered only if tricyclic antidepressants have failed.

Phenelzine has proved to be therapeutically active in personal depressions accompanied by anxiety, phobic fears and irritability. The other MAO inhibitors have not been tested in this respect.

The use of MAO inhibitors is justifiable only if one has an adequate knowledge of the ins and outs of these agents and the ability to give the patient adequate guidance during medication. It is not uncommon, after all, that a patient consults several doctors (especially the depressive patient, who often has somatic complaints) and receives medication from each (one doctor being insufficiently informed of the other's activities). This may lead to mishaps; MAO inhibitors cannot be combined with just any other compound without problems.

When a MAO inhibitor is used in the treatment of a patient with a history of liver disease, regular liver function tests are imperative.

3) The results of medication with tricyclic antidepressants are good-to-satisfactory in some 65% of patients with vital depressions. EST is indicated within the same range of indications, and the improvement rate with this method is even more favourable. Nevertheless antidepressants are a major asset because their use is not too drastic and entails few risks, while they can be prescribed to walking patients. As to the risks: in actual practice only (orthostatic) hypotension is to be feared, particular in dealing with elderly patients. In toxic doses, these compounds endanger the heart in particular. An attempted suicide with tricyclic antidepressants calls for admission to an intensive care unit.

4) No immediate effect can be expected of an antidepressant of the tricyclic series. Only after about 10-24 days can an effect become manifest. The decision that a compound is ineffective cannot be

made until after at least a month. During the latent period, the suicide risk persists undiminished, and can in fact be increased if mood improvement lags behind improvement in activity and initiative. On the other hand, a limit must be placed on therapeutic expectations. If a patient fails to respond after four weeks, the dose is increased. If no effect becomes apparent in the next four weeks, then a different (tricyclic or tetracyclic) compound can be tried. If this, too, is unsuccessful, then it is advisable to hospitalize the patient for treatment with a MAO inhibitor or by EST.

5) In order to prevent an abrupt decrease in blood pressure, antidepressants should be gradually introduced. Once an optimal therapeutic effect is obtained, the dose is gradually reduced to the minimum effective dosage. The "ceiling" should be maintained as briefly as possible.

Antidepressants with an activating action component should be preferably administered twice daily, mornings and afternoons.

6) The rate of inactivation of a given tricyclic antidepressant is subject to marked interindividual variations. The same applies to MAO inhibitors. In other words, the dosage required to achieve an effective concentration is highly variable. This means that individual dosage is a prerequisite in antidepressant medication.

It looks as if blood concentrations of tricyclic and tetracyclic antidepressants, and the degree of MAO inhibition in blood platelets following administration of MAO inhibitors are to become important variables in determining adequate dosage.

7) A vital depressive syndrome can be provoked by a wide variety of psychological and somatic factors. Once developed, the syndrome takes an autonomous course, independent of the provoking factors. The duration of a vital depressive phase averages six months. Unlike EST, antidepressants do not so much arrest as bridge the depressive phase. Premature discontinuation of this medication leads to relapse. With these compounds one provides what may be described as substitution therapy. This is why treatment should be continued for at least four months (assuming that the patient does not immediately seek medical advice as soon as symptoms heralding a depression occur). After this period, medication is gradually reduced under careful monitoring of the psychological

condition, and discontinued if possible. Reduction of dosage is postponed whenever symptoms return.

8) The use of antidepressants in the prophylaxis of (unipolar and bipolar) depressions is discussed in chapter XVII.

9) Some authors recommend combining electroshock therapy with antidepressant medication, the rationale being that fewer EST sessions would then suffice. However, this combination is not entirely devoid of danger. In such cases severe hypotension can develop shortly after the convulsion. This risk can be reduced by refraining from antidepressant medication on the morning of the EST day, and by confining the patient to bed for a few hours after the EST session.

10) Combinations of tricyclic antidepressants with MAO inhibitors, although probably more effective than each of these compounds separately, entail risks. They should be used only for therapy-resistant patients and under careful clinical supervision.

11) Although there are no reports on a teratogenic effect of antidepressants, these compounds (like any other drugs) are to be used with great prudence during pregnancy, and especially during the first three months.

XV

Antidepressants III: Specific Part

In the chapter XVIII the various categories of antidepressants were discussed. This chapter discusses the individual compounds. Deviations from the general pattern of effects and side effects, if any, will be mentioned under the heading "Particulars." The dosages indicated are averages, not optima, for the optimal dose varies from patient to patient, as do the doses of all psychotropic drugs.

1. Dimethyl compounds of the tricyclic series (Table 12)

Amitriptyline (Tryptizol, Saroten, Sarotex, Elavil)

Chemical structure. 1-(3′-dimethylaminopropylidene) 2-3,6-7, dibenzocycloheptadiene-2,6-hydrochloride. Apart from replacement of the central nitrogen atom by a carbon atom, the structure of this compound is identical to that of imipramine, the prototype of the series.

Table 12. Dimethyl compounds of the tricyclic series

Chemical structure	Generic name	Trade name	Daily oral dose in mg	
			Average	Maximum
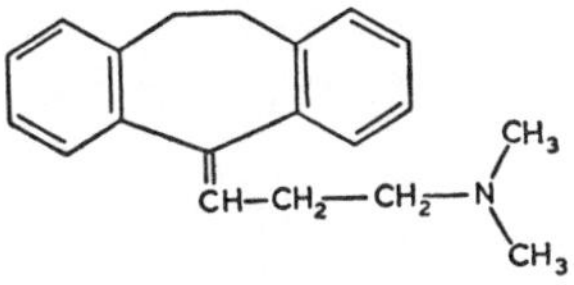	Amitrip-tyline	Elavil Saroten Sarotex Tryptizol	150-225	300
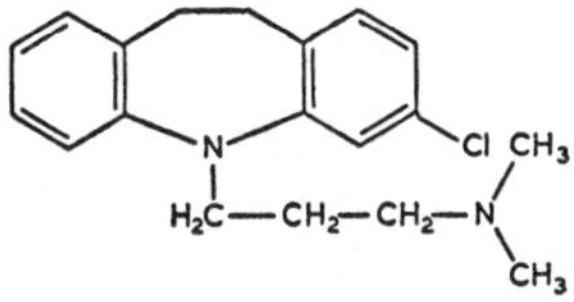	Clomi-pramine	Anafranil	150-225	300
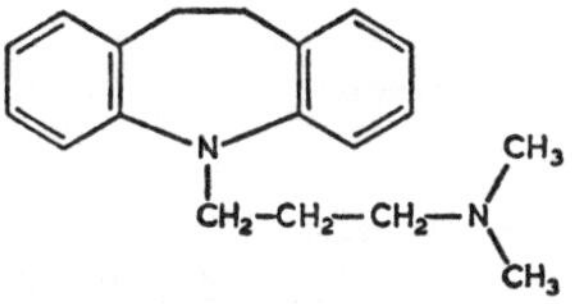	Imi-pramine	Presamine Tofranil	150-225	300
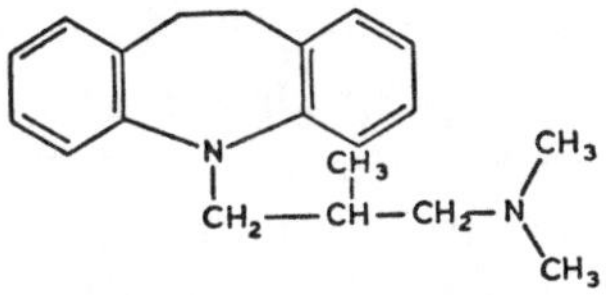	Trime-primine Trimi-pramine	Stangyl Surmontil	100-250	400

Dosage. The daily oral dose is 150-225 mg. In severe cases treatment can be started by intramuscular injection. This mode of administration is subject to the same rules as those given for imipramine. Four intramuscular injections of 20-30 mg each are given per day, and after a few days one switches to oral administration, cautiously increasing the dose to a maximum of 300 mg per day under constant monitoring of the blood pressure.

Particulars. The anxiolytic, relaxing action component of this agent is very pronounced; this is why it is suitable par excellence for the treatment of agitated vital depressions, the more so because, unlike the mood-improving effect, the sedative effect ensues quickly and sleep is also facilitated. In view of the last-mentioned effect it can be useful to give a large fractional dose of amitriptyline shortly before bedtime (dosage scheme, for example, 50-50-150 mg).

It is to be noted that amitriptyline strongly potentiates the effects of alcohol and of sedatives. Its anticholinergic effects are pronounced, like those of imipramine, but often do not become inconvenient until the daily dose exceeds 200 mg.

There are long-acting amitriptylines (e.g. *Sarotex Retard*), which need be given only once a day. Combined compounds are *Mutabon* (amitriptyline and perphenazine), *Limbritol* and *Limbatril* (both of which combine amitriptyline with chlordiazepoxide).

Clomipramine (Anafranil)

Chemical structure. 3-chloro-5-(3-dimethylaminopropyl)-10,11-dihydro-5H-dibenz(b,f)azepine. Clomipramine is chlorinated imipramine.

Dosage. The daily oral dose is 150-225 mg. Parenteral administration is also possible. Infusion has become especially popular: 25-50 mg clomipramine in 500 ml physiological saline per day for 1-2 weeks, whereupon treatment is continued by oral administration. The infusion should be of the slow-drip type (3-4 hours) in order to prevent side effects (e.g. hypotension). This mode of administration is believed to make clomipramine more quickly effective, but this has not been demonstrated with certainty. It is uncertain, moreover, whether acceleration (if any) is based on a pharmacological mechanism or on suggestion.

Particulars. This is an effective antidepressant which is "neutral" in its influence on anxiety and activity; this is to say that it has hardly any sedative or activating effect. This means that it can be prescribed both in retarded and in agitated vital depressions. Compulsive syndromes are believed to be a second range of indications, but this has not been adequately studied. Compulsive symptoms can occur or be aggravated in the context of a vital depressive phase. In such cases antidepressants (not only clomipramine) are undoubtedly very useful. With the depression, the compulsive symptoms disappear. However, it has not been demonstrated that clomipramine has a specific therapeutic effect also in non-depressive compulsive syndromes. It is believed that clomipramine provokes a change to a hypomanic phase more often than other tricyclic antidepressants.

Imipramine (Tofranil, Presamine)

Chemical structure. 1-(3′-dimethylaminopropyl)2-3,6-7,dibenzo-1-azacycloheptadiene-2,6.

Dosage. The agent can be given by mouth or by intramuscular injection. The usual daily oral dose is 150-225 mg. In severe cases treatment can be started parenterally, beginning with 3 × 25 mg intramuscularly per day and increasing the dosage by 25 mg per day up to a daily dose of 200 mg. Next, the dose is reduced by 50 mg per day, and at the same time oral medication is started with 50 mg per day. The oral dose is then increased by 50 mg per day up to a daily dose of 200-300 mg. In view of the risk of orthostatic hypotension the patient should be confined to bed for an hour after each injection.

The above dosage scheme calls for careful monitoring of the blood pressure; it should be used only in a clinical setting and is precluded in the case of poor heart function.

Parenteral administration can accelerate the therapeutic activity of imipramine but it is uncertain whether this is a pharmacological or a placebo effect.

Particulars. Imipramine is the prototype of the tricyclic antidepressants. In addition to an antidepressant effect, it is slightly activating. In terms of its influence on psychomotor activity, it is placed between amitriptyline on the one hand, and MAO inhibitors and demethylated tricyclic compounds on the other. It is indicated in retarded vital depressions but, in combination with an ataractic or neuroleptic, can also be used in agitated vital depressions. It has pronounced anticholinergic properties, and atropine-like side effects are accordingly pronounced.

Trimeprimine, Trimipramine (Surmontil, Stangyl)

Chemical structure. 5-(3-methylamino-2-methylpropyl)-5H-10,11-dihydrodibenzazepine. The central structure of this compound is identical to that of imipramine, but the side chain is identical to that of laevomepromazine.

Dosage. This agent can be given by mouth (tablets or droplets) or parenterally. The daily oral dose is 100-250 mg. In severe cases trimeprimine can be given intramuscularly for a few days: 4 × 25-50 mg per day.

Particulars. This is a strongly sedative antidepressant, which does not essentially differ from amitriptyline except for the fact that its side effects are believed to be slightly less marked.

2. Demethylated (monomethyl) compounds of the tricyclic series (Table 13)

The monomethyl derivatives have no sedative effect and stimulate motor activity; the intensity of the latter effect shows fairly marked interindividual variations. All these compounds can provoke or intensify anxiety and restiveness. In biochemical terms they have in common the ability more or less selectively to block the uptake of noradrenaline into the central noradrenergic neurons. The final dose should not be given after 1600 hrs.

Table 13. Monomethyl compounds of the tricyclic series

Chemical structure	Generic name	Trade name	Daily oral dose in mg	
			Average	Maximum
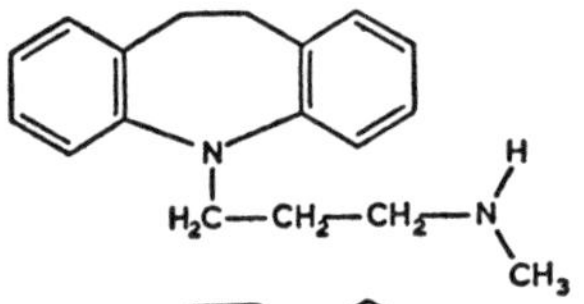	Desipramine	Norpramine Pertofran Pertofrane	100-200	250
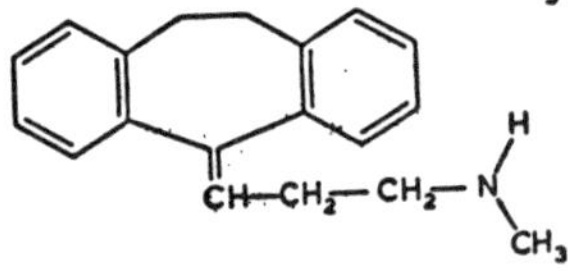	Nortrip-tyline	Aventyl Nortrilen Nortriptyline	100-200	250
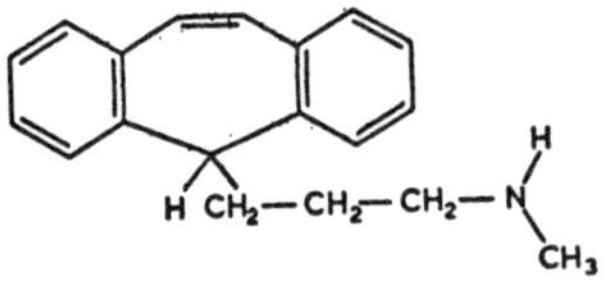	Protrip-tyline	Concordin Maximed Vivactyl	15-60	75

Desipramine (Pertofran, Pertofrane, Norpramine)

Chemical structure. 5-(3-methylaminopropyl)-5H-10,11-dihydroxibenzazepine.

Dosage. The usual daily oral dose is 100-200 mg. In severe cases, treatment can be started parenterally: 25-50 mg intramuscularly twice daily (morning and afternoon). After a few days, treatment is continued by oral administration.

Particulars. This activating antidepressant is indicated in retarded vital depressions. It is an (active) metabolite of imipramine, but there are no indications that it acts more quickly than the mother substance. In terms of vegetative side effects it also resembles the mother substance.

Nortriptyline (Aventyl, Nortrilen)

Chemical structure. 5-(3-methylaminopropylidene)-dibenzocyclohepta-1,4-diene.

Dosage. The usual daily oral dose is 100-200 mg. Treatment can be started by intramuscular injection in severe cases: 2 × 20-40 mg per day. After a few days treatment is continued orally.

Particulars. Nortriptyline is an (active) metabolite of amitriptyline. Its effect does not differ from that of desimipramine.

Protriptyline (Concordin, Maximed, Vivactyl)

Chemical structure. 5-(3-methylaminopropyl)-5H-dibenzocycloheptatriene.

Dosage. The daily oral dose is 15-60 mg.

Particulars. Protriptyline has few side effects and is believed to have the most marked activating effect of the three monomethyl compounds.

3. Other tricyclic antidepressants (Table 14)

Dibenzepine (Noveril)

Chemical structure. 5-methyl-10-(2-dimethylaminoethyl)-10,11-dihydro-11-oxo-5H-dibenzo(b,e) (1,4)diazepine. The structure of this antidepressant is related to that of the neuroleptic clozapine.

Dosage. The daily oral dose is 240-480 mg; in severe cases it is 3 × 240 mg. If necessary, treatment can be started by intramuscular injection: 3-4 × 40 mg.

Particulars. The action profile of this compound corresponds with that of imipramine, but its anticholinergic side effects are believed to be less marked.

Table 14. Other tricyclic antidepressants

Chemical structure	Generic name	Trade name	Daily oral dose in mg	
			Average	Maximum
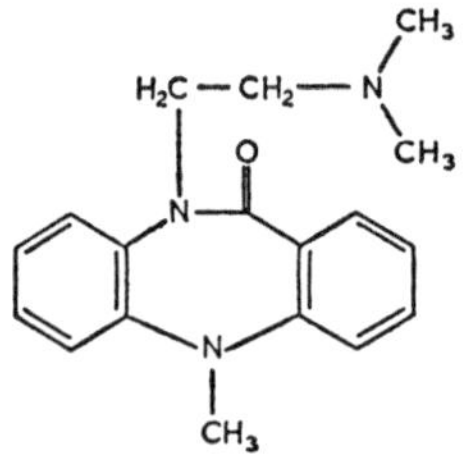	Dibenzepine	Noveril	240-480	720
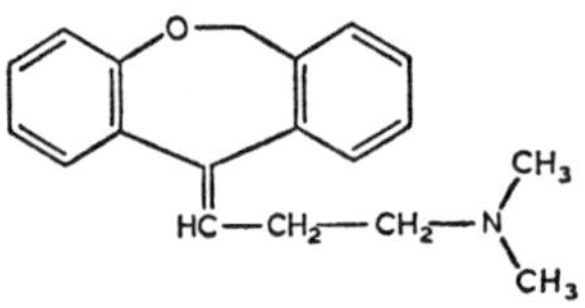	Doxepine	Aponal Quitaxon Sinequan	150-225	300

Doxepine (Sinequan, Aponal, Quitaxon)

Chemical structure. 11-(3-dimethylaminopropylidene)-6,11-dihydrodibenz(b,e)oxepine.

Dosage. The daily oral dose is 150-225 mg. The intramuscular dose is 3-4 × 25-50 mg per day, but no more than 150 mg/24 hours.

Particulars. The properties of this antidepressant resemble those of amitriptyline and trimipramine, i.e. it has a marked sedative effect and is therefore suitable for the treatment of agitated vital depressions. Since the sedative effect ensues quickly (unlike the antidepressant effect), it is useful to start treatment parenterally. Anticholinergic side effects are common. In parenteral treatment one should beware of hypotension. As always after intramuscular administration of tricyclic antidepressants, the patient should be confined to bed for an hour after each injection.

The group of the modified tricyclic antidepressants comprises yet other compounds, of which I mention *melitrancen* (Trausabun), *dimetacrin* (Istonil, Linostil) and *noxiptiline* (Agedal). There are no indications that these differ essentially from the original compounds imipramine and amitriptyline. In fact the same applies to the two compounds which I have discussed in some detail, by way of example.

4. Tetracyclic antidepressants (Table 15)

Maprotiline (Ludiomil)

Chemical structure. N-[3-(dibenzo[b,e]bicyclo[2.2.2]octa-2,5-diene-1-yl)-propyl]-N-methylamine.

Dosage. The daily oral dose is 150-225 mg.

Particulars. Maprotiline was the first tetracyclic compound to be used as an antidepressant. It is chemically related to the tetracyclic ataractic benzoctamine. Its characteristic biochemical feature is that it inhibits the uptake of noradrenaline into noradrenergic neurons in the brain while exerting no influence on that of serotonin into the serotonergic neurons. It is a so-called selective noradrenaline reuptake inhibitor. Its selectivity exceeds that of the monomethyl derivatives in the tricyclic series.

Table 15. Tetracyclic antidepressants

Chemical structure	Generic name	Trade name	Daily oral dose in in mg	
			Average	Maximum
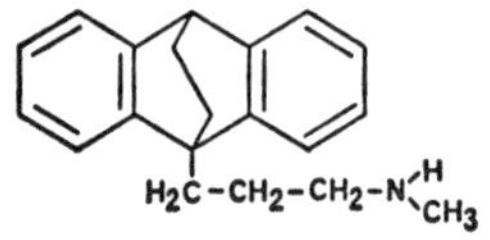	Maprotiline	Ludiomil	150-225	300
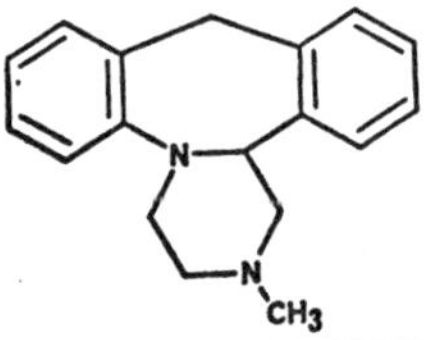	Mianserine	Tolvin Tolvon Bolvidan	40-120	?

Maprotiline is a slightly activating antidepressant with a therapeutic efficacy comparable to that of imipramine, and with relatively few vegetative side effects. So far as we know, its indications are the same as those for tricyclic antidepressants. There may be a biochemically classifiable group of vital depressions for which this selective noradrenaline agonist is a specific therapeutic agent (chapter XVI); however, no pertinent research has so far been carried out.

Mianserine (Tolvin, Tolvon, Bolvidan)

Chemical structure. 1,2,3,4,10,14-b-hexahydro-2-methyldibenzo (c,f)pyrazino-(1,2-a)-azepine.

Dosage. The daily oral dose is 40-120 mg.

Particulars. The action profile of this tetracyclic compound corresponds with that of amitriptyline. Unlike the tricyclic compounds, however, mianserine has no anticholinergic properties, and therefore produces substantially fewer side effects. The most striking feature of this compound is that, in the classical pharmacological screening tests in animals, it did not impress as a potential antidepressant. Biochemically, too, it is an "outsider" because it does not inhibit MAO and is not a classical reuptake inhibitor. Possibly, and hopefully, mianserine could be the first of a new series of antidepressants, even in biochemical terms.

5. Monoamine oxidase (MAO) inhibitors with a hydrazine group (Table 16)

Phenelzine (Nardelzine, Nardil, Stinerval)

Chemical structure. β-phenylethylhydrazine.

Dosage. The daily oral dose is 45-90 mg.

Particulars. The indications for phenelzine are believed to differ from those for all other antidepressants, i.e., the "atypical depressions." In these syndromes it is not so much motor inhibition and sadness that predominate as anxiety feelings—"free floating" or of a more phobic character—and various somatic symptoms (headaches, myalgia, palpitations, etc.). This theme is discussed on page 235. Whether other MAO inhibitors are likewise effective in these atypical depressions is unknown.

Mebanazine (Actomol)

Chemical structure. α-methylbenzylhydrazine.

Dosage. The daily oral dose is 20-30 mg.

Particulars. Mebanazine is the therapeutically most effective of the group of MAO-inhibiting hydrazines (in the group of the vital depressions). It is an activating antidepressant, and therefore indicated in retarded vital depressions. Doses exceeding 20 mg per day frequently lead to hypotension, and daily doses up to 30 mg are often required for an optimal therapeutic result. This is why the blood pressure should be carefully monitored during the first weeks of medication. The final dose each day should not be given after 1600 hours.

6. MAO inhibitors without hydrazine group (Table 16)

An attempt to reduce the side effects of MAO inhibitors has been made by eliminating the hydrazine group. However, this has not (yet?) been achieved.

Tranylcypromine (Parnate)

Chemical structure. trans-1-amino-2-phenylcyclopropane.

Dosage. The daily oral dose is 30-50 mg.

Particulars. Because it has a phenylethylamine group, tranylcypromine is chemically related to the amphetamine derivatives. Clinically, however, it is a typical antidepressant of the activating category, suitable for the treatment of retarded vital depressions. It

Table 16. MAO inhibitors

Chemical structure	Generic name	Trade name	Average daily dose in mg by mouth
1. Compounds with a hydrazine group			
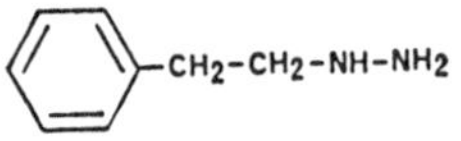	Phenelzine	Nardelzine Nardil Stinerval	45-80
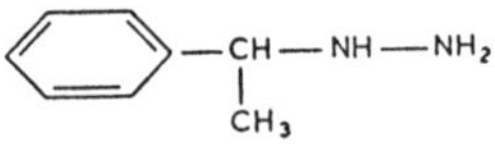	Mebanazine	Actomol	20-30
2. Compounds without hydrazine group			
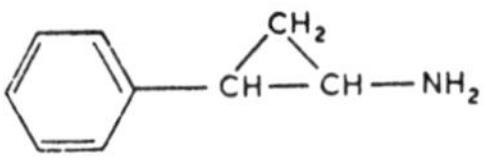	Tranylcypromine	Parnate	30-50

acts relatively quickly: A therapeutic effect (if any) as a rule becomes manifest in the first week. The famed "cheese reaction" described on page 234 was discovered in patients treated with this compound.

BIBLIOGRAPHY

BLASHKI, T. G., R. MOWBRAY AND B. DAVIES (1971). Controlled trial of amitriptyline in general practice. *Brit. Med. J.* I, 133.

Ciba Foundation Symposium 39 (New Series) (1976). *Monoamine Oxidase and Its Inhibition.* Amsterdam, Oxford, New York: Elsevier, Excerpta Medica, North Holland.

ESCOBAR, J. I., A. FLEMENBAUM AND B. C. SCHIELE (1973). Chlorimipramine: a double-blind comparison of intravenous versus oral administration in depressed patients. *Psychopharmacologia* 33, 111.

JOHNSON, D. A. W. (1974). A study of the use of antidepressant medication in general practice. *Brit. J. Psychiat.* 125, 186.

KLERMAN, G. L. AND J. O. COLE (1965). Clinical pharmacology of imipramine and related antidepressant compounds. *Pharmacol. Rev.* 17, 101.

LAURITSEN, B. J., AND H. MADSEN (1974). A multinational, double-blind trial with a new antidepressant maprotiline (Ludiomil[R]) and amitriptyline. *Acta Psychiat. Scand.* 50, 192.

MOIR, D. C., W. B. CORNWELL, I. DINGWELL-FORDYCE, J. CROOKS, K. O'MALLEY, M. J. TURNBULL AND R. D. WEIR (1972). Cardiotoxicity of amitriptyline. *Lancet* II, 561.

MORRIS, J. B. (1974). The efficacy of antidepressant drugs. *Arch. Gen. Psychiat.* 30, 667.

MURPHY, J. E. (1975). A comparative clinical trial of Org. GB 94 and imipramine in the treatment of depression in general practice. *J. Int. Med. Res.* 3, 251.

RASKIN, A. (1974). A guide for drug use in depressive disorders. *Amer. J. Psychiat.* 131, 181.

RASKIN, A. (1974). Depression subtype and response to phenelzine, diazepam and a placebo. *Arch. Gen. Psychiat.* 30, 66.

SHOPSIN, B. AND N. S. KLINE (1975). What's new in psychopharmacology. In: S. Arieti and G. Chrzanowski (Eds.)., *New Dimensions in Psychiatry.* New York, London:.John Wiley.

SIMPSON, G. M., M. AMIN, J. W. S. ANGUS et al. (1972). Role of antidepressants and neuroleptics in the treatment of depression. *Arch. Gen. Psychiat.* 27, 337.

VOGEL, H. P., D. BENTE, J. FEDER, H. HELMCHEN, B. MUELLER-OERLINGHAUSEN, N. BOHACEK, M. MIHOVILOVIC, A. BRANDLI, J. FLEISCHHAUER AND W. WALCHER (1976). Mianserine versus amitriptyline. A double-blind-trial evaluated by the AMP system. *Int. Pharmacopsychiat.* 11, 25.

WITTENBORN, J. R. AND N. KEREMITEI (1975). A comparison of antidepressive medications in neurotic and psychotic patients. *Arch. Gen. Psychiat.* 32, 1172.

XVI

Some Biological Aspects of Depressions and Their Treatment

1. Antidepressants and central monoamine metabolism

The prototypes of the current antidepressants—the monoamine-oxidase (MAO) inhibitor iproniazid (Marsilid) and the tricyclic compound imipramine (Tofranil)—were discovered in 1958. Although unrelated in terms of chemical structure, they proved to be similar in two respects. In psychopathological terms: they have a beneficial effect on depressions, particularly on vital depressions. In biochemical terms: in the brain they behave like monoamine (MA) agonists, albeit via different mechanisms. MAO inhibitors inhibit the enzyme MAO and therefore the degradation of MA inside and outside the neuron. Tricyclic antidepressants are assumed to inhibit re-uptake of the transmitter substance from the synaptic cleft into the neuron after impulse transmission. In both cases the amount of transmitter substance available at the postsynaptic receptors increases, and transmission is believed to be facilitated (chapter IV).

Tricyclic antidepressants exert no or hardly any influence on the re-uptake of DA, and have varying effects on the re-uptake of 5-HT and NA. The tertiary amines such as clomipramine (Anafranil) chiefly block the re-uptake of 5-HT, whereas the secondary amines such as desipramine (Pertofran) and nortriptyline (Sensaval) chiefly block that of NA. The former group is assumed to potentiate 5-HT in particular, whereas the latter group mainly potentiate NA. Compounds with a much more selective inhibitory effect on 5-HT (re-) uptake than clomipramine have been recently introduced. Their effect on the NA metabolism is minimal. Their antidepressant efficacy is now being studied.

The group of the MAO inhibitors is less homogeneous in terms of their effect on central MA than was originally believed to be the case. MAO has been demonstrated not to be a homogeneous enzyme but a complex of related enzymes which differ in substrate specificity, i.e. in the facility with which they oxidize a given amine, and in their sensitivity to given MAO inhibitors. In other words, different MAO inhibitors inhibit the different components of the MAO complex to different extents. The clinical significance of this fact is still obscure. Efforts are being made to evolve selective MAO inhibitors—compounds with a marked inhibitory effect on certain components of the MAO complex, and no or a much less marked inhibitory effect on other components.

The relation between antidepressants and central MA metabolism raised two questions: 1) Does MA potentiation underlie (certain components of) the therapeutic effect of antidepressants, and 2) are depressive patients, particularly those who show a favourable response to antidepressants, suffering from a functional deficiency of 5-HT and/or CA in the brain?

The relevance of the second question was further enhanced when it was found that reserpine (Serpasil), and probably also methyldopa (Aldomet) can induce true vital depressions, especially in patients with a history of this type of depression. These antihypertensives are both counterparts of antidepressants, in biochemical terms also: they *reduce* the amount of 5-HT and/or CA available in the brain. Reserpine inhibits the uptake of 5-HT and CA into the intraneuronal stores, and consequently they fall victim to MAO and their concentration diminishes. Methyldopa is converted to methyl-NA via methyl-DA. In CA-ergic neurons, these substances can act as false transmitters, causing diminution of their activity.

The following is a brief outline of the results of research into the two questions formulated above. Chapter IV discusses impulse transmission in central MA-ergic synapses as well as the methods used to study the human central MA metabolism.

2. Disorders in central NA metabolism in depressions

Chemical research

Noradrenaline (NA) in the human CNS is oxidized for a small part to vanillylmandelic acid (VMA), but for the most part reduced to 3-methoxy-4-hydroxyphenyl-glycol (MHPG). At the periphery this proportion is reversed. In a series of 25 patients with so-called primary depressions, the National Institute of Mental Health (NIMH) group found a decreased concentration of MHPG (Fig. 25) and of VMA (Fig. 26) in the CSF (Post et al. 1973; Jimerson et al. 1975). Shopsin et al. (1973) reported normal values, but their group of patients was small (n = 8) and heterogeneous.

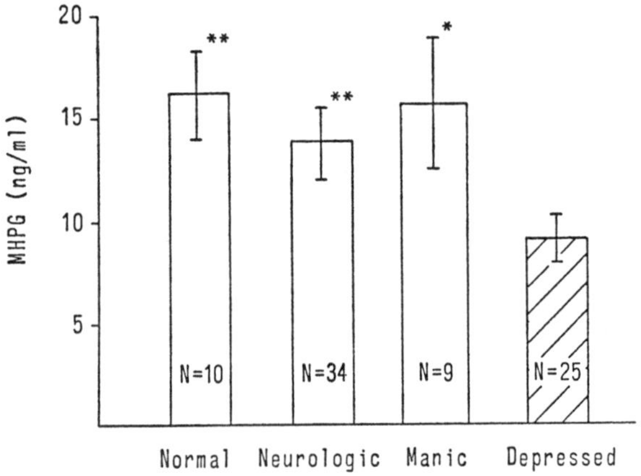

Figure 25. Low MHPG concentration in CSF in depressed patients. Levels of MHPG in depressed patients were significantly lower than those in other groups (*, P<0.05; **, P<0.01; Student's t-test, two-tailed) (Post et al., 1973).

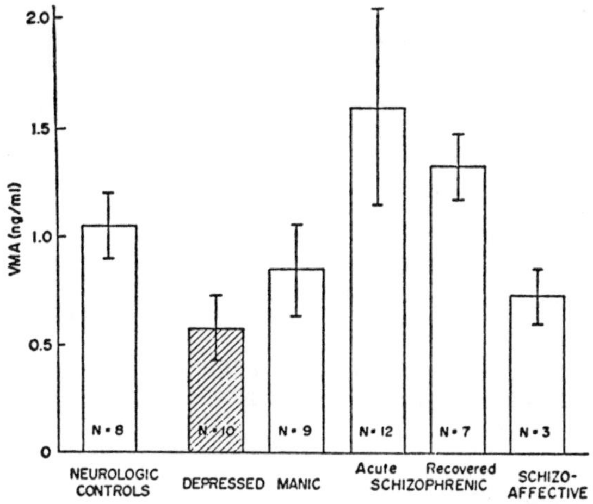

Figure 26. Mean (± S.E.) baseline VMA levels in ng/ml in lumbar CSF from different psychiatric groups and neurological controls. Mean VMA for the depressed patients is lower than that for the controls ($P<0.05$), acute schizophrenics ($P<0.01$), or recovered schizophrenics ($P<0.05$) (Jimerson et al., 1975)

Patients with primary depressions also had a smaller urinary excretion of MHPG than a control group, and also smaller than after their recovery (Table 17). This applies in particular to patients with a history of (hypo)manic phases, i.e. bipolar type of depression (Maas 1975). The phenomenon was observed in patients with motor retardation as well as in agitated patients and the decreased MHPG excretion is therefore not likely to be a phenomenon of peripheral origin, determined by the patient's motor inactivity. Since renal MHPG is regarded as a gross indicator of extraneuronal NA degradation in the CNS, the abovementioned phenomenon might indicate a reduced release of NA in central NA-ergic neurons.

The transport of MHPG from the CNS is not probenecid-sensitive. The probenecid technique is therefore unsuitable for a study of central NA metabolism.

Postmortem findings have failed to support the hypothesis that NA deficiency plays a role in the pathogenesis of depressions. The concentrations of NA and a few enzymes involved in its synthesis were normal.

Table 17. Excretion of MHPG in depressed patients with primary and secondary affective disorder and in a healthy control group (Deleon-Jones et al., 1975).

Group	Number	Excretion of MHPG per 24-hour urine (μg)* Mean	SEM
Primary affective disorder patients			
bipolar patients	5	911	154
recurrent unipolar patients	9	1066	86
single-episode unipolar patients	7	1073	140
Undiagnosed affective disorder patients	11	1280	185
Healthy subjects	21	1348	67

*An analysis of variance indicated significant differences between groups, and each of the patient groups differed significantly from the control group ($p<0.05$, Duncan's Multiple Range Test).

Pharmacological research

If NA depletion plays a role in the pathogenesis of certain types of depression, then it may be expected that an exogenously induced NA depletion has a depressogenic effect, while enhancement of the NA supply should have an antidepressant effect, at least in NA-deficient patients. α-Methyl-p-tyrosine (α-MT) inhibits tyrosine hydroxylase and therefore NA synthesis. In subhuman primates it induced behaviour changes reminiscent of depressivity. In humans this has not been unequivocally demonstrated, but then the agent has been used on only a limited scale. In manic phases it is therapeutically effective.

Of course α-MT inhibits not only the synthesis of NA but also that of DA. Exclusive inhibition of NA synthesis calls for an inhibitor of DA-β-hydroxylase. Fusaric acid is such a compound. It aggravates the condition of manic patients rendering human subjects not so much depressive as psychotic. It is not clear whether this is an effect of fusaric acid or a result of the fact that the patient is deprived of effective medication.

Since tyrosine hydroxylase is normally saturated with substrate, administration of tyrosine does not lead to an increase in NA synthesis. DOPA stimulates DA production in particular, but little of it is transformed to NA. Dihydroxyphenylserine (DOPS), an amino-acid which is not naturally present in the human organism, is directly decarboxylated to NA without intermediate DA synthesis. In depressive patients, however, this agent has not been tested.

3. NA metabolism and treatment of depressions

If decreased MHPG concentrations in CSF and urine denote reduced degradation of NA in the brain, and if this reduced degradation is of importance in the pathogenesis of depression, then a therapeutic effect can be expected from enhancement of central NA activity. This expectation would seem to be corroborated by empirical findings, and the postulates preceding this expectation therefore gain plausibility.

Maas (1975) found, and Beckmann and Goodwin (1975) confirmed, that the therapeutic efficacy of imipramine and desipramine (Pertofran) is greater when pre-therapeutic urinary excretion of MHPG is low than when pre-therapeutic MHPG excretion is normal or high (Table 18; Fig. 27). Moreover, the low MHPG excretors

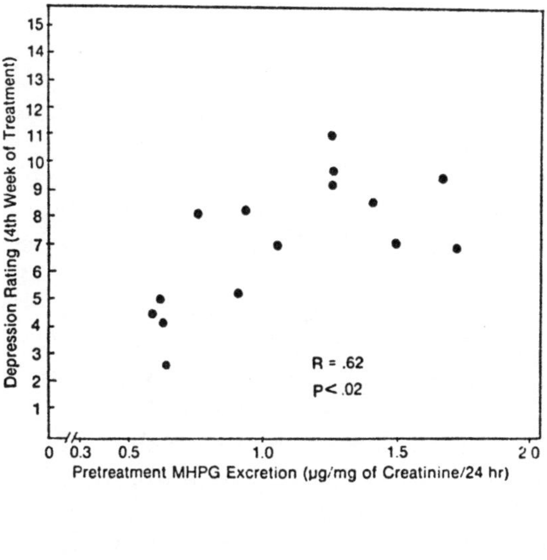

Figure 27. Micrograms of MHPG per milligram of creatinine excreted in urine per 24 hours prior to drug treatment plotted against depression ratings during the fourth week of treatment with imipramine (Maas et al., 1972, see Maas, 1975).

Table 18. Relation between tricyclic response and 24-hour urinary MHPG excretion in unipolar patients (Beckman and Goodwin, 1975)

	24-hour urinary MHPG excretion (mg/24 hr)		
	responders	non-responders	Difference†
Amitriptyline	2.17 ± 0.9 (n = 4)	1.21 ± 0.9 (n = 4)	$p<0.01$
Imipramine	1.10 ± 0.7 (n = 9)	1.93 ± 0.13 (n = 7)	$p<0.001$

†student t-test, two-tailed

responded to d-amphetamine by an improved mood, while the normal excretors showed an unchanged mood or a change in the dysphoric direction.

The compounds used can be assumed capable of relatively selective potentiation of central NA. Imipramine and desipramine have a more marked inhibitory effect on re-uptake of NA into the neuron than on re-uptake of 5-HT (Carlsson et al. 1969a,b). This is more evident for desipramine than for imipramine, but the latter is demethylated to desipramine in the organism. We may, therefore, assume that these compounds enhance central noradrenergic activity more than they do central serotonergic activity. Via different mechanisms (MAO inhibition, inhibition of re-uptake and CA release), amphetamines increase the amount of CA available at the central receptors; their influence on the 5-HT system is only marginal.

Depressive patients with a high or normal MHPG excretion show a better response to amitriptyline (Tryptizol; Elavil) than patients with a low MHPG excretion (Table 18). Amitriptyline is an antidepressant which inhibits re-uptake of 5-HT more markedly than that of NA. It is conceivable that less favourable results in low MHPG excretors are based on the relatively slight NA-potentiating effect of amitriptyline, while the favourable effect in normal or high MHPG excretors is based on its relatively marked influence on 5-HT. The second term of this hypothesis would become plausible only if it could be demonstrated that a central 5-HT deficiency probably existed before treatment in the patients showing the favourable response. Pertinent studies have not yet been made. Nor have any studies been devoted to the question whether variations in renal

MHPG excretion in these patients are reflected in the MHPG concentration in the CSF.

As imipramine is demethylated in the organism to desipramine, so also is amitriptyline demethylated to nortriptyline (Sensaval). As pointed out, amitriptyline exerts no marked influence on NA uptake, but nortriptyline does. This fact does not automatically devaluate the abovementioned hypothesis, for it is quite possible that transformation of amitriptyline to the secondary amine is slower than its inactivation, so that no effective concentration of nortriptyline can be built up (Maas 1975).

The above discussed data warrant the following *conclusions*.

1) The disorders of central NA metabolism present in certain categories of depression probably play a role in the pathogenesis of these syndromes. This conclusion is based on two observations: a) depressive patients showing indications of a central NA deficiency show a more favourable response to NA-potentiating antidepressants than depressive patients with no indications of such deficiency; b) the former group shows a less favourable response to antidepressants with relatively little NA-potentiating capacity than the latter group.

2) Disorders of the NA metabolism are not characteristic of depression in general but only of certain categories of depression.

3) Renal MHPG excretion supplies information which is of importance in determining indications for antidepressant medication.

4. Disorders of central DA metabolism in depressions

Chemical research

In rats, HVA and 3,4-dihydroxyphenylacetic acid (DOPAC) are the principal degradation products of DA. In the human individual, DA is largely converted to HVA. In the human CSF at least, DOPAC is found in only very small quantities, even after preceding acute or chronic l-DOPA administration. HVA in lumbar CSF largely originates from the brain: the spinal cord contains hardly any DA.

The largest contribution is probably made by the nigrostriatal DA system.

Several investigators have reported a decreased HVA concentration in the CSF in depressions, although the finding was not always statistically significant. Moreover, the probenecid-induced HVA accumulation in the CSF was decreased, and this is also indicative of a decreased central DA turnover (van Praag, 1976). An additional argument in favour of a disturbed DA turnover was supplied by Sjöström and Roos (1972), who administered methylperidol as well as probenecid to a number of test subjects. Methylperidol is a neuroleptic of the butyrophenone series, which greatly stimulates the DA turnover in the brain, probably secondarily to postsynaptic DA receptor block. Given an undisturbed DA production, this compound can be expected to cause a marked increase of the probenecid-induced HVA accumulation in the CSF. This was in fact observed, except in the depressive group where the extra increase caused by methylperidol was much less marked.

According to Goodwin et al. (1973), the disorder of DA metabolism is most marked in vital depressions with a unipolar course. We ourselves found that the decreased HVA accumulation is not a characteristic of vital depression but a phenomenon related to

Table 19. Concentration of HVA in CSF in depressive patients and controls before and after probenecid adminstration (in ng/ml) (van Praag and Korf, 1971, see van Praag, 1977).

	no. of test subjects	Before probenecid	After probenecid	Difference
Depression (retarded and non-retarded)	20	39 ± 16 (14 – 67)	82 ± 43 (27 – 185)	44 ± 38 (0.0 – 130)
retarded depression	8	32 ± 8 (20 – 46)	53 ± 32 (27 – 114)	20 ± 28 (0.0 – 74)
non-retarded depression	12	43 ± 17 (14 – 67)	106 ± 36 (40 – 185)	63 ± 37 (10 – 130)
Control	12	42 ± 16 (21 – 73)	91 ± 26 (59 – 151)	50 ± 33 (23 – 122)

Results are given as means ± s.d. (with range)

the state of motor retardation (Table 19). Since motor retardation is much more common in vital than in personal depressions, the disorder of DA metabolism *seems* to be a characteristic of vital depression. However, the phenomenon is also observed in personal depressions in which motor retardation is a prominent feature.

Postmortem studies have failed to reveal any abnormalities in DA metabolism.

Pharmacological research

The effect of inhibition of CA synthesis on behaviour has been discussed in section 4, and the effect of increased DA synthesis is discussed in section 5.

5. DA metabolism and treatment of depressions

In the CNS, exogenous l-DOPA is for the most part converted to DA, but a small amount is converted to NA. Its therapeutic effect in a psychopathologically and biochemically undifferentiated group of depressions is unspectacular, particularly if evaluated on the basis of differences in total scores, disregarding changes in certain components of the depressive syndrome. Different findings are obtained when biochemical variables are considered in the test arrangement and profiles rather than total scores are compared.

Ten depressive patients were selected on the basis of a biochemical criterion: the response to probenecid of HVA in the CSF (van Praag 1976). In 5 patients it was more, and in 5 it was less than 100 ng/ml. Motor retardation, measured by two independent raters using a 10-point scale, was more marked in the second than in the first group. Mood scores in the two groups were not significantly different. All patients were treated with l-DOPA and a peripheral decarboxylase inhibitor for two weeks. At the end of this period, motor retardation had virtually disappeared in the patients with a low HVA response (Table 20), while in patients with a normal response the motor status remained unchanged. This was to be expected because in this group pre-therapeutic motor activity had been hardly abnormal. The mood scores were not significantly influenced by l-DOPA. In both groups, finally, the HVA response to probenecid during treatment was about twice the pre-therapeutic response. The

Table 20. DA metabolism before treatment and response to l-DOPA in depression (van Praag, 1974, see van Praag, 1977).

	no. of patients	HVA accumulation* (ng/ml)	Motor retardation* before treatment	after treatment
DA deficient patients	5	74 (65 – 90)	6.8 (4 – 8)	2.7 (0 – 3)
non-DA-deficient patients	5	121 (107 – 143)	2.1 (0 – 3)	2.4 (0 – 3)

*Group mean and range

low responders, too, were evidently able to convert l-DOPA to DA. In practical terms, l-DOPA is not an acquisition in any case because its influence on mood is too slight. Moreover, the activating effect of l-DOPA in depressions is not superior to that of tricyclic antidepressants with an activating component.

In a second experiment, clomipramine (Anafranil) was compared with nomifensine in a double-blind study of a group of patients with vital depressions. Nomifensine is a compound with a relatively selective stimulating effect on postsynaptic DA receptors. It was significantly more effective in patients with a subnormal than in those with a normal HVA response to probenecid before treatment. In the clomipramine group this difference was not observed (van Scheyen et al., 1977).

My *conclusion* from these data is a dual one:

1) Since DOPA has a favourable effect on certain (motor) components of the depressive syndrome in DA-deficient patients, and fails to produce this effect in patients with a normal DA metabolism, I regard it as plausible that the biochemical disorder plays a role in the pathogenesis of these components.

2) The current antidepressants, i.e. roughly speaking the so-called tricyclic and tetracyclic antidepressants, exert only a slight influence on central DA metabolism. Consequently, in patients with indications of central DA deficiency, one should consider administering a DA agonist, such as l-DOPA or nomifensine, at the same time.

6. Disorders of central 5-HT metabolism in depressions

CSF studies

The principal degradation product of the central 5-HT metabolism is 5-hydroxyindoleacetic acid (5-HIAA). This applies to human and animal subjects alike. The human CSF contains only traces of the corresponding alcohol, 5-hydroxytryptophol. Part of the 5-HIAA found in lumbar CSF is of spinal origin, and another part originates from higher levels.

Data on the baseline concentration of 5-HIAA in CSF are not unequivocal. Decreased values have been reported but there have also been reports on normal values. However, since the psycho-

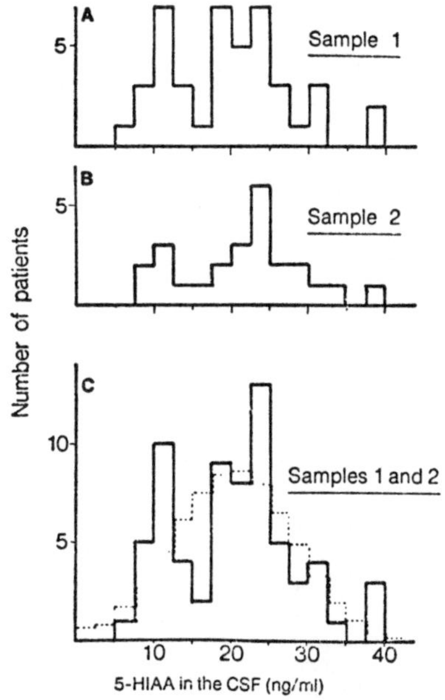

Figure 28. Distribution of 5-HIAA in depressed patients: (A) sample 1, N = 43; (B) sample 2, N = 25; (C) samples 1 and 2 combined. The dashed line represents the expected normal distribution (mean ± standard deviation = 20.36 ± 7.77). The deviation from normality is significant (X^2 = 19.76, 9 d.f., P = 0.02) (Åsberg et al., 1976)

pathological classification of the syndromes studied was often rather imperfect, it is conceivable that characteristics inherent to certain subcategories were overlooked. Åsberg et al. (1976) demonstrated that this is a very real possibility. Within a group of patients with endogenous depressions, some showed a normal and others a decreased 5-HIAA concentration in the CSF. The 5-HIAA concentrations measured (by means of gas chromatography/mass spectrometry) showed a bimodal distribution (Fig. 28). This suggests that the group of endogenous depressions, although tending towards homogeneity in terms of symptomatology, is a heterogeneous group in biochemical terms, i.e. in terms of pathogenesis. A few years earlier van Praag and Korf (van Praag 1977) had reached a similar conclusion on the basis of results of the probenecid test. Within a group of patients with vital depressions, the 5-HIAA response to

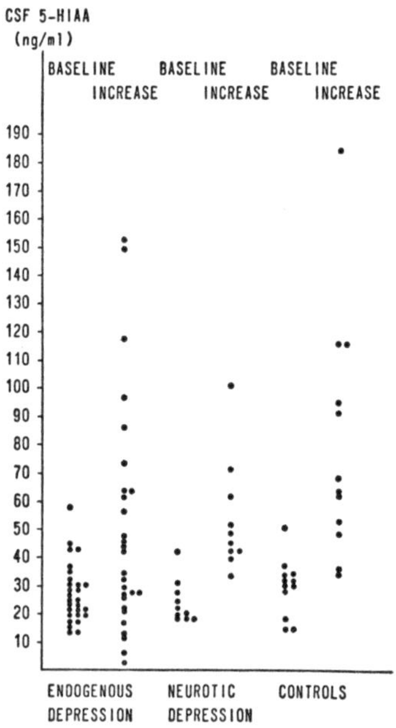

Figure 29. Baseline 5-HIAA concentration in CSF and increase of concentration after probenecid in endogenous (vital) depressions, neurotic (personal) depressions and controls (van Praag et al., 1973, see van Praag, 1977).

probenecid was decreased in about 40% of patients (Fig. 29). On the basis of this finding they formulated the postulate of the biochemical heterogeneity of the group of vital depressions; this group was believed to include forms with and forms without demonstrable central 5-HT deficiency. The decreased 5-HIAA accumulation in vital depressions has been confirmed by several groups of investigators. Only Bowers (1972) reported normal values, but this may have been due to the syndromal heterogeneity of the group of patients studied: the group of personal depressions, it should be borne in mind, shows virtually no instances of decreased 5-HIAA accumulation.

Postmortem studies

The results of postmortem studies in suicide victims are not unequivocal but do point in the same direction: a tendency of the 5-HT and 5-HIAA concentrations in the brain, more particularly in the raphe nuclei, to decrease; the raphe nuclei are the site of predilection of 5-HT in the brain (Table 21). This phenomenon might indicate that 5-HT synthesis was decreased prior to death. The different results reported by different investigators can possibly be explained on the basis of the fact that the histories of these suicide victims were not always known; moreover, suicide is also committed by patients in diagnostic categories other than that of pathological depressions.

Pharmacological research

Human central serotonergic activity can be suppressed in two different ways: with the aid of p-chlorophenylalanine (PCPA), an inhibitor of tryptophan hydroxylase, and with the aid of methysergide (Deseril), a 5-HT antagonist. In this context it is to be noted that, although this is often assumed, it is not certain that reduction of 5-HT synthesis causes decreased serotonergic function. Depressions have not been described after these two compounds. On the other hand, PCPA abolishes the therapeutic effect of imipramine (Tofranil) within a few days (Shopsin et al. 1975). It can therefore not be stated that suppression of serotonergic activity effected by pharmacological means has no effect on mood regulation.

The possibilities of relatively selective stimulation of human

Table 21. Concentrations of 5-HIAA and 5-HT in the raphe nuclei of controls and suicides (Lloyd et al. 1974).

	5-HIAA (μg/g)				5-HT (μg/g)			
Raphe nuclei	Controls Mean ± SEM	n	Suicides Mean ± SEM	n	Controls Mean ± SEM	n	Suicides Mean ± SEM	n
Centralis superior	12.37 ± 0.65 (11.25 –14.53)	5	12.39 ± 0.91 (9.19 – 14.61)	5	2.25 ± 0.19 (1.88 – 2.97)	5	1.86 ± 0.16 (1.41 – 2.26)	5
Dorsalis	7.04 ± 0.59 (5.85 – 8.63)	5	6.14 ± 0.52 (5.00 – 7.79)	5	2.22 ± 0.13 (1.92 – 2.56)	5	1.55 ± 0.12[a] (1.23 – 1.90)	5
Pontis	7.66 ± 0.57 (6.21 – 8.92)	5	7.12 ± 0.68 (5.42 – 9.55)	5	1.34 ± 0.21 (0.80 – 1.89)	5	1.04 ± 0.13 (0.65 – 1.38)	5
Centralis inferior	4.49 ± 0.43 (3.63 – 5.77)	5	4.01 ± 0.32 (3.14 – 4.67)	5	1.32 ± 0.12 (0.94 – 1.47)	5	0.95 ± 0.07[b] (0.69 – 1.09)	5
Obscurus	2.86 ± 0.24 (2.00 – 3.46)	5	3.36 ± 0.31 (2.46 – 4.24)	5	1.07 ± 0.14 (0.62 – 1.39)	5	1.02 ± 0.14 (0.75 – 1.56)	5
Pallidus	2.28 ± 0.16 (1.85 – 2.67)	5	2.25 ± 0.20 (1.90 – 2.74)	4	0.61 ± 0.09 (0.44 – 0.91)	5	0.42 ± 0.12 (0.28 – 0.76)	4

n is the number of brains examined. Ranges are given in parentheses. Significantly different from controls: [a]$p<0.01$; [b]$p<0.05$.

Table 22. 5-HIAA accumulation in CSF after probenecid, before treatment and during treatment with l-5-HTP (200 mg per day) in combination with a peripheral decarboxylase inhibitor (MK 486 150 mg per day) (van Praag and Korf, 1975, see van Praag, 1977).

	no. of patients	CSF 5-HIAA after probenecid (ng/ml) before treatment	after treatment	CSF probenecid μg/ml
Low 5-HIAA response	5	26 ± 11.1	63 ± 22.5	8.7 ± 1.9
Normal 5-HIAA response	5	90 ± 32.3	150 ± 40.8	9.80 ± 3.0

central 5-HT activity are limited. The 5-HT precursors tryptophan and 5-hydroxytryptophan (5-HTP) increase 5-HT synthesis, as demonstrated by the increased 5-HIAA accumulation in response to probenecid. The effect of 5-HTP is shown in Table 22. The effects of tryptophan and 5-HTP in depressions are discussed in section 7. The influence of chloramphetamines on central 5-HT is a fairly selective but complex one, which comprises at least four components: 1) inhibition of 5-HT synthesis; 2) release of 5-HT from the synaptic vesicles; 3) inhibition of 5-HT re-uptake; 4) MAO inhibition. At least in acute experiments, the net effect is reported to be enhancement of central 5-HT activity. When used in depressive patients, they produce a therapeutic effect which differs from that of the non-chlorated amphetamine derivatives, and closely resembles that of the conventional antidepressants.

7. 5-HT metabolism and treatment of depressions

Hypotheses

Assuming that: a) a low 5-HIAA response to probenecid indeed indicates a diminished 5-HT turnover in the brain, and b) the suspected 5-HT deficiency plays a role in the pathogenesis of (certain components) of the (vital) depression, the following hypothesis are justifiable.

1) 5-HT-potentiating antidepressants will be therapeutically effective in "5-HT-deficient depressions" but not, or in a lesser

degree, in depressive patients without a demonstrable central 5-HT deficiency.

2) Antidepressants with a mainly NA-potentiating effect will produce little effect in "5-HT-deficient depressions."

Precursor studies

The 5-HT precursors tryptophan and 5-HTP stimulate central 5-HT synthesis in test animals. That they do the same in human individuals is apparent from the increased 5-HIAA response to probenecid which they produce. It has been demonstrated that low 5-HIAA responders, too, are capable of converting 5-HTP to 5-HT.

The antidepressant activity of l-tryptophan is controversial; some authors described it as effective while others regarded it as a placebo. So far, however, clinical studies have not been related to data on the central 5-HT metabolism. It remains possible, therefore, that a 5-HT-deficient subgroup exists which is susceptible to tryptophan. This could explain the variability of results reported so far. The observation that a combination of a MAO inhibitor with tryptophan is more effective than a MAO inhibitor alone has not been contradicted so far.

The still scanty research so far done with 5-HTP indicates that my plea in favour of considering biochemical data in the interpretation of therapeutic results obtained with new, potential antidepressants has not been groundless. For van Praag et al. (1972) found that 1-5-HTP can be therapeutically effective in depressions and that this effect occurs in particular in low 5-HIAA responders to probenecid (Table 23). Good results obtained with 5-HTP have also been reported by Sano (1972) and Takahashi et al. (1975). However, theirs were open studies. That the 5-HTP effect in depressions is not a non-specific one but is really produced via 5-HT is probable in view of the fact that the 5-HTP effect is potentiated by the relatively selective 5-HT re-uptake inhibitor clomipramine (Anafranil) in doses which as such are not effective. However, a "mirror" experiment concerning the question whether a relatively selective NA re-uptake inhibitor such as nortriptyline lacks this effect of clomipramine has not been carried out. The combination of l-tryptophan and clomipramine has also been reported to produce a more marked antidepressant effect than clomipramine alone. In normal test subjects, too, a positive effect of l-5-HTP on the mood level has been reported.

Table 23. Increase of CSF 5-HIAA in response to probenecid and effectiveness of l-5-HTP in patients with vital depressions (van Praag et al., 1972, see van Praag, 1977).

	CSF 5-HIAA level (ng/ml)			CSF probenecid level (μg/ml)
	Before probenecid	After probenecid	Increase	
5-HTP, improved*	18 (16-22)	35 (28-48)	16 (11-26)	7.2 (5.0-10.7)
5-HTP, not improved*	17 (13-22)	71 (61-81)	50 (39-68)	6.5 (5.5-7.5)
Placebo**	25 ± 9 (13-33)	72 ± 33 (51-129)	47 ± 39 (20-116)	12.6 ± 6.2 (4.0-19.0)
Non-depressive** control group	21 ± 14 (21-66)	112 ± 46 (60-179)	80 ± 49 (26-153)	9.1 ± 3.5 (3.0-16.5)

*Group mean and range
**Group mean with standard deviation and range

There is as yet no certainty about the value or lack of value of 5-HT precursors in depressions. I consider it to be of essential importance that future studies account for the patient's pre-therapeutic biochemical status.

CSF 5-HIAA and nortriptyline

Åsberg et al. (1972) studied the question whether there is a relation between the 5-HIAA concentration in CSF and the therapeutic response to nortriptyline. They found that the therapeutic effect of nortriptyline was less pronounced in depressive patients with a CSF 5-HIAA concentration of less than 15 ng/ml than in patients with higher 5-HIAA concentrations (Table 24). The plasma nortriptyline concentration was within the therapeutic range in both groups.

Nortriptyline is a relatively selective inhibitor of the "NA pump" (Carlsson et al. 1969a, 1969b). It seems a plausible hypothesis that the group with low 5-HIAA shows little response because nortriptyline potentiates chiefly NA. In that case it might be expected that such patients would benefit more from an antidepressant which chiefly potentiates 5-HT, e.g. clomipramine. Research into this hypothesis is now in progress (see next section).

Table 24. Relation between pre-therapeutic CSF 5-HIAA and clinical improvement during nortriptyline medication (150 mg per day), as measured with the aid of the Cronholm-Ottosson scale in 20 patients suffering from vital ("endogenous") depressions (Åsberg et al., 1972).

		Severity of depression (rating score)		
5-HIAA in CSF (ng/ml)	Number of patients	Before treatment, mean ± S.D.	During treatment, mean ± S.D.	Amelioration (reduction in rating score) mean ± S.D.
6.0 – 14.6	7	14.0 ± 3.1*	10.0 ± 8.3	4.0 ± 7.7**
17.7 – 37.5	13	11.7 ± 3.1*	3.9 ± 3.1	7.8 ± 2.8***

*t to compare means = 1.55 (N.S.)
**does not differ significantly from zero; t = 1.38
***significantly different from zero; t = 10.26, $p<0.001$

CSF 5-HIAA and clomipramine

In 30 patients with vital depressions, van Praag and co-workers studied the relation between post-probenecid 5-HIAA accumulation (interpreted as an indicator of central 5-HT turnover) prior to medication and the therapeutic effect of clomipramine, a mainly 5-HT-potentiating antidepressant. The course of the depression was unipolar in 16 and bipolar in 7 patients, the remaining patients being in their first depressive phase. The drug was administered during 3 weeks at a daily dosage of 225 mg. A negative correlation was established between the two variables in the sense that the therapeutic effect of medication increased by as much as pre-therapeutic 5-HIAA accumulation had been lower (Fig. 30).

After 3 weeks, 8 patients were considered not to have improved at all. Clomipramine was discontinued in these cases and replaced by a placebo for one week. The placebo period was followed by 3 weeks of daily administration of 150 mg nortriptyline, a mainly NA-potentiating antidepressant. Placebo and nortriptyline were given in capsules identical to those in which clomipramine had been administered. Neither raters nor patients were aware of the switch to placebo and then to nortriptyline. Of these 8 patients, 5 were considered to have markedly improved at the end of the third week of nortriptyline medication (Table 25). No correlation was found between pre-therapeutic CSF MHPG concentration and therapeutic effect of medication. Renal MHPG excretion was not measured.

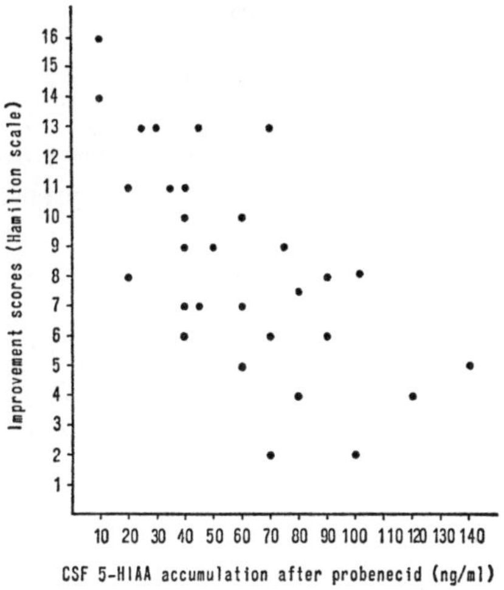

Figure 30. Relation between pre-therapeutic 5-HIAA response to probenecid and clinical improvement during clomipramine medication (225 mg daily) as measured with the aid of the Hamilton scale in 30 patients with vital ("endogenous") depressions. Bravais-Pearson correlation coefficient $r = -0.40$, $p<0.05$.

Table 25. Pre-therapeutic CSF MHPG concentration and effect of nortriptyline medication (3 × 50 mg daily) in 8 clomipramine-resistant depressive patients.

Patient	CSF MHPG before treatment (ng/ml)	Improvement score after 3 weeks (Hamilton scale)	Clearly improved
1	6.5	0	no
2	7.6	+ 5	no
3	8.2	+10	yes
4	8.9	+ 2	no
5	9.8	+16	yes
6	10.1	+11	yes
7	14.7	+17	yes
8	15.9	+13	yes

Combined precursor/clomipramine studies

Finally we studied the combined effect of two 5-HT potentiating drugs—i.e. l-5-HTP and clomipramine—in a group of patients suffering from vital depression with uni- or bipolar course. For this purpose we compared, double-blind, the antidepressant potency of l-5-HTP, clomipramine, l-5-HTP in combination with clomipramine and placebo. l-5-HTP was always administered together with a peripheral decarboxylase inhibitor.

The three treatment modalities were significantly superior to placebo. The therapeutic effect of 5-HTP was inferior to that of clomipramine, but not significantly so. The outcome of the combined

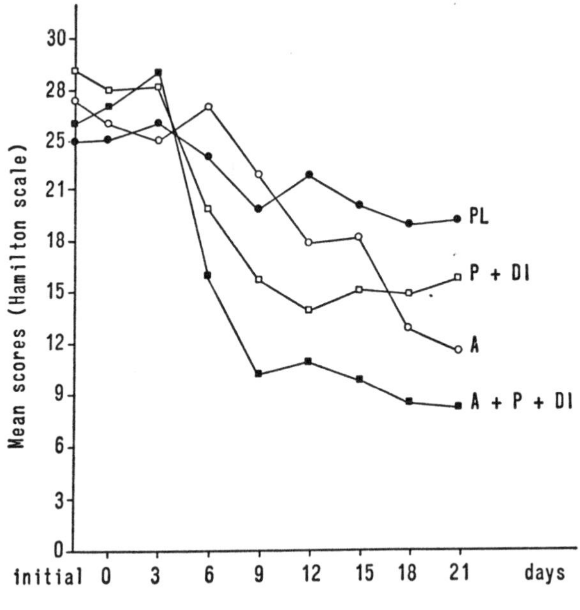

Figure 31. Hamilton scores in 4 groups of patients suffering from vital depression with uni- and bipolar course, before and during a 3-week treatment period with serotonin-potentiating compounds.

The groups consisted of 10 patients each, treated respectively with clomipramine alone (225 mg per day; A), 5-HTP alone (P; 200 mg per day, in combination with 150 mg MK 486, a peripheral decarboxylase inhibitor; DI), the combination of clomipramine with 5-HTP and placebo (Pl). The design was double blind.

treatment was significantly better than that with 5-HTP and clomipramine alone (Fig. 31).

Next we compared the efficacy of the three 5-HT potentiating treatments in patients with subnormal and normal 5-HIAA responses to probenecid before treatment. It appeared that the treatment results were superior in the former group: the group with decreased central 5-HT "turnover" (Fig. 32).

Conclusions

The data discussed warrant the following conclusions:

1) The disorders of central 5-HT metabolism which have been observed in certain depressive syndromes are not a secondary phenomenon but probably play a role in the

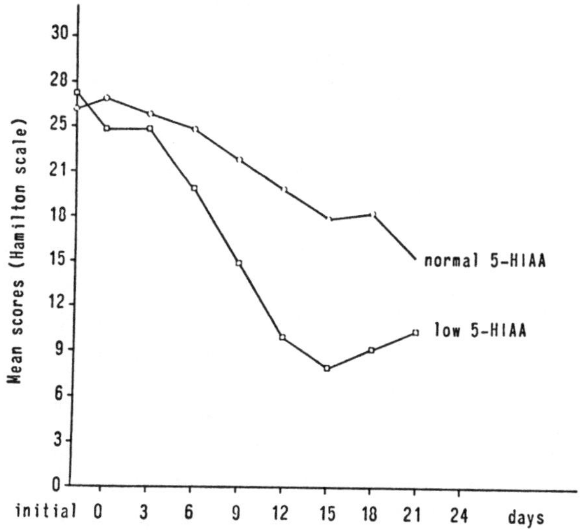

Figure 32. Hamilton scores of 30 patients suffering from vital depression with uni- and bipolar course before and during a 3-week treatment period with serotonin-potentiating compounds, i.e.: clomipramine alone, 5-HTP (together with a peripheral decarboxylase inhibitor) alone, and those drugs in combination.

The lower curve depicts treatment results in patients with subnormal pretreatment 5-HIAA response to probenecid (n = 13), the upper curve those in patients with normal pretreatment 5-HIAA responses (n = 17).

pathogenesis of these depressions. This conclusion is based on the following data: a) "5-HT-deficient depressions" improve in response to compounds considered to increase the amount of 5-HT available in the brain; their therapeutic effect is more pronounced than that in patients without a demonstrable central 5-HT deficiency. b) In "5-HT-deficient depressions," the therapeutic effect of an antidepressant with a mostly NA-potentiating effect (e.g. nortriptyline) is less marked than that in patients without a demonstrable defect in central 5-HT metabolism. It is logical to expect these nortriptyline-susceptible patients to be NA-deficient. However, CSF studies have failed to corroborate this expectation. Renal MHPG excretion was not determined in these patients. The finding of a decreased excretion would elegantly clinch the hypothesis.

2) Disorders of 5-HT metabolism are characteristic, not of depressions in general, but of certain types of (vital) depression.

3) Determination of the CSF 5-HIAA concentration (preferably after probenecid administration) supplies data which can be of significance in the choice of an optimal antidepressant.

8. MA metabolism and treatment of depressions. General conclusions

I believe that the above discussed relations between MA metabolism and treatment results with compounds which influence MA lend support to two concepts: the concept that disorders of central MA metabolism can play a role in the pathogenesis of (vital) depressions, and the concept that the group of vital depressions is a heterogeneous one in biochemical terms. At least two types of vital depression exist; 5-HT deficiency plays a role in the pathogenesis of one, while NA deficiency is important in the pathogenesis of the other. These types of depression are indistinguishable in psychopathological terms.

Patients of the first group seem to respond best to antidepressants with a strong ability to potentiate 5-HT and less to NA-potentiating compounds, while the reverse applies to the NA-deficient patient. The CSF supplies no reliable information on the presence or absence of a central NA deficiency; according to Maas

(1975), renal MHPG excretion is more instructive in this respect (section 3 above). It was already known that renal MHPG and CSF MHPG show a poor correlation. A possible explanation is that MHPG in the lumbar CSF is chiefly of spinal, not of cerebral, origin.

This conclusion raises three new questions.

1. What exactly is the relation between renal MHPG and MHPG in CSF?
2. Can both 5-HT and NA metabolism be disturbed in the same patient, or are (vital) depressions either chiefly 5-HT-deficient or chiefly NA-deficient?
3. What is the therapeutic efficacy of various (biochemical) types of antidepressants in patients with vital depressions who show no demonstrable disorders of central MA metabolism?

It is to these questions that answers must now be found.

9. Specific chemoprophylaxis

Let us assume that: 1) the reported disorders of MA metabolism are an expression of a central MA deficiency, and 2) this deficiency contributes to the development of the depressive syndrome. This assumption raises the question whether this deficiency is of causal importance or is merely a predisposing factor, i.e. a factor which increases the risk that a balance of mood will change in a negative direction under certain less favourable circumstances. Longitudinal studies of the biochemical disorders can provide an answer to this question. If the biochemical disorders gradually disappear with the psychopathological disturbances, then this argues in favour of their causal significance; if they persist after abatement of the depression, then they are more likely to be a predisposing factor.

Few longitudinal studies have so far been made. Their results so far can be summarized as follows. The subnormal HVA response to probenecid returns to normal after normalization of motor activity. The decreased renal MHPG concentration is likewise syndrome-dependent: the phenomenon disappears as the depression disappears. No data are available on MHPG in CSF.

The data on 5-HIAA accumulation in response to probenecid

point in a different direction. In slightly less than 50% of patients with a low pre-therapeutic 5-HIAA response, the response returns to normal after clinical recovery. In the remaining patients the 5-HIAA response does not increase, or not to normal values. The second probenecid test was carried out after the patient had been free from symptoms for six months, and without medication for at least one month (van Praag 1977).

If a persistently decreased 5-HIAA accumulation is indeed a factor predisposing to depressions, then chronic administration of 5-HT precursors might have a prophylactic effect. We studied the prophylactic value of 5-HTP in 5 patients suffering from recurrent vital depressions with a) a high rate of recurrence, and b) a low 5-HIAA response to probenecid during the depressive phase and after clinical recovery. The depression was of the bipolar type in 3 and of the unipolar type in 2 of these patients. They were successfully treated with tricyclic antidepressants and, one month after discontinuation of this treatment, daily administration of 200 mg l-5-HTP and 100 mg of a peripheral decarboxylase inhibitor (MK 486) was started. After a month, the 5-HIAA response to probenecid was found to be quite above normal, demonstrating their ability to convert 5-HTP to 5-HT. No recurrences have so far been observed during a follow-up of one year (Fig. 33). In view of these patients' histories this is a striking result, but it is still to be verified by insertion of placebo periods.

I *conclude* that, at least in a number of patients, the decreased 5-HT turnover seems to have the characteristics of a predisposing factor. It might be the biological expression, so to speak, of the increased tendency of some individuals to respond to threatening endogenous or exogenous stimuli by a pathological deterioration of mood.

10. Four-dimensional psychiatric diagnosis and some of its consequences

The principal conclusion which I have drawn from the data discussed is that disorders of central MA metabolism can play a role in the pathogenesis of depressions. If correct, this conclusion would add a fourth criterion, a fourth dimension, to the three criteria already

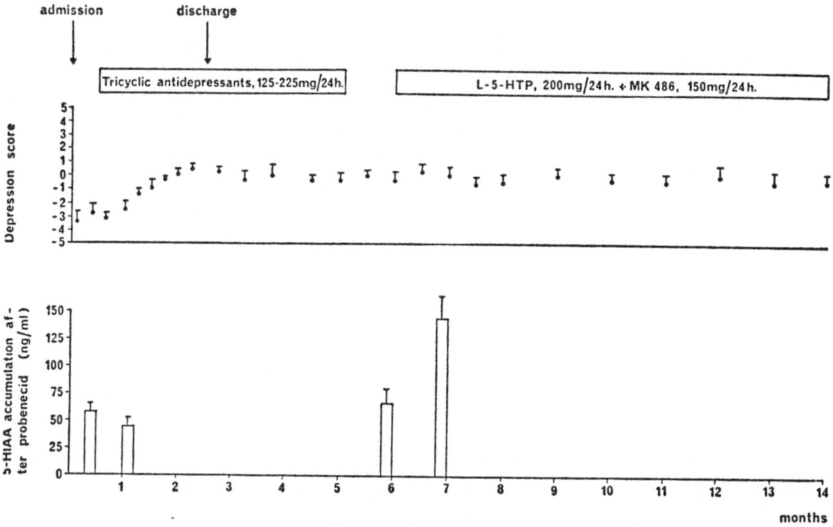

Figure 33. Depression scores and 5-HIAA accumulation in response to probenecid in 5 depressive patients during therapeutic administration of a tricyclic antidepressant and prophylactic administration of l-5-HTP combined with a peripheral decarboxylase inhibitor.

applied in the diagnosis of depression: symptomatology, aetiology and course. This fourth criterion would be pathogenesis, in the sense I have attached to this concept in chapter V. This observation is important for several reasons.

1) In my opinion it heralds the approach of an era in which biochemical variables will come to play a role in the diagnosis and treatment of psychiatric disorders; an era in which physical examination of the psychiatric patient will not be confined to general neurological and medical screening.

2) Today, the training programme of future psychiatrists is still all too often dominated by psychological and sociological approaches. If the above expectation is justified, then equal attention will have to be focused on discussions of the biological determinants of disturbed human behaviour. The subject "biological psychiatry" in the curriculum will then have to comprise more than the knowledge gained from a few talks on prescribing psychotropic drugs.

3) The prototypes of the current psychotropic drugs were all discovered by accident. Their derivatives are not products of

purposeful research, but result from random variations on existing basic structures. If the above discussed metabolic disorders should indeed prove to be of pathogenetic significance, then they might guide the development of new psychotropic drugs. There are unmistakable indications that this change has already begun. For example, the development of selective 5-HT re-uptake inhibitors would not have been undertaken without the theory that a central 5-HT deficiency can play a role in the pathogenesis of depression—a theory based on clinical studies. This means that psychopharmacology has entered a new phase in its development.

11. Conclusions

So far, three criteria have been available for classification of psychiatric syndromes: symptomatology, aetiology and course.

Medicine recognizes a fourth principle of classification: that based on pathogenesis, i.e. the pathological substrate underlying the disease symptoms. This principle can be applied in psychiatry also. I define the pathogenesis of behaviour disorders as the complex of cerebral functional disorders which creates the instrumental conditions for the development of behaviour disorders. While until recently this was merely a theoretical possibility, there are now indications that this principle of classification can be made operational in psychiatry also. As regards disturbed behaviour this applies in particular to the group of the depressions, and as regards the cerebral substrate it applies to MA metabolism.

A survey is presented of disorders of central MA metabolism observed in depressions, and of their diagnostic and therapeutic significance. It is concluded that the existence of two subtypes of vital ("endogenous") depression is likely: a 5-HT-deficient and a NA-deficient subtype. These subtypes cannot be differentiated in psychopathological terms. The distinction is not an "academic" one, but has its consequences for the treatment to be instituted.

It seems probable that this development will not be confined to the depressions and that, in addition to psychological and environmental factors, biological determinants of disturbed behaviour will come to play a role in diagnosis in other psychiatric fields as well. I have no doubt that the reliability and validity of psychiatric diagnoses will increase as a result.

BIBLIOGRAPHY

ÅSBERG, M., L. BERTILSSON, D. TUCK, B. CRONHOLM AND F. SJÖQVIST (1972). Indoleamine metabolites in the cerebrospinal fluid of depressed patients before and during treatment with nortriptyline. *Clin. Pharmacol. Ther.* 14, 277.

ÅSBERG, M., P. THORÉN, L. TRÄSKMAN, L. BERTILSSON AND V. RINGBERGER (1976). Serotonin depression—a biochemical subgroup within the affective disorders? *Science* 191, 478.

BECKMANN, H. AND F. K. GOODWIN (1975). Antidepressant response to tricyclics and urinary MHPG in unipolar patients. *Arch. Gen. Psychiat.* 32, 17.

BOWERS, M. B. JR. (1972). Cerebrospinal fluid 5-hydroxyindoleacetic acid (5-HIAA) and homovanillic acid (HVA) following probenecid in unipolar depressives treated with amitryptyline. *Psychopharmacologia* (Berl) 23, 26.

CARLSSON, A., H. CORRODI, K. FUXE AND T. HÖKFELT (1969a). Effect of antidepressant drugs on the depletion of intraneuronal brain 5-hydroxytryptamine stores caused by 4-methyl- -ethyl-meta-tyramine. *Europ. J. Pharmacol.* 5, 357.

CARLSSON, A., H. CORRODI, K. FUXE AND T. HÖKFELT (1969b). Effects of some antidepressant drugs on the depletion of intraneuronal brain catecholamine stores caused by 4-methyl-α-ethyl-meta-tyramine. *Europ. J. Pharmacol.* 5, 357.

CARLSSON, A., H. CORRODI, K. FUXE AND T. HÖKFELT (1969b). Effects of some antidepressant drugs on the depletion of intraneuronal brain catecholamine stores caused by 4-methyl-α-ethyl-meta-tyramine. *Europ. J. Pharmacol.* 5, 357.

DELEON-JONES, F., J. W. MAAS, H. DEKIRMENJIAN AND J. SANCHEZ (1975). Diagnostic lumbar CSF: The question of their origin in relation to clinical studies. *Brain Res.* 79, 1.

GOODWIN, F. K., R. M. POST, D. L. DUNNER AND E. K. GORDON (1973). Cerebrospinal fluid amine metabolism in affective illness: the probenecid technique. *Amer. J. Psychiat.* 130, 73.

GORDON, E. K., J. OLIVIER, F. K. GOODWIN, T. N. CHASE AND R. M. POST (1973). Effect of probenecid on free 3-methoxy-4-hydroxyphenylethylene glycol (MHPG) and its sulphate in human cerebrospinal fluid. *Neuropharmacology* 12, 391.

GORDON, M. (1974). *Psychopharmacological Agents*. New York, San Francisco, London: Academic Press.

JIMERSON, D. C., E. K. GORDON, R. M. POST AND F. K. GOODWIN (1975). Central noradrenergic function in man: vanillylmandelic acid in CSF. *Brain. Res.* 99: 434.

LLOYD, K. G., I. J. FARLEY, J. H. N. DECK AND O. HORNYKIEWICZ (1974). Serotonin and 5-hydroxyindoleacetic acid in discrete areas of the brainstem of suicide victims and control patients. In: *Serotonin New Vistas. Biochemistry and behavioral and clinical studies*. Vol. 11. (Eds.) E. Costa, G. L. Gessa and M. Sandler. New York: Raven Press.

MAAS, J. W. (1975). Biogenic amines and depression. Biochemical and pharmacological separation of two types of depression. *Arch. Gen. Psychiat.* 32, 1357.

MENDELS, J., J. L. STINNET, D. BURNS AND A. FRAZER (1975). Amine precursors and depression. *Arch. Gen. Psychiat.* 32, 22.

POST, R. M., E. K. GORDON, F. K. GOODWIN AND W. E. BUNNEY JR. (1973). Central norepinephrine metabolism in affective illness: MHPG in the cerebrospinal fluid. *Science* 179, 1002.

PRAAG, H. M. VAN (1974). Therapy-resistant depressions. Biochemical and pharmacological considerations. *Psychother. Psychosom.* 23, 169.

PRAAG, H. M. VAN (1977). *Depression and schizophrenia. A contribution on their chemical pathology*. New York: Spectrum Publications.

PRAAG, H. M. VAN (1977a). Indoleamines in depression. In: *Neuroregulators and hypotheses of psychiatric disorders*. Edited by: J. D. Barchas, D. A. Hamburg and E. Usdin. Oxford University Press.

PRAAG, H. M. VAN (1977b). The vulnerable brain. Biological factors in the diagnosis and treatment of depression. In: *Psychiatric diagnosis*. Edited by: V. M. Rakoff, H. C. Stancer and H. B. Kedward. New York: Brunner/Mazel.

PRAAG, H. M. VAN AND J. KORF (1973). 4-Chloramphetamines. Chance and trend in the development of new antidepressants. *J. Clin. Pharmacol.* 13: 3.

PRAAG, H. M. VAN AND J. KORF (1971). Retarded depression and the dopamine metabolism. *Psychopharmacologia* 19, 199.

PRAAG, H. M. VAN, J. KORF, L. C. W. DOLS AND T. SCHUT (1972). A pilot study of the predictive value of the probenecid test in application of 5-hydroxytryptophan as an antidepressant. *Psychopharmacologia* 25: 14.

SACK, R. L. AND F. K. GOODWIN (1974). Inhibition of dopamine-ß-hydroxylase in manic patients. *Arch. Gen. Psychiat.* 31, 649.

SANO, I. (1972). L-5-hydroxytryptophan (l-5-HTP)-therapie bei endogener depression. *Münch. Med. Wschr.* 144, 1713.

SCHEYEN. J. D. VAN, J. H. VAN PRAAG AND J. KORF (1977). A controlled study comparing nomifensine and clomipramine in unipolar depression, using the probenecid technique. *Brit. J. Clin. Pharmacol.* 4, 1795.

SCHILDKRAUT, J. J. (1975). Depressions and biogenic amines. In: *American Handbook of Psychiatry*, VI. D. Hamburg (Ed.) New York: Basic Books.

SHOPSIN, B., S. WILK, S. GERSHON, K. DAVIS AND M. SUHL (1973). Cerebrospinal fluid MHPG. An assessment of norepinephrine metabolism in affective disorders. *Arch. Gen. Psychiat.* 28, 230.

SHOPSIN, B., S. GERSHON, M. GOLDSTEIN, E. FRIEDMAN AND S. WILK (1975). Use of synthesis inhibitors in defining a role for biogenic amines during imipramine treatment in depressed patients. *Psychopharmacol. Communic.* 1, 239.

SJÖSTRÖM, R. AND B-E. ROOS (1972). 5-Hydroxyindoleacetic acid and homovanillic acid in cerebrospinal fluid in manic-depressive psychosis. *Europ. J. Clin. Pharmacol.* 4, 170.

TAKAHASHI, S., H. KONDO AND N. KATO (1975). Effect of l-5-hydroxytryptophan on brain monoamine metabolism and evaluation of its clinical effects in depressed patients. *J. Psychiat. Res.* 12, 177.

YOUDIM, M. AND K. TIFTON (1976). *Monoamine Oxidase Inhibition*. Elsevier Excerpta Medica, North Holland.

XVII

Lithium

1. Profile of the lithium ion

The lithium ion (henceforth simply referred to as lithium) has a therapeutic effect on states of agitation of a psychotic nature, without exerting an untoward influence on the level of consciousness. In this respect, therefore, its action is similar to that of neuroleptics. However, there are important differences clinically, as well as in animal experiments. To begin with, the range of indications for lithium is well defined, and largely restricted to maniacal agitation. It has no antipsychotic effect in the sense described in chapter VII, and no or hardly any affinity for the extrapyramidal system. As a final difference, I mention the inability of lithium to inhibit conditioned reflexes in test animals. Neuroleptics do have this ability; in fact it is one of their highly characteristic properties, which is utilized in pharmacological screening of neuroleptics. A characteristic difference from the ataractics is that lithium has no or hardly any sedative effect on non-psychotic anxious individuals. Finally, lithium is unique in its prophylactic effect against unipolar and bipolar depressions.

All in all, there are therefore sound reasons for devoting a separate chapter to lithium.

2. History

Modern psychopharmacology is usually assumed to have started in 1952—the year of the discovery of chlorpromazine. This, however, is an error. Three years earlier Cade (1949), an Australian psychiatrist, had discovered lithium as an effective agent against the manic syndrome. The discovery was quite accidental. Cade was interested in the possible importance of metabolic factors in the pathogenesis of manic-depressive syndromes. In this context he studied urea—a compound which induces a state of hyperexcitability in guinea pigs. In an effort to establish whether uric acid potentiates this effect, he administered urea in combination with lithium urate (the most readily soluble urate). Against expectations, this was found not to enhance but to attenuate the excitant effect of urea. Cade noted: "The animals, although fully conscious, became extremely lethargic and unresponsive to stimuli for one to two hours before once again becoming normally active and timid." Lithium carbonate likewise had a protective effect, and from this fact Cade concluded that the lithium ion itself must be responsible for the sedative effect.

In view of the anti-excitant effect, Cade administered lithium to 18 manic patients, obtaining results which he described as "impressive." The manic symptoms disappeared within 7-10 days in all cases. Six schizophrenic patients with symptoms of agitation failed to respond. No effect on depressive symptoms was observed. Cade therefore regarded lithium as a specific agent, with the manic syndrome as its range of indications.

Cade's report should have caused a stir, but did not. I can see two possible causes for this: the first is that a wide variety of sedatives were available at the time, so that no new compounds were really needed. Cade's claim concerning the circumscribed range of indications was not taken seriously, and in fact was not incontrovertibly indicated by the research results. Another possible cause lies in the fact that lithium salts, used in the forties as NaCl substitute in salt-restricted diets, had become discredited because of their toxicity. At the time of Cade's publication, they had just been taken off the market, and the climate was therefore unfavourable for their re-introduction.

Cade discontinued his research. Some of his Australian colleagues confirmed his observations in open studies. Nothing else happened until 1954, when Schou and co-workers in Aarhus resumed this line of investigation (which they have since continued without interruption). They corroborated Cade's observations and found indications that lithium has a prophylactic effect in manic-depressive conditions; in addition they pointed out that: a) lithium is not transformed in the organism, and all its effects must consequently be attributed to the ion itself; b) lithium is not bound to plasma proteins; c) its concentration in serum can be determined without difficulty, and the compound is therefore suitable par excellence for studying the relation between serum concentration and effect. Theirs was a unique series of observations which, in the latter half of the sixties, placed lithium in the centre of psychopharmacological attention.

3. Lithium in mania

Lithium salts are therapeutically effective in the manic syndrome. The best results are obtained if hyperactivity and agitation are not too pronounced and if the symptoms are confined to the affective and motor spheres. In these cases lithium is superior to chlorpromazine. However, if the agitation is vehement and if the syndrome is "impure" (i.e. if it includes symptoms not characteristically found in the manic syndrome, e.g. hallucinatory symptoms, paranoid ideas and disturbed consciousness), then lithium is generally less effective than chlorpromazine. Such mixed syndromes are not infrequently encountered in schizophrenic, schizoaffective and psychogenic psychoses. In the case of agitation based on organic cerebral lesions, too, neuroleptics are to be preferred. This means that lithium has a limited range of indications but, within this range, often produces striking results.

The effect of lithium differs in quality from that of chlorpromazine. Lithium does not merely reduce motor hyperactivity, impulsiveness and irritability. Unlike chlorpromazine and other neuroleptics, it does not act exclusively on the motor root of the manic syndrome, but also has a mood-leveling effect. It attenuates the manic wave over its entire width, so to speak. Chlorpromazine, moreover, often has to be given in high doses in order to arrest manic disinhibition, and inconvenient side effects may consequently occur, neurological (hypokinesia and rigidity) as well as psychological (bradyphrenia, drowsiness, etc.). The side effects of lithium are generally slight and transient.

Why then has not lithium superseded chlorpromazine in the treatment of *all* states of motor hyperactivity? Because Cade's claim concerning the selectivity of lithium in manic conditions proved to be correct. In non-manic agitation, chlorpromazine is superior. Lithium is also unsuitable in the treatment of non-psychotic anxiety and tension.

The butyrophenone derivative haloperidol is an excellent drug in the case of motor agitation, also, if this occurs in the context of mania. In this respect it is even superior to lithium. As pointed out, however, the great advantage of lithium is that it also normalizes the mood.

Lithium has one major disadvantage: as a rule its effect does not become apparent until after a few days or a week. In the case of a florid mania, this interval is too long, for the patient as well as for the environment. In these cases it is advisable to combine lithium, during the first week, with a motor-inhibitory neuroleptic such as haloperidol at a daily dosage of 3 × 1-5 mg orally or intramuscularly. These compounds do not potentiate each other's side effects.

The latter recommendation should be qualified. Cohen and Cohen (1974) described four patients who, during combined lithium/haloperidol medication, developed severe neurological symptoms including a lowered level of consciousness, an increased body temperature and a wide variety of motor changes. The lithium concentration was rather high, although below 2 mEq/l, and the haloperidol dosage was above average in three of the four patients (up to 70 mg per day). The relation to medication has not been established with certainty. Moreover, the combination in question has been tolerated by numerous patients without problems. Nevertheless, prudence is necessary and determined efforts should be made to establish the minimal effective doses.

4. Lithium as a prophylactic agent in the group of manic-depressive conditions

So-called manic-depressive psychosis is a common disease which, if untreated, carries a poor prognosis, the risks of relapse and suicide being substantial. The relapse rate, moreover, increases with increasing age, which means that the duration of the free interval between two phases diminishes.

In any case, the term manic-depressive psychosis is misleading, firstly because the manic and the depressive phases often assume no psychotic form, and secondly because patients who show (hypo)-manic as well as depressive phases (so-called bipolar depression) are a minority versus those who develop only depressive phases (so-called unipolar depression). Unipolar and bipolar depressions also differ in other respects, e.g. family taint, relapse rate and premorbid personality. The concept "manic-depressive psychosis" therefore encompasses at least two different syndromes, and is best avoided.

Curative measures against the depressive phases (antidepressant medication, and EST if necessary) and the manic phases (lithium salts, combined with neuroleptics if necessary, and in severe cases EST) are generally quite effective. Recovery from one phase, however, does not reduce the risk of a subsequent phase. The necessity of preventive treatment is therefore evident, but until recently such treatment was an illusion. Lithium has changed this situation. Although initially disputed, its prophylactic effect can now be regarded as firmly established.

The prophylactic action becomes manifest in two ways. The *frequency* of the depressive as well as of the manic phases diminishes, but the *depth* of the phases diminishes also. This means that the phases occur less often and, if they do occur, are less severe. The prophylactic effect occurs in unipolar as well as in bipolar depressions. It can be expected in some 65% of cases and, contrary to what was initially believed, the chances in bipolar depression are not better than those in unipolar depression.

The question whether lithium is equally effective prophylactically in manic and in depressive phases cannot yet be answered with certainty. Some authors maintain that the effect is most pronounced with regard to manic phases. Others found that manic and depressive phases are equally influenced.

Several methods have been used in research into the prophylactic value of lithium. First of all the classical double-blind placebo experiment: within a group of patients with unipolar and bipolar depressions, the one receives a placebo and the other lithium; or the same patient is given lithium during one period and a placebo during the next. The effects of the two treatments are then compared. Another arrangement calls for a group of patients treated with lithium, which in 50% of the patients is then replaced by a placebo while the follow-up on their condition continues. In a variant of the firstmentioned method, a number of patients were given either lithium or a placebo and the attending physician (unaware of the nature of the tablets) was given the freedom to institute any antidepressant or antimanic treatment he considered necessary, with the exception of lithium. After a certain period, the need for supplementary treatment in the two groups was studied for possible differences.

Table 26 summarizes the results of 8 studies in which lithium was compared with a placebo. The data were taken from the excellent study reported by Davis (1976). It is this type of study that warrants the conclusion that the value of lithium as a prophylactic agent in unipolar and bipolar depressions is beyond doubt.

5. Lithium in depression

Is lithium an antidepressant? The answer to this question has long been uncertain. Some authors denied it, while others were inclined to believe that it was, but their studies were of the "open" type (i.e. without controls) and could have been influenced by wishful thinking; after all, absence of an antidepressant activity would hardly have been consistent with the status of lithium as a prophylactic against manic as well as depressive periods.

Controlled studies have been published only since 1968 and so far indicate that lithium can be active also in depressions. Probably, however, its range of indications differs from that of the conventional antidepressants in that lithium is therapeutically effective especially in depressions with a bipolar course. However, the number of observations is still small. It is unknown, moreover, how the effect of lithium compares with that of the tricyclic antidepres-

Table 26. Effectiveness of lithium versus placebo in preventing relapse (from Davis, 1976).

Study*	Patients in Lithium Group		Patients in Placebo Group		
	Number Relapsed	Number Not Relapsed	Number Relapsed	Number Not Relapsed	Significance**
Baastrup et al.	0	45	21	18	$p=2.0 \times 10^{-9}$
Coppen et al.	3	24	33	3	$p=4.0 \times 10^{-11}$
Hullen et al.	1	17	6	12	$p=4.4 \times 10^{-2}$
Stallone et al.	12	24	27	9	$p=4.0 \times 10^{-4}$
Prien et al. study 1	53	48	94	10	$p=1.0 \times 10^{-9}$
Prien et al. study 2	26	19	36	3	$p=2.6 \times 10^{-4}$
Melia	4	4	7	2	$p=2.46 \times 10^{-1}$
Cundall et al.	7	9	13	3	$p=3.3 \times 10^{-2}$
Persson	11	22	25	8	$p=5.7 \times 10^{-4}$

*Most of the studies used a noncrossover design with random assignment and blind evaluation; however, the study of Cundall et al. used a crossover design, and Persson's study used a matched design (control patients were matched with lithium patients).
**By Fisher exact test.

sants. For the time being, therefore, it is advisable to treat (vital) depressions with (tricyclic) antidepressants.

6. Lithium in atypical manic-depressive syndromes

In view of the success of lithium prophylaxis in unipolar and bipolar depressions, lithium has also been tried out in other psychiatric syndromes with a phasic course, and particularly in conditions known in the USA as schizo-affective psychoses and referred to on the European continent as degenerative psychoses, cycloid psychoses, or schizophreniform psychoses. These patients show affective changes, either of a manic or of a depressive type, as well as symptoms known from the group of schizophrenic psychoses, e.g. delusions, hallucinations, etc. They frequently relapse, spontaneously or in response to psychogenic provocation, and usually recover without personality defects.

Several authors have found that in this category of patients, too, lithium can be of prophylactic value, albeit less pronounced than in unipolar and bipolar depressions. Such patients, if they relapse frequently, undoubtedly provide a good indication for long-acting neuroleptics. The latter's prophylactic efficacy is an established fact. Whether lithium can compete with the long-acting neuroleptics remains to be seen.

There is a limited literature which would seem to indicate that lithium is valuable in the treatment of periodical non-psychotic behaviour disorders in children. In some cases, the course of the condition was suggestive of a manic-depressive condition and/or the family history contained evidence of manic-depressive syndromes. Most of these children were referred to as hyperactive. These reports, however, are not based on sound methods of investigation, and the same applies to many communications on the effect of psychotropic drugs in children. In anticipation of more reliable data, the use of lithium for this indication should be regarded as an experiment.

7. Dosage

General aspects

Lithium is nearly always administered as lithium carbonate—a lithium salt with a relatively low ability to absorb moisture (Calmcolit, Eskalith, Lithane, Lithonate). The margin between therapeutic and toxic dose is narrow. Morever, there is a relation between the lithium concentration in the blood and its clinical (side) effects. For these reasons lithium dosage is determined on the basis of the blood level. The dose required to maintain a given serum level is determined chiefly by the ability of the kidney to excrete lithium. The lithium clearance in a given individual is remarkably constant, but interindividual differences may amount to as much as 100-200%. This means that doses should be determined individually.

A serum concentration of 2 mEq/l must not be exceeded if toxic symptoms are to be avoided. The lithium level is best determined in a fasting patient and 12 hours after the last dose. All values mentioned in this section were determined at this time. The lithium concentration can be measured by emission flame photometry and by absorption flame photometry. Although the latter method is more sensitive and more reliable than the former, emission flame photometry is quife acceptable for clinical purposes. If local laboratory facilities are inadequate, blood samples can be sent elsewhere without undue difficulty for haemolysis does not interfere with the determination.

Lithium carbonate is usually given in tablets three times daily. According to Schou et al. (1970) the 24-hour dose can also be given in two fractions. Such a regimen enhances reliability of ingestion but also increases the risk of side effects, for absorption of lithium in the intestine is not constant, and the serum lithium level therefore shows a peak after each administration. Side effects are observed in particular during these "peak hours." A larger dose means a higher peak, which in turn implies more side effects. Two *slow-release lithium preparations* are commercially available: *Priadel* and *Phasal*. They can be given in a single daily dose, and their gradual absorption reduces side effects. Phasal is believed to be more completely absorbed than Priadel.

There are no fundamental objections to starting lithium therapy or prophylaxis in outpatients, provided they are carefully monitored for side effects and for changes in the serum lithium level. This should be avoided, however, in the following situations:

1) disturbed renal function (lithium is cleared almost entirely by renal excretion);
2) age over 60 (renal function decreases with increasing age);
3) dehydration (reduction of the dilution factor);
4) salt-restricted diet and/or use of thiazide diuretics (sodium deficiency stimulates re-absorption of lithium in the kidney);
5) medication with chlorpromazine, a compound which reduces renal lithium excretion.

Outpatients given lithium medication should be instructed about the early symptoms of lithium intoxication and about the necessity of reporting for examination as soon as these symptoms are noticed. This is a necessary supplement to the periodical determinations of the serum lithium level.

Lithium therapy

Efforts are made to ensure a lithium concentration of 1.5 mEq/l serum, which usually requires daily administration of 1200-2400 mg lithium carbonate (occasionally more: 2400-3000 mg). Higher serum levels do not enhance the therapeutic effect. On the other hand, underdosage should be avoided also. At a serum level of less than 0.8 mEq/l, the effectiveness of treatment probably diminishes quickly. The therapeutic effect usually becomes apparent after 5-10 days.

The initial daily dose is 3 × 400 mg lithium carbonate; larger initial doses often cause nausea, vomiting and diarrhoea. The fasting lithium concentration attains its maximum after 2-4 days, during which period the dosage must not be increased. If the required serum concentration is not attained after 4 days, the dose can be increased by a maximum of 300 mg daily. Initial doses should always be smaller in the five abovementioned situations.

There are indications that the amount of lithium required to attain a given serum level is as much larger as the patient is more manic and that, inversely, lithium tolerance diminishes with subsidence of symptoms. This would imply that symptomatic improvement calls for correction of the dosage.

The serum level should be determined twice weekly until stabilization is attained, and subsequently once a week. If medication is continued prophylactically, then the dosage is reduced (vide infra) and monthly check-ups are sufficient.

Lithium prophylaxis

The required serum level of about 1 mEq/l calls for an average daily dose of 1000-1500 mg lithium carbonate. A suitable initial dose is 3 × 300 mg daily. After a minimum of 4 days, the dose can be increased by a maximum of 300 mg daily. Serum levels below 0.8 mEq/l are probably ineffective or insufficiently effective.

For prophylactic use of lithium following its therapeutic use, a guideline has been given above. If prophylaxis is the primary indication, then the serum level should be determined twice weekly until stabilization, and then once a week. If the level has remained stable for a minimum of 4 weeks, monthly determinations suffice.

If a (hypo)manic phase develops during lithium prophylaxis,

then medication should not be discontinued but in fact the dosage should be increased. A neuroleptic may be prescribed in addition. If a depressive phase develops, then lithium medication is likewise continued, but in combination with an antidepressant. According to Lingjaerde et al. (1974), lithium potentiates the therapeutic effect of tricyclic antidepressants.

At which time should lithium prophylaxis be resorted to? My personal rule of thumb is: after at least three phases requiring clinical treatment in the past 5 years. However, each case has to be individually assessed, and of course the patient's willingness to cooperate also plays an important role.

Lithium prophylaxis, if effective, should be long continued. How long? This question cannot yet be answered with certainty. It would seem logical to say "for life," because the frequency of manic-depressive phases is more likely to increase than to decrease with increasing age. On the other hand, a lifelong regimen of medication can be a heavy burden. This is why I consider it permissible to discontinue medication tentatively and with continued check-ups after a 4-year period without attacks (the duration of this period is an entirely arbitrary choice). I would revise this opinion immediately if it were shown that resumption of lithium medication has a reduced chance of efficacy. In cases in which attacks have decreased in frequency and/or severity but have not disappeared, medication should always be continued. Reduction of the dosage is useless because this would reduce the blood level to below the effective value.

When can one decide to discontinue medication as ineffective? This depends on the phase frequency during the pre-therapeutic period. If during this period the patient relapsed about twice a year or more frequently, then medication should be continued for at least a year before it can be regarded as ineffective. With a lower pre-therapeutic relapse rate, the period of assessment should be increased accordingly.

8. Combination with other psychotropic drugs

Lithium can be combined with a neuroleptic, and in severe manias such a combination is in fact often a necessity, particularly during the first week of medication. Chlorpromazine is less suitable in these cases because it reduces the renal excretion of lithium. In my view a suitable adjuvant is haloperidol at a daily dosage of 3 × 1-5 mg orally or intramuscularly.

Whenever a depressive phase develops during lithium prophylaxis, a tricyclic antidepressant can be prescribed without hesitation, e.g. imipramine or amitriptyline. In that case lithium medication should not be discontinued. A combination of lithium with a MAO inhibitor, too, has so far produced not untoward interactions.

9. Side effects and toxic symptoms

Side effects

These are untoward effects which occur in spite of adequate dosage. During the initial phase of lithium medication, patients may complain of nausea, xerostomia, gastric pain, diarrhoea, fatigue, reduced powers of concentration, a fine tremor in the hand, polyuria and thirst. These symptoms can be alleviated by giving the 24-hour dose in four instead of three fractions. In any case, these symptoms disappear after a few days to maximally 3-4 weeks, with the exception of polyuria and the tremor which can be persistent and inconvenience patients in occupations that require manual dexterity. Anti-parkinson drugs have no effect on this tremor, which according to Kirk et al. (1972) should show a favourable response to propranolol at a daily dosage of 30-80 mg. Kellett et al. (1975), however, were unable to confirm this.

The persistence of recurrence of one of the other symptoms is suggestive of overdosage and calls for (extra) determination of the serum level.

According to Shopsin and Gershon (1975), lithium can in the long run induce a cogwheel phenomenon which, unlike the "genuine" cogwheel phenomenon, fails to respond to anticholinergic anti-parkinson medication. No other extrapyramidal (?) symptoms have been described.

Symptoms of overdosage

These usually occur when the serum lithium level exceeds 2 mEq/l, but occasionally even at lower concentrations. The cause of this higher sensitivity is unknown. Perhaps the intracellular/extracellular lithium distribution in these patients has shifted in favour of the first compartment, leading to a high intracellular concentration at relatively low serum levels. Lithium intoxication as a rule develops gradually (except in the presence of renal damage) and can therefore be recognized in due time. Early identifying signs are the following.

1) Gastrointestinal symptoms, especially anorexia, vomiting and diarrhoea. Vomiting may be violent and is not always accompanied by nausea.
2) Neuromuscular symptoms: muscular weakness; increased fatigability; coarse tremors, particularly in the hands; muscle twitching and slow, sometimes slightly dysarthric speech.
3) Cardiovascular symptoms: decreased pulse rate and ECG changes, e.g. reduction of the QRS complex, flattening of the T-wave and, in some cases, bundle-branch block. No characteristic changes in blood pressure have been reported. The cardiac symptoms are reversible and disappear after discontinuation of medication or adjustment of the dosage.
4) Renal symptoms: polyuria with urine of low specific gravity and complaints of thirst. These symptoms are reversible. There are no reports of permanent renal damage caused in human individuals by lithium overdosage.*

The occurrence of one or several of the abovementioned symptoms calls for immediate determination of the serum lithium level. Interpretation should take into account that the serum level diminishes by about 50% per day after discontinuation of lithium. In previously well-balanced patients, the cause of the decrease in tolerance should be traced (e.g. decreased uptake or increased loss of sodium or fluid; reduced renal function) before the decision to continue lithium medication is made.

---

*There is now suggestive evidence that this statement may be incorrect; that lithium can cause permanent renal damage (J. Hestbech et al., *Kidney International*, in press). This question is now being studied in several centres.

In more advanced stages of intoxication, ataxia develops and there may be some—initially periodical—clouding of consciousness. During periods of decreased consciousness, thinking shows delusional disturbances and sometimes hallucinations occur. In elderly patients such a delirious syndrome can be the first symptom of intoxication.

If lithium intoxication continues unrecognized or if there is an acute overdosage (attempted suicide), then the patient enters (sub)-coma. The muscles become hypertonic, and tremors and fasciculations may occur. The tendon reflexes are intensified. More or less characteristic is intermittent hyperextension of arms and legs, sometimes accompanied by growling and panting, with the eyes opened wide. The attacks last a few seconds (up to 30 sec) and can occur either spontaneously or in response to exogenous (e.g. sonic) stimuli. Epileptic seizures can occur.

Chronic toxicity

Under this heading I shall describe a number of symptoms which can occur after protracted lithium medication in spite of an adequate serum level.

To begin with, lithium can interfere with *thyroid function*. The most common changes are a decreased serum thyroid-stimulating hormone (TSH) concentration and an intensified TSH response after injection of thyrotropin-releasing hormone (TRH). Once present, these changes persist during treatment. The serum concentrations of the thyroid hormones T_3 and T_4 can also decrease, but this change is usually a transient one. Enlargement of the thyroid gland occurs in some 4% of patients, but clinical symptoms of hypothyroidism are rare. In such cases, thyroxine can be administered or medication discontinued or interrupted. Palpation of the thyroid should be a routine monitoring procedure during lithium prophylaxis. Should determination of serum TSH or T_3 and T_4 levels be a routine procedure? I do not think so. These determinations are expensive and the abnormality they disclose is rare. Rather than in routine determinations, guidance should be sought in the patient's clinical condition and the size of the thyroid gland. The thyroid changes are dependent on the presence of lithium and disappear when medication is continued. There have been no reports on irreversible damage to the thyroid.

Further, a number of patients have been described who developed a *disorder of renal function* during adequate lithium prophylaxis, with production of excessive amounts of urine of low specific gravity. There was no other evidence of lithium intoxication. The features resembled those of diabetes insipidus but failed to respond to vasopressin. A renal biopsy specimen showed morphological changes in the distal convoluted tubules (see also note, p. 301). In the patients so far described, renal function returned to normal without residual symptoms after discontinuation of lithium. (In my opinion, this complication necessitates discontinuation of lithium.)

Many patients, finally, show a *weight gain* during protracted lithium medication. According to Vendsborg et al. (1976), the increase amounted to about 10 kg in more than 50% of patients. The weight gain was most pronounced in patients who had been overweight prior to medication. The phenomenon is probably based, not on increased appetite but on increased thirst, which is quenched with high-caloric drinks. The patient should be advised to abstain from such drinks.

Treatment of lithium overdosage

There is no specific therapy. Of course lithium administration must be discontinued, and gastric lavage is indicated if the stomach is likely still to contain a significant amount of lithium. The water and electrolyte balance should be checked and corrected if necessary. Theoretically, infusions of NaCl ought to increase lithium excretion. The amount of NaCl required, however, exceeds the toxic limit. Danish investigators, including Schou (1968), advise administration of osmotic diuretics (e.g. a hypertonic glucose solution or mannitol) in combination with measures to alkalize the urine. In this way it should be possible to double lithium excretion. Haemodialysis is required in serious cases.

It should be borne in mind that an initial fall of the serum level can be followed by another rise as a result of gradual release of intracellular lithium into the blood. Treatment, therefore, should not be stopped too quickly.

10. Contraindications

There are no absolute contraindications to lithium administration. Under certain circumstances, however, lithium medication is less desirable or requires exceedingly careful monitoring. These circumstances are the following.

1) A saltless or salt-restricted diet and/or the use of thiazide diuretics. Since the lithium and the sodium ion compete for the same renal reabsorption mechanism, lithium retention in these cases is abnormally large and the risk of intoxication accordingly high, at least if one omits reducing the dosage in accordance with blood levels.
   Similar considerations apply to situations associated with marked sodium loss, either pathological (high fever) or physiological (excessive sweating during strenuous exercise). In these cases it can be advisable to prescribe some NaCl repletion (about 1-4 g per day).

2) Pregnancy. Until recently, data on the occurrence of teratogenic effects of lithium either in human individuals or in test animals have not been unequivocal. Congenital anomalies can occur in rats and mice, but not in all strains. Similar abnormalities have been observed in "lithium babies," but their frequency was not evidently above the expected rate. It has meanwhile been established with certainty, however, that lithium can be responsible for congenital anomalies of the cardiovascular system. In a group of 120 mothers who had used lithium during the first 3 months of pregnancy, 8 gave birth to children with congenital heart diseases such as ventricular septal defect, mitral atresia, coarctation of the aorta, tricuspid atresia, and Epstein syndrome. This incidence of heart disease is far in excess of the expected, and this applies in particular to the Epstein syndrome which was found in 4 of the 8 lithium babies (the normal incidence in our population is about 1 in 20,000 births [Nora et al. 1974]). Lithium should therefore be considered contraindicated during the first half of pregnancy. Nothing is known about the effect of lithium on breast-fed neonates, but it is advisable to avoid this medication as long as breast-feeding continues.

3) Disorders of renal function. Some 90% of the lithium is eliminated from the organism via the kidneys. Undiagnosed renal insufficiency is a frequent cause of lithium intoxication.

4) Decreased thyroid function. Lithium can reduce the secretion of thyroid hormones and cause decompensation of a marginally functioning thyroid gland (section 9).

11. Precautions

The following laboratory data should be available before lithium is prescribed.

1) Renal function. As already pointed out, decreased renal function increases the risk of intoxication.
2) Thyroid function. In rare cases, long-term lithium medication leads to thyroid enlargement and reduction of thyroid function. Hypothyroidism is not an absolute contraindication to lithium medication, but does call for careful monitoring of thyroid function and, if necessary, correction by substitution therapy.
3) Serum electrolytes. These need to be determined only if a low serum sodium content is suspected; this markedly increases the toxicity of lithium, and medication should not be started until the electrolyte balance has been restored.
4) ECG. Lithium can lead to reduction of the QRS-complex and flattening or inversion of the T-wave. These changes are stable and not progressive. No cases of cardiac decompensation have so far been reported. The cardiac patient who requires lithium should be carefully supervised; the cardiologist should be consulted before it is decided whether medication can be continued.

12. Mechanism of action

As already pointed out in chapter VII, most psychotropic drugs are used for syndromal or symptomatic treatment. Lithium, as used prophylactically, is an exception to this rule. It is used more as an agent against a given disease entity or "morbus" (in this case, manic-depressive disease) or, in more modern terms, against the group of the unipolar and bipolar depressions. This selectivity of action has greatly intensified the interest taken in its mechanism of action. Elucidation of this mechanism can be reasonably expected to enhance our understanding of the pathophysiology of the periodical affective disturbances. There are hypotheses which relate disorders in the cerebral metabolism of catecholamines (noradrenaline and dopamine) and 5-hydroxytryptamine (serotonin) to the disturbances of mood and motor activity observed in (vital) depressions. It is, therefore, logical that many lithium studies focus on the monoamine metabolism in the CNS. Indications have been found that lithium reduces the amount of noradrenaline available at the central postsynaptic receptors by inhibiting its release and increasing its reuptake. The release of serotonin, too, is believed to be reduced.

Considerable research has been devoted also to the influence of lithium on the water and salt metabolism. Lithium supersedes (if incompletely) extracellular (NA^+) and intracellular (K^+) cations and, possibly as a consequence, interferes with various processes in which cyclic AMP is involved. To give an example: the antidiuretic hormone (ADH) from the posterior hypophyseal lobe stimulates the enzyme adenylcyclase in the kidney, causing synthesis of cyclic AMP to increase. It is regarded as likely that lithium inhibits the activity of the ADH-activated adenylcyclase. In the thyroid, too, lithium is believed to interfere with the activity of adenylcyclase, which in this case is activated by the hypophyseal hormone TSH. In this way, less cyclic AMP is produced, and this phenomenon is believed to underlie the reduced secretion of T_4.

It is conceivable that inhibition of hormone-activated adenylcyclase plays a role also in lithium effects on the CNS. In the activation of postsynaptic receptors by such neurotransmitters as acetylcholine, serotonin and the catecholamines, activation of adenylcyclase with increased production of cyclic AMP plays an important role. Another possibility is that the process of neurotransmission is upset because Na^+ ions are replaced by Li^+ ions in the axons.

These brief notes should be sufficient. A survey of this fundamental research is not within the scope of this book, particularly since it has not yet led to a comprehensive understanding of the central actions of lithium.

13. The prophylactic value of tricyclic antidepressants

Finally, let us consider the question whether maintenance therapy with (tricyclic) antidepressants in unipolar and bipolar depressions has a prophylactic effect and, if so, the question of its value as compared with that of lithium prophylaxis. Only imipramine and amitriptyline have so far been studied in this respect. Double-blind comparative studies with a placebo have demonstrated that these antidepressants have a prophylactic effect in *unipolar depressions*. The prophylactic effect of the antidepressant was superior not only to that of the placebo but, according to Paykel et al. (1975), also to that of psychotherapy alone. The latter did improve the level of adjustment between phases but did not prevent the phases. This result is analogous to that reported in psychotics treated with neuroleptics and/or by psychotherapy (chapter VII).

The efficacy of tricyclic antidepressants as compared with that of lithium prophylaxis has not yet been studied. The value of tricyclic compounds in *bipolar depressions* is less certain. They probably prevent depressive but not manic phases. This is why in bipolar depressions lithium prophylaxis is probably to be preferred, partocularly because tricyclic antidepressants can induce manic phases as a side effect. In unipolar depressions, maintenance medication with tricyclic antidepressants certainly merits consideration. For the time being I myself prefer lithium, for this indication also, because our knowledge of the chronic toxicity of tricyclic antidepressants is still imperfect.

14. Conclusions

1) Lithium is a drug with a relatively specific effect. It is therapeutically active in the manic syndrome and, to a lesser degree, in states of agitation of a different nature. Moreover, it regulates motor activity as well as mood; it attenuates the manic wave over its entire width, so to speak.

2) Its principal practical importance lies in its prophylactic effect in manic-depressive syndromes. In an important proportion of cases, it reduces the severity and/or frequency of the phases. This applies both to unipolar (only depressions) and to bipolar (depressive and (hypo)manic phases) forms. There is as yet no certainty that lithium can be equally effective in preventing manic and in preventing depressive phases.

3) Lithium is an important but "difficult" agent. Its therapeutic range is limited, and its toxicity high. Fortunately, dosage can be adjusted to the serum level, and overdosage can

therefore be avoided. One of the reasons for having each lithium patient report regularly for a follow-up is determination of the serum lithium level. Another reason is that suicidal tendencies must be recognized in time, because lithium intoxication is very dangerous. Moreover, with all drugs used over long periods with which experience is still relatively limited, one should beware of chronic toxicity despite an adequate dosage scheme.

The final but certainly not least important reason is that lithium is not a substitute for psychotherapy and social guidance. It reduces affective instability, but of course exerts no influence on the social and psychological factors which threaten to upset the affective balance. These factors should be eliminated or attenuated by psychotherapy and social intervention. The necessity of keeping a close watch on lithium medication affords an excellent opportunity for systematic protracted application of these methods.

4) In my opinion, it is highly recommendable to give the lithium patient his combined therapy (the pretentious term integral therapy is best avoided at this time) at a separate outpatient clinic with a permanent staff, e.g. one physician, one social worker and one nurse, who can thoroughly familiarize themselves with the somatic, psychological and social problems of patients of this type.

In another area of psychiatry, excellent results have been obtained with such a set-up. I am referring to the so-called depot clinics where chronic (recurrent) psychotic patients are regularly treated with long-acting neuroleptics but, for the same money (literally and figuratively), receive psychotherapy and social guidance (chapter VII). In this situation, the relapse rate proved to diminish quite drastically. Analogous to this set-up, specialized lithium clinics have been organized, and already there are convincing indications that they save expense as well as much suffering.

BIBLIOGRAPHY

Baastrup, P., K. S. Poulsen, M. Schou, K. Thomsen and A. Amdisen (1970). Prophylactic lithium: double-blind discontinuation in manic-depressive and recurrent-depressive disorders. *Lancet*, II, 326.

Bakker, K. (1977). *The Influence of Lithium Carbonate on the Hypothalamic-Pituitary-Thyroid-Axis*. Thesis, Groningen.

Baron, M., E. S. Gershon, V. Rudy, W. Z. Jonas and M. Bucksbaum (1975). Lithium carbonate response in depression. *Arch Gen. Psychiat.* 32, 1107.

Bech, P., P. B. Vendsborg and O. J. Rafaelsen (1976). Lithium maintenance treatment of manic-melancholic patients: its role in the daily routine. *Acta Psychiat. Scand.* 53, 70.

CADE, J. F. J. (1949). Lithium salts in the treatment of psychotic excitement. *Med. J. Aust.* 36, 349.
CADE, J. F. J. (1970). The story of lithium. In: *Discoveries in Biological Psychiatry*. Ed. F. J. Ayd, Jr. Philadelphia: Blackwell, pp. 218.
COHEN, W. J. AND N. H. COHEN (1974). Lithium carbonate, haloperidol, and irreversible brain damage. *J. Amer. Med. Ass.* 230, 1283.
COPPEN, A., R. NOGUERA, J. BAILEY, B. H. BURNS, M. S. SWANI, E. H. HAIR, R. GARDINER, AND R. MAGGS (1971). Prophylactic lithium in affective disorders. *Lancet* II, 275.
CUNDALL, R. L., P. W. BROOKS, AND L. G. MURRAY (1972). A controlled evaluation of lithium prophylaxis in affective disorders. *Psychol. Mel.* 2, 308.
DAVIS, J. M. (1976). Overview: maintenance therapy in psychiatry: II. Affective disorders. *Amer. J. Psychiat.* 133, 1.
EDITORIAL (1976). Bioavailability of lithium preparations. *Drug and Therapeutics Bulletin.* 14, 30.
FIEVE, R. R. (1975). The lithium clinic: a new model for the delivery of psychiatric services. *Amer. J. Psychiat.* 132, 1018.
GERSHON, S. AND B. Shopsin (1973). *Lithium: Its Role in Psychiatric Research and Treatment.* New York-London: Plenum Press.
HULLEN, R. P., R. MCDONALD, M. N. E. ALLSOPP (1972). Prophylactic lithium in recurrent affective disorders. *Lancet* I, 1044.
JOHNSON, F. N. (1975). *Lithium Research and Therapy*. New York, London, San Francisco: Academic Press.
KELLETT, J. M., M. METCALFE, J. BAILEY AND A. J. COPPEN (1975). Beta blockade in lithium tremor. *J. Neurol. Neurosurg. Psychiat.* 38, 719.
KIRK, L., P. C. BAASTRUP AND M. SCHOU (1972). Propranolol and lithium-induced tremor. *Lancet* I, 839.
KLERMAN, G. L., A. DIMASCIO AND M. WEISSMAN (1974). Treatment of depression by drugs and psychotherapy. *Amer. J. Psychiat.* 131, 186.
LACROY, G. H. AND H. M. VAN PRAAG (1971). Lithium salts as sedatives. An investigation into the possible effect of lithium on acute anxiety. *Acta Psychiat. Scand.* 47, 163.
LINGJAERDE, O., A. EDLUND, C. A. GORMSEN, C. G. GOTTFRIES, A. HAUGSTAD, I. L. HERMANN, P. HOLLNAGEL, A. MÄKIMATTILA, K. E. RASMUSSEN, J. REMVIG AND O. H. ROBAK (1974). The effect of lithium carbonate in combination with tricyclic antidepressants in endogenous depression. *Acta Psychiat. Scand.* 50, 233.
MELIA, P. I. (1970). Prophylactic lithium: a double-blind trial in recurrent affective disorders. *Brit. J. Psychiat.* 116, 621.
MENDELS, J. (1976). Lithium in the treatment of depression. *Amer. J. Psychiat.* 133, 373.
MINDHAM, R. H. S., D. HOWLAND, AND M. SHEPHERD (1973). An evaluation of continuation therapy with tricyclic antidepressants in depressive illness. *Psychol. Med.* 3, 5.
NORA, J. J., A. H. NORA AND W. H. TOEWS (1974). Lithium, Epstein's anomaly, and other congenital heart defects. *Lancet* I, 594.
PAYKEL, E. S., A. DIMASCIO, D. HASKELL AND B. A. PRUSOFF (1975). Effects of maintenance amitriptyline and psychotherapy on symptoms of depression. *Psychol. Med.* 5, 67.
PERSSON, G. (1972). Lithium prophylaxis in affective disorders: an open trial with matched controls. *Acta Psychiat. Scand.* 48, 462.
PRIEN, R. F., E. M. CAFFEY, JR. AND C. J. KLETT (1973). Prophylactic efficacy of lithium carbonate in manic-depressive illness. *Arch. Gen. Psychiat.* 28, 337.
PRIEN, R. F., C. J. KLETT AND E. M. CAFFEY, JR. (1973), Lithium carbonate and imi-

pramine in prevention of affective episodes. *Arch. Gen. Psychiat.* 29, 420.

SCHOU, M. (1968). Lithium in psychiatric therapy and prophylaxis. *J. Psychiat. Res.* 6, 67.

SCHOU, M., P. C. BAASTRUP, AND P. GROF (1970). Pharmacological and clinical problems. *Brit J. Psychiat.* 116, 615.

SHOPSIN, B., AND S. GERSHON (1975). Cogwheel regidity related to lithium maintenance. *Amer. J. Psychiat.* 132, 536.

SINGER, I. AND D. ROTENBERG (1973). Mechanisms of lithium action. *New Engl. J. Med.* 24, 254.

STALLONE, F., E. SHELLEY, J. MENDLEWICZ (1973). The use of lithium in affective disorders: III. A double-blind study of prophylaxis in bipolar illness. *Amer. J. Psychiat.* 130, 1006.

VENDSBORG, P. B., P. BECH AND O. J. RAFAELSEN (1976). Lithium treatment and weight gain. *Acta Psychiat. Scand.* 53, 139.

XVIII

Stimulants

1. Definition

Stimulants are compounds with a central stimulating effect which becomes manifest mostly in motor activity. They are also known as stimulant amines. Some authors confine the latter term to the amphetamine derivatives, but others use it with reference to all sympathicomimetic compounds with a central stimulating effect.

The stimulating effect of the compounds in question is only one among several effects. They are also anorectics, possibly via an influence on central regulatory mechanisms. They impede initiation of sleep and reduce the depth of sleep. In addition, they produce a whole range of sympathicomimetic effects such as: vasoconstriction (resulting in hypertension), tachycardia, bronchodilatation and mydriasis. Since larger doses are required to produce these additional effects, they are generally not troublesome in actual practice.

The stimulants are usually distinguished from the group of the *analeptics*—compounds which likewise have a stimulant effect but primarily not on motor activity but on centres of the autonomic nervous system, e.g. those involved in regulation of respiration and circulation. They have therefore been used in the treatment of intoxications with barbiturates or other compounds with a central depressant effect. The analeptics include compounds of diverse chemical structure such as: pentylenetetrazole (Metrazole), pentetrazole (Cardiazole), nikethamide (Coramine), cocaine, strychnine and caffeine. However, the boundary between analeptics and stimulants is not sharply defined. Caffeine, for example, can be clinically called an analeptic with as much justification as it can be described as a stimulant. If given in sufficiently large doses, all analeptics in fact behave as stimulants. With the large doses required, however, there is a grave risk of convulsions. On the other hand, parenterally given amphetamine derivatives can serve as analeptics. The group of the analeptics will not be further discussed here.

2. Classification of stimulants

On the basis of their chemical structure, stimulants can be divided into two groups:

1) amphetamine derivatives, i.e. compounds with a phenylethylamine ring: 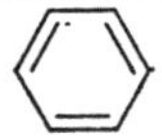 $-CH_2-CH_2-NH_2$;

2) compounds with a piperidine ring: 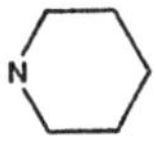

The group of the *amphetamine derivatives* is represented first of all by the oldest known stimulant amine: ephedrine—an alkaloid contained in several plants of the genus Ephedra. For more than 5000 years Chinese medicine has made use of Ephedra vulgaris. An extract from this plant, known as Ma Huang, was used as antipyretic, analeptic and antitussive agent.

In the thirties of this century ephedrine was introduced in the treatment of narcolepsy. Its stimulant effect was feeble, however, and after a few years it was therefore replaced by amphetamine, which was much more effective in this respect. This compound had been synthesized at the end of the 19th century, but its stimulant effect remained unnoticed until it was reported by Alles in 1933.

Table 27. Amphetamine derivatives

Chemical structure	Generic name	Trade name	Average daily oral dose in mg
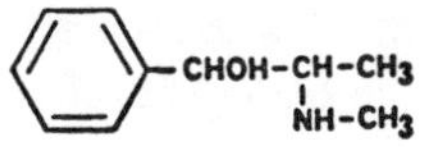 1-phenyl-2-(methylamino)-propanol-1	Ephedrine	–	–
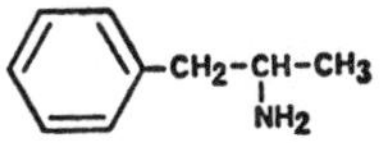 1-phenyl-2-aminopropane	d,l-Amphetamine	Benzedrine	5-20
As amphetamine	Dextro-amphetamine	Dexedrine	5-20
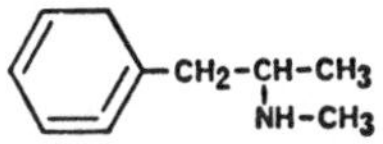 1-phenyl-2-(methylamino)-propane	Methamphetamine	Desoxyn Methedrine Pervitin	3-12

The principal amphetamine derivatives used as stimulants are the following (Table 27):

1) amphetamine

2) dextro-amphetamine

3) methamphetamine.

Amphetamine is a racemic mixture, dextro-amphetamine is the dextrorotatory isomer of this compound, and methamphetamine is its methyl derivative.

If given for the stimulant effect, amphetamine as well as dextro-amphetamine is given by mouth in a daily dose of 5-20 mg. If reduction of the depth of sleep is required (in enuresis nocturna), then about 5 mg is given shortly before turning in. Methamphetamine is the strongest of the three amphetamine derivatives: 5 mg corresponds to about 8 mg (dextro-)amphetamine.

The *stimulants with a piperidine ring* are synthetic compounds of relatively recent date. They differ from the amphetamine derivatives in three ways: they are less euphoretic (which may reduce the risk of addiction), they exert less influence on appetite, and their peripheral sympathicomimetic activity is less marked. Their side effects are consequently less disturbing, but their stimulant effect equals that of the amphetamines. The principal compounds of this group (Table 28) are:

1) Methylphenidate, of which the daily oral dose is 20-30 mg.

2) Pipradol, of which the daily oral dose is 3-7.5 mg.

3. Clinical effects of stimulants

Stimulants reduce fatigue and increase the clarity of consciousness, which results in an increased degree of alertness. In addition

Table 28. Stimulants with a piperidine ring

Chemical structure	Generic name	Trade name	Average daily oral dose in mg
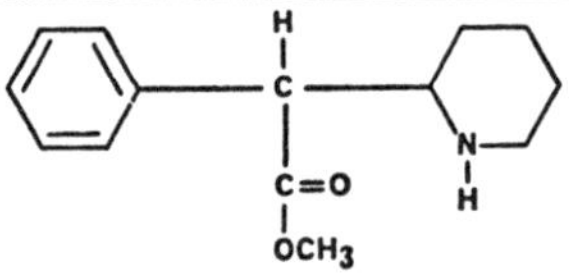 phenyl-(2-piperidyl) acetic acid methyl ester	Methylphenidate	Ritalin	20-30
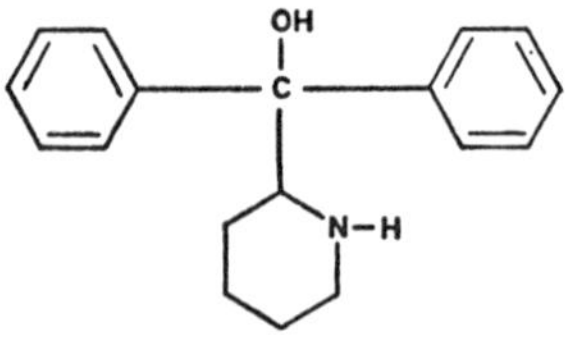 2-piperidyl-benzhydrol	Pipradol	Meratran Alertol	3-7.5

there is an increase in motor activity; motor performance is stimulated in a quantitative sense, but only if for some reason performance has suffered (as a result of fatigue, depressed mood, etc.). The limit of performance is not changed, but depressions in performance are corrected, at least in part—the habitual level is not, as a rule, reached again. The quality of performance cannot be improved with stimulants. In terms of actual practice, therefore, performance is not better than normal in response to these agents, but a given performance can be continued longer than normal. The stimulant effect on endurance has led to abuse in certain sports ("doping").

The effect of stimulants on affective life is not very pronounced, not constant and not protracted. The most common effect is a degree of euphoria, with increased self-confidence and resoluteness and some loss of self-criticism; but a more dysphoric change of mood may also occur.

With most of these compounds, the stimulant effect lasts 4-6 hours, after which the user feels tired and depressed—"done in," as they say. Fatigue is a physiological alarm signal of the organism. To disregard it with the aid of stimulant amines can lead to exhaustion.

4. Dangers and side effects

"Trips" and their dangers

Prescribing stimulants entails considerable risks. The principal risk simply lies in the fact that these drugs are brought into circulation. Medical channels can readily develop "leaks." I am alluding to the fact that, in the past decades, stimulants have become fashionable as a means to become "high." For this purpose, much larger doses are generally used than those required for the traditional stimulant effect, up to hundreds of milligrammes per "trip," often given parenterally. A "trip" that turns out well involves a state of euphoria and increased clarity of consciousness. All sorts of details are perceived with unusual clarity, and intensity of experience is enhanced. This applies both to exogenous impressions (colours seem to have become more vivid, sounds more melodious, shapes more baroque, etc.) and to the world of inner experience. Sexual feelings, for example, can be intensified as well as prolonged. The scope of consciousness can also increase, in which case the periphery can be so obtrusive that concentration on a particular subject becomes difficult. In brief: amphetamine derivatives can produce states which show a striking resemblance to those provoked by LSD.

A bad "trip," on the other hand, involves dysphoric states with feelings of anxiety, or manifest aggressiveness, or combinations of these. In some cases a paranoid psychosis develops: the patient hears voices, feels threatened, and can become very panicky. Since consciousness remains unclouded, these states can show marked similarities to paranoid forms of schizophrenia.

Anxiety states and dysphoria provoked by stimulants respond very well to treatment with ataractics, e.g. 10-20 mg diazepam intramuscularly, repeated after 30-60 minutes if necessary. Amphetamine psychoses generally disappear quickly after administration of neuroleptics, e.g. 50-75 mg chlorpromazine or 2-5 mg haloperidol, both by intramuscular injection, repeated after an hour if necessary. Once the acute symptoms abate, the medication can be continued with oral doses for one to a few weeks.

The "true" amphetamine psychosis, characterized by paranoid delusions while consciousness remains unclouded, is usually caused by acute parenteral administration of large doses of stimulants. Chronic abuse can lead to the development of delirious syndromes with a lowered level of consciousness and disorders of orientation, perception (hallucinations, illusions) and cognition (delusions). Apart from the intoxicating factors, chronic lack of sleep and deficient nutrition (due to anorexia) may play a role in this context. Treatment consists of withdrawal of amphetamines and administration of neuroleptics.

Habituation and addiction

Habituation to stimulants develops quickly (within a few weeks); this means that a given dose becomes less and less effective, and that ever-increasing doses are required in order to obtain a given stimulant effect. Addiction to these agents, moreover, is also a very real danger. By addiction I mean a state of chronic or intermittent intoxication produced by repeated use of a given drug, and characterized by psychological and/or physical dependence on this drug. *Psychological dependence* means that the craving for this drug is overwhelming and uncontrollable. *Physical dependence* means that the organism has adjusted itself to the state of chronic intoxication so that a (pathological) equilibrium has been established. If in such cases the drug is abruptly withdrawn, a series of so-called withdrawal symptoms develop which differ with different drugs and which in some cases can assume a vitally dangerous character. A withdrawal course is therefore always a clinical procedure. The phase of abstinence after abuse of stimulants is characterized by an intensive feeling of weakness, despondency, irritable dysphoria, tremors and gastrointestinal disorders.

Not infrequently, addiction to stimulants is associated with addiction to narcotics. The hangover which develops when the narcotic drug has lost its effect is alleviated with the aid of stimulants in such cases. The resulting insomnia in turn causes the patient to resort to the narcotic drug again. A disastrous vicious circle can result. The problem of addiction and its treatment will be discussed in chapter XXIII.

Side effects

The other inconveniences of amphetamine use are nothing if compared with the above. Sleep disturbances are a common occurrence even if the stimulant is not used after 1500 hours, as prescribed. Restive, tense people can enter a state of dysphoria. In other cases anxieties may be provoked or actualized. In these cases one readily resorts to a sedative. Combined specifics are in fact commercially available (e.g. *Drinamyl*).

Since the central stimulant effect of these compounds exceeds their peripheral sympathicomimetic activity, symptoms such as increased blood pressure, increased pulse rate, constipation and dilatation of the pupils are not too troublesome in actual practice, always assuming that the proper dosages are not exceeded. The influence of stimulants on the appetite, however, becomes manifest even when they are used in therapeutic doses. With the exception of massive doses, amphetamine derivatives exert no influence on the convulsion threshold.

5. Are there still indications for stimulants?

The use of amphetamine derivatives in the treatment of depressions dates back to the years shortly before World War II. As antidepressants, however, these compounds have never been successful. There are several reasons for this. The main reason is that they exert little influence on pathologically depressed mood, whereas their psychomotor activating effect can be very pronounced but is of only short duration. Activation while affective life remains uninfluenced increases the suicide risk. Moreover, the stimulant effect is often followed by a degree of exhaustion. Add the risk of habituation and addiction (reason to limit medication with these compounds to at best a few weeks), and it becomes understandable that they became obsolete soon after the introduction of antidepressants. A positive reason for the obsoleteness of these compounds is the fact that, in controlled studies, they were found to be inferior to tricyclic antidepressants (Overall et al. 1962; Wheatley 1969).

Stimulants are contraindicated in inert, apathetic patients of the chronic schizophrenic group. In these patients the use of stimulants entails a substantial risk of reactivating various anomalies of perception and experience (e.g. hallucinations and delusions). It is also possible that inactivity disappears, but only to be replaced by motor agitation and anxiety.

In principle, the stimulant effect of these compounds could be of some incidental use in healthy individuals of whom a more-than-normal effort is required within a well-defined time span. On the basis of the dangers discussed in the preceding section, however, prescription of stimulants for this indication is absolutely to be discouraged.

Amphetamine derivatives have been used in nocturnal enuresis, on the assumption that sleep is so deep that a full bladder is insufficient as a waking stimulus. The stimulants are used in an attempt to reduce the depth of sleep. In view of the rapidly developing tolerance, however, the efficacy of this treatment is very doubtful. There have been no reports on addiction to these compounds in preadolescent children.

To put it briefly: the range of indications for stimulants has really become very small. Their use is still justifiable only in the following conditions: a) narcolepsy; b) control of the hypnotic effects of certain anti-epileptic agents; c) treatment of children with a hyperkinetic syndrome (an indication discussed in detail in chapter XXV); d) as adjuvant to narco-analytic (or thiopental) treatment. For the lastmentioned purpose, both methamphetamine and methylphenidate have been recommended. Intravenous administration of 5-10 mg of either of these compounds is believed to potentiate the disinhibiting effect of the narcotic. The rationale of narco-analytic treatment is briefly explained on page 354.

6. Anorexigenic agents

Stimulants with a piperidine ring demonstrate the possibility of suppressing the anorexigenic effect without changing the central stimulant effect. The same has been achieved in reverse, resulting in compounds used mainly as anorexigenic agents. The principal representatives of this category are: phentermine (Mirapront), chlorphentermine (Lucofen), phenmetrazine (Preludin), and facetoperanum (Lidepran). The first two are amphetamine derivatives, while the last two are compounds with a piperidine ring.

My only purpose in discussing these compounds here is to point out that, although the stimulant effect of these anorexigenic agents has been reduced, it has not disappeared. A compound such as phenmetrazine, for example, is a potentially addictive drug.

BIBLIOGRAPHY

Alles, G. A. (1933). Comparative physiological actions of dl-β-phenylisopropylamines; pressor effect and toxicity. *J. Pharmacol.* 47, 339.

Cameron, J. S., P. G. Specht and G. R. Wendt (1965). Effects of amphetamine on moods, emotions and motivations. *J. Psychol.* 61, 93.

Connell, P. H. (1958). *Amphetamine Psychosis.* London: Chapman and Hall.

Freed, H. (1958). The use of Ritalin intravenously as a diagnostic adjuvant in psychiatry. *Amer. J. Psychiat.* 114, 944.

Garattini, S. and E. Costa (Eds.) (1970). *Amphetamines and Related Compounds.* New York: Raven Press.

Overall, J. E., L. E. Hollister, A. D. Pokorny, J. F. Casey and G. Katz (1962). Drug therapy in depressions: controlled evaluation of imipramine, isocarboxazide, dextroamphetamine-amobarbital, and placebo. *Clin. Pharmacol.* 3, 16.

Praag, H. M. van (Ed.) (1972). Amphetamine derivates. *Psychiat. Neurol. Neurochir.* 75, 163.

Praag, H. M. van (1968). Abuse of, dependence on and psychoses from anorexigenic drugs, in: Drug Induced Diseases, *Excerpta Medica Foundation* 3, 281.

Sjöqvist, F. and M. Tottre (1969). *Abuse of Central Stimulants*. New York: Raven Press.

Wheatley, D. (1969). Amphetamines in general practice: Their use in depression and anxiety. *Seminars in Psychiatry* 1, 163.

PART FOUR

Pharmacotherapy of Neurotic Changes and Other Personality Disorders

The Moisture of our Air, the Variableness of our Weather (from our situation amidst the Oceans), the Rankness and Fertility of our Soil, the Richness and Heaviness of our Food, the Wealth and Abundance of the Inhabitants (from their universal Trade), the Inactivity and sedentary Occupations of the better Sort (among whom this Evil mostly rages), and the Humour of living in a great, populous and consequently unhealthy Town, have brought forth a Class and Set of Distempers, with atrocious and frightful symptoms, scarce known to our Ancestors, and never rising to such fatal Heights, nor afflicting such Numbers in any other known Nation. These nervous Disorders being computed to make almost one third of the Complaints of the People of Condition in England.

George Cheyne. The English Malady: or a treatise of nervous disorders of all kinds, as spleen, vapours, lowness of spirits, hypochondriacal and hysterical distempers, etc. G. Strahand and J. Leahe, London 1733.

XIX

Ataractics I: General Part

1. Definition

Ataractics are compounds with a tranquillizing, relaxant effect, which is to say they are sedatives. Unlike the classical sedatives, however, they exert little influence on clarity of consciousness and intellectual performance. Although they are not hypnotics in the strict sense of the word, ataractics with their relaxant effect can greatly facilitate natural sleep. In the *absence* of anxiety and tension, ataractics in therapeutic doses are usually somnifacient.

Ataractics differ from neuroleptics in the following respects:

1) They have no antipsychotic effect.
2) They exert little or no influence on the level of initiative.
3) They have no affinity for the extrapyramidal system.
4) Their influence on central vegetative regulatory mechanisms is small. Hypotension in particular rarely is a problem.

Even when given in large doses, ataractics do not become

neuroleptics, but instead behave more like hypnotics. They are alternatively known as *anxiolytics* because, more selectively than the classical sedatives, they resolve feelings of anxiety and tension. Another synonym is *minor tranquillizers*—a terminology in which neuroleptics are known as major tranquillizers, and ataractics and neuroleptics are lumped together as tranquillizers.

2. Classification

On the basis of their chemical structure, four groups of ataractics can be distinguished:

1) Substituted dioles (prototype: meprobamate).
2) Diphenylmethane derivatives (prototype: hydroxyzine).
3) Benzodiazepine derivatives (prototype: chlordiazepoxide).
4) Tricyclic and tetracyclic compounds (so far with two representatives: benzoctamine and opipramol).

The benzodiazepines are undoubtedly the most widely used ataractics. The first two groups are no longer much used in psychiatric pharmacotherapy; their importance is mostly historical. The last-mentioned group is chronologically the youngest. In chemical structure, these compounds are related to the tricyclic and tetracyclic antidepressants, but the claim that they are ataractics with antidepressant properties has not been adequately documented. They nevertheless merit greater attention than they have so far received. All ataractics entail a risk of addiction, whereas addiction to antidepressants is exceedingly rare. It is, therefore, worthwhile to establish whether the tricyclic and tetracyclic central ring has reduced the addictive potency of these ataractics.

There is a *fifth group of ataractics*, classified not according to chemical structure but on the basis of biochemical action. They are the so-called beta-blockers. The use of these compounds as ataractics is of recent date, and experience with them has been limited. This development seems promising, however, because there are some indications that they combat anxiety and tension on two fronts: peripheral as well as central.

3. Pharmacology

In animal experiments, potential antidepressants and neuroleptics can be recognized with a fair degree of probability. More or less characteristic of (tricyclic) antidepressants, for example, are the following effects: inhibition of spontaneous motor activity in combination with increased irritability; antagonism of reserpine and tetrabenazine effects; potentiation of various catecholamine effects and central anticholinergic activity. A compound tested is probably a neuroleptic if it: provokes catalepsy, antagonizes the effects of amphetamine and apomorphine, and inhibits conditioned reflexes, including conditioned flight reactions.

There is no such thing as a more or less reliable battery of screening tests for ataractics. Whether a compound will produce ataractic effects in a human individual cannot be predicted with confidence on the basis of the results of animal experiments. In other words: the principal effects of ataractics in test animals are not specific, as will be shown in the following enumeration (which is limited to the benzodiazepines, but their action profile is not markedly different in quality from that of the other ataractics).

Muscle-relaxant effect

This property is based on inhibition of so-called interneurons. To explain this briefly: the afferent impulse which enters the spinal cord reaches the motor anterior horn cell either directly (monosynaptic reflex, e.g. knee tendon reflex) or via one or several interposed neurons, the so-called interneurons (polysynaptic reflex, e.g. flexion and extension reflexes). The compounds under discussion block the interneurons, and therefore the polysynaptic reflexes. This results in reduction of muscle tonus. With larger doses, the monosynaptic reflex arc can be interrupted as well.

Because of their influence on spinal impulse conduction, these compounds are used not only as sedatives but also as muscle relaxants in hypertonic states of pyramidal or myogenic origin. Evidently their sedative effect cannot be (exclusively) explained by inhibition of spinal reflexes, but suggests an influence on a higher central nervous level.

Anticonvulsant effect

Convulsions caused by strychnine or by electro-shocks are attenuated or prevented. This is why a compound like diazepam has come to occupy such a prominent position in the treatment of epilepsy, more specifically in that of status epilepticus. It is to be noted that neuroleptics, on the other hand, have epileptogenic properties.

Anti-aggressive effect

Aggression is inhibited. Pugnacity diminishes even though the animals are not sedated. This applies both to "naturally aggressive" animals and to those made aggressive, e.g. by isolation or by lesions of certain parts of the brain (septum pellucidum).

Anti-anxiety effect

A state perhaps to be compared with human anxiety can be induced in test animals by placing them in a conflict situation. A hungry animal quickly approaches food offered but, if it is then punished by an electric shock, the speed at which it approaches food and the frequency of its approaches diminish. In response to ataractics, speed and frequency increase again, probably because they reduce the fear of the punitive shock.

No inhibition of conditioned flight reactions

This is a negative characteristic (the inhibitory effect is typical of neuroleptics).

4. Biochemical action mechanism

Benzodiazepines

Whereas there are well-documented and verifiable theories on the biochemical action mechanism of antidepressants and neuroleptics, the biochemical substrate of the ataractic effects is still almost entirely obscure. I can therefore be brief about it, and confine myself to mentioning a few lines of research.

In view of the great interest taken in the relation between central monoamines (MA) and behaviour, the benzodiazepines have been studied in this context. Evidence has been obtained of their influences, not so much on the absolute MA concentration as on the MA turnover. These compounds reduce the turnover of noradrenaline (NA) as well as that of dopamine (DA) and serotonin (5-HT), and they reduce the stress-induced increase in central NA turnover. Barbiturates, however, have virtually the same activity, and the particular therapeutic "profile" of the benzodiazepines is therefore not explained by it. Moreover, the changes in MA metabolism occur only if the benzodiazepines are given in large doses.

A second line of research is that into the influence of benzodiazepines on central GABA (gamma-aminobutyric acid) and glycine neurons. GABA, which is present in large parts of the CNS, is believed to be a transmitter with an inhibitory effect which is thought to be based on two mechanisms (Fig. 34):

1) depolarization of presynaptic nerve endings and inhibition of transmitter release from the synaptic vesicles (a mechanism known as presynaptic inhibition);
2) hyperpolarization of the postsynaptic membrane, reducing the chance that an in-coming depolarizing impulse evokes an action potential (postsynaptic inhibition).

Benzodiazepines are believed to potentiate effects of GABA-ergic neurons. This effect is believed to be involved in at least three benzodiazepine activities: a) muscle relaxation; b) anticonvulsant activity (it is at least a certainty that reduced availability of GABA is a convulsant factor); c) ataxia, which can be a side effect of benzodiazepines given in large doses. The lastmentioned effect is believed to be based on intensified postsynaptic inhibition in the cerebellum. Whether the anxiolytic effect is related to enhanced GABA activity is unknown.

Like GABA, glycine is considered to be an inhibitory transmitter chiefly localized in brain stem and spinal cord. Glycine neurons are believed to reduce the excitability of the postsynaptic membranes (i.e. to hyperpolarize them). In this respect they correspond with GABA neurons. Unlike the latter, however, they do not de-

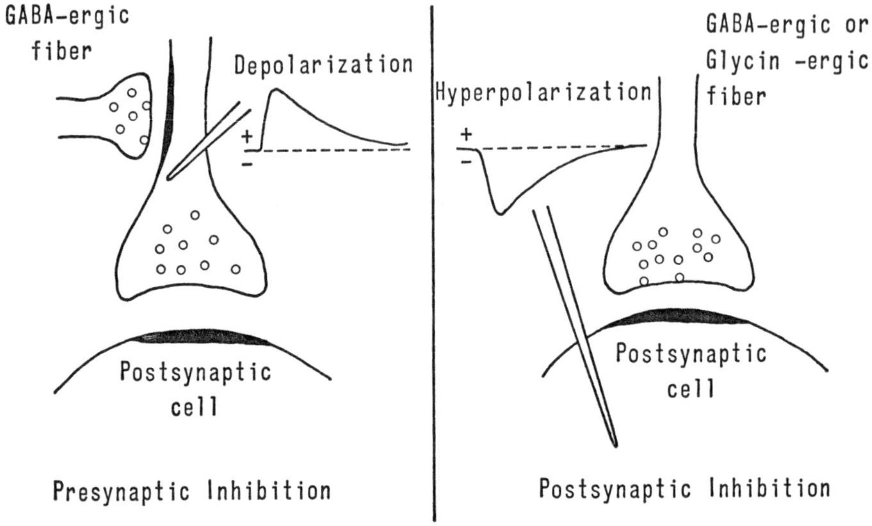

Figure 34. Schematic representation of presynaptic inhibition (*left*) (GABA-ergic fibres) with depolarization of terminal afferents to postsynaptic cells, and postsynaptic inhibition (*right*) with hyperpolarization of postsynaptic cells produced by glycinergic and GABA-ergic axon terminals (according to Costa et al. 1975).

polarize the presynaptic terminals. There are indications that benzodiazepines can activate the postsynaptic glycine receptors; the significance of this ability for their clinical effects is now under investigation.

Beta-blockers

On the basis of pharmacological criteria, the receptors of the peripheral sympathetic nervous system are divided into those of the "alpha" and those of the "beta" type. These criteria will not be discussed here. Suffice it to say that beta-receptors are present in abundance in heart, skeletal muscles, blood vessels and bronchial muscles, and that their stimulation at these sites leads to an increased pulse rate, increased myocardial contractility, dilatation of muscular vessels, and bronchodilatation.

Beta-blockers block peripheral β-adrenergic receptors and, so far as they reach them, central noradrenergic receptors. They are thought to exert little influence on the central dopaminergic systems. These compounds have been in use for some considerable time in internal medicine: in hypertension, angina pectoris and arrhythmia. It has recently become clear that there is a psychiatric indication as well: anxiety, specifically if the clinical picture is dominated by associated somatic manifestations such as palpitations, tremors, precordial pseudo-anginous pains, diarrhoea, etc. These compounds can also be useful in combating incidental tensions produced by anticipation of a particular performance and with an untoward effect on the quality of this performance (e.g. an examination to be passed, a speech to be delivered, etc.). It is to be noted, however, that clinical experience with these agents is still rather limited.

The anxiolytic effect of these compounds probably has two roots. The first is peripheral block of sympathetically innervated functions which have become over-activated. Such "anxiety equivalents" can deeply alarm the patient and, in turn, become a source of anxiety and tension. The second root could be reduction of the activity of central noradrenergic systems. Little is known about this possible action component. In any case, not all beta-blockers enter the brain: propranolol does, for example, but practolol practically does not. It seems plausible a priori that a beta-blocker which combines a peripheral with a central action should be superior as an anxiolytic to one which has only a peripheral action.

5. Indications

Uncertainties

Ataractics are used in states of anxiety and tension of a nonpsychotic nature. They are unsuitable as a therapeutic in psychoses (apart from an occasional indication, still to be discussed), because they exert little influence on seriously disturbed cognitive and experiential modalities, and because in terms of their influence on psychomotor agitation they are also inferior to neuroleptics.

In spite of this restriction, ataractics cover an ample range of indications—a range so wide that in fact it can be described as vague. In principle, they cover the entire field between psychosis and normality; and it is precisely this field that has so far been only very inadequately charted in psychopathological terms. The abundance of aetiological theories in this context contrasts sharply with the primitiveness of the syndromal classification.

Anxiety and neurosis

Anxiety is an essential symptom of the neuroses. In psychoanalytic theory it is interpreted as an alarm signal which anticipates imminent danger. This danger can be from outside or from inside and in the latter case may be either conscious or unconscious. Interpreted as an inside danger is imminent manifestation of suppressed, unacceptable impulses.

Anxiety can be consciously experienced. It can also be unconscious and manifest itself in symptoms which appear to bear little or no relation to anxiety, e.g. conversion phenomena, various somatic complaints (palpitations, pseudo-anginous pains, moist hands, sweating, gastric symptoms, frequent micturition, etc.) and compulsive symptoms. Such manifestations are interpreted as attempts to prevent the development of manifest anxiety. This is very obvious so far as compulsive symptoms are concerned. Whenever the patient is hampered in the execution of his ritual activities, he can become panicky. "Anxiety equivalents" are as a rule experienced as unpleasant and lead the patient to the doctor's office.

Consciously experienced anxiety can be linked to a particular situation (e.g. agoraphobia), to a particular object (e.g. phobic fear of knives), or not linked to any particular situation or object. In the former two cases the word phobia is appropriate, while the lastmentioned type of anxiety is described as "free-floating." The former types of anxiety can be avoided, but the latter type is unavoidable. Free-floating anxiety can either be permanent or occur intermittently in "bursts" which last from a few minutes to several days. If such bursts of anxiety are accompanied by somatic symptoms which as such are alarming (e.g. dyspnoea, palpitations and paraesthesias), then anxiety usually assumes the character of mortal fear (panic attacks). Such attacks of panic can be preceded by hyperventilation.

Anxiety control is more than symptom control

Ataractics can be prescribed in non-psychotic syndromes with manifest anxiety or if it is suspected that anxiety generates the symptoms. If one succeeds in reducing anxiety, one has done more than simply control the symptoms. One has done more for several reasons. 1) Anxiety focuses the attention of the person who experiences it on the origin of the anxiety (so far as this is known, or partly known). This in turn intensifies the anxiety. In this manner anxiety potentiates itself; and, inversely, reduction of the anxiety reduces the activity of the "anxiety generator." 2) "Anxiety equivalents," e.g. somatic symptoms, can as such inspire anxiety and this potentiates the original anxiety. 3) Reduction of the anxiety level enables the patient to be less anxious in coping with a situation which, in principle, inspires anxiety. When the threat does not materialize, he can gradually learn to be less hasty in activating the alarm signal (anxiety). To phrase it differently: reduction of the anxiety produces (some) extinction of the anxiety "reflex."

Limitations of treatment with ataractics

The above arguments are not by any means intended to suggest that ataractic medication could be regarded as a superior form of neurosis treatment. It is not. Treatment of neuroses should focus in principle on elimination of the source of anxiety and tension, and only psychotherapy is a suitable means of achieving this. Within the context of a psychotherapeutic approach, however, ataractics can be useful adjuvants. Moreover, it is no more than realistic to recognize that: a) not all neuroses can be effectively treated by the types of psychotherapy now available; b) there are simply not enough trained psychotherapists to meet the demands. While ataractics may be second choice in these cases, for the patient with his disabling symptoms a second choice is better than none.

When, exactly, are ataractics indicated? There are no generally valid guidelines, but they certainly should not be prescribed too readily. Transiently increased tension in a normal personality structure is generally no more an indication for ataractics than a common respiratory infection is an indication for antibiotics. The use of ataractics can be contemplated if: a) chronic anxiety is present; b) anxiety is acutely evoked and the patient's defence threatens to be insufficient; c) psychotherapy or social intervention is not likely quickly to lead to a solution to the problems. These agents should be used with great prudence in the treatment of individuals with addictive tendencies.

Before prescribing ataractics, the purpose of the prescription should be discussed with the patient in realistic terms. He must not expect a miracle drug, nor should he regard the prescription as a "sop." The medication is intended as a means to bridge a period of increased anxiety and tension. It is important to stress that the medication is temporary: a "course of treatment" of limited duration, e.g. one or two months. If this is omitted, it may be difficult to discontinue the medication—which is the more risky because habituation and addiction to ataractics can develop.

Nothing is known with certainty about the specificity of these compounds, i.e. the question whether a particular ataractic has a better effect on a particular anxiety syndrome than another ataractic. I do not mean to say that such differences do not exist, but the question has not yet been systematically studied. What is worse: they can hardly be studied in the absence of a reliable syndromal classification.

It is therefore not surprising that the results of ataractic medication are variable: success in the one patient and failure (against expectation) in the other; a given patient can prove to show no response to one ataractic and a good response to the other. Pharmacokinetic factors probably play a role in this respect. There are indications that the blood concentration of an ataractic in a given dose differs widely from one individual to the next, and that a given minimum concentration is required to obtain a therapeutic effect. For the time being, therefore, prescribing ataractics is a matter of trial and error.

Finally, ataractics are *not* antidepressants, even though they can have a favourable effect on the mood. The latter effect, however, is secondary to their relaxant, anxiolytic effect. Primary improvement of the mood, as produced by antidepressants, cannot be achieved with ataractics.

As explained in chapter VII, neuroleptics are not indicated in neurotic states of anxiety and tension, unless they are given in very small doses (in which case their effect can be compared with that of an ataractic).

Benzodiazepines and alcohol abstinence

Benzodiazepines, more specifically chlordiazepoxide and diazepam, are successfully being used in the treatment of delirium tremens and its prevention after acute withdrawal of alcohol. For this indication they are usually given in large doses, parenterally to begin with and subsequently by mouth. Other withdrawal symptoms such as anxiety, motor unrest and somatic manifestations (e.g. nausea and vomiting) also commonly show a favourable response to these agents.

Which of the two benzodiazepines is to be preferred has not been established with certainty. Diazepam has a more marked sedative and somnifacient effect than chlordiazepoxide. It is the compound of choice in the case of severe restiveness and markedly disturbed sleep. The fact that its anticonvulsant potency is higher is another advantage in these cases.

The net therapeutic effect of benzodiazepines in delirium tremens is probably not superior to that obtained with neuroleptics, but it starts surprisingly quickly (often within 6-12 hours) and is not accompanied by many side effects.

Benzodiazepines and sleep disorders

Benzodiazepines are effective hypnotics which influence the sleep pattern in several ways. They can increase the total duration of sleep, shorten the period required to attain sufficient depth of sleep, reduce the frequency of interruption of sleep, and improve the subjectively experienced quality of sleep. Sleep phases 3 and 4 are usually shortened (at least if benzodiazepine medication is protracted), but the amount of REM sleep is hardly influenced, and no REM rebound occurs upon withdrawal.

The benzodiazepine derivatives flurazepam and nitrazepam are prescribed exclusively as hypnotics. Benzodiazepines used as ataractics, however, can also favourably influence sleep via their general relaxant effect. Benzodiazepines are prescribed in all kinds of sleep disorders: difficulty in getting to sleep, restless sleeping and early awakening.

Since benzodiazepines suppress phase 4 sleep, Fisher et al. (1973) tested diazepam (5-20 mg before bedtime) in patients suffering from nightmares (which are believed mainly to occur in phase 4). This treatment was successful: the complaints disappeared after 1-2 weeks and the compound remained effective for a considerable time.

Benzodiazepines have advantages over barbiturates: much lower toxicity; no suppression of REM sleep; no or much less REM rebound; no enzyme induction; less quickly addictive. Some authors consequently believe that barbiturates are obsolete as hypnotics.

Indications outside clinical psychiatry

Diazepam in particular has been used as an anticonvulsant. In status epilepticus, whether of the grand mal or of the petit mal type, intravenously injected diazepam is regarded as a very effective compound.

The muscle-relaxant effect of ataractics, more specifically of benzodiazepines and meprobamate, is utilized in conditions with increased muscle tonus, of myogenic or of central origin. These agents may also be considered in tetanus.

Benzodiazepines are also frequently used to reduce acute situational tensions, e.g. in patients who anticipate an operation or a disagreeable (e.g. endoscopic) examination. In these cases the compound—often diazepam—is given intravenously about 30 minutes before the intervention. In principle, preoperative administration of a benzodiazepine has a dual advantage: the anxious patient feels calmer, and consequently he needs a smaller dose of anaesthetics. Premedication with, say, barbiturates has the disadvantage that respiration and circulation are much more influenced and that the respiratory depressant effects of anaesthetics are potentiated. Benzodiazepines are valuable also in (non-psychotic) postoperative agitation and restiveness. In the surgical clinic, diazepam is by far the most widely used benzodiazepine. Very few comparative studies with other ataractics are available.

6. Dosage

Ataractics, like all psychotropic drugs, require individualized dosage. The optimal dose of a given compound can vary in different patients by as much as factor 10. We do not know exactly why this is so. The nature of the syndrome can play a role, as well as the characteristics of the patient's personality, the setting in which the compound is given, and the expectations of patient and/or therapist. Perhaps the complex of pharmacokinetic factors is the most important factor. A given dose leads to different steady-state blood concentrations in different individuals, and a relation has been established between blood concentration and therapeutic efficacy. Routine determination of blood concentrations, however, is precluded by the complexity of the chemical methods.

In view of these considerations, it is advisable to start with a small dose, which can then be gradually increased on the basis of the ratio between therapeutic effect and side effects. The distribution of the dose in fractional doses through the day also requires flexibility. Benzodiazepines have a fairly long half-life (12-30 hours), and therefore leave the organism slowly. Moreover, the metabolites of some compounds (e.g. diazepam) are active whereas those of others (e.g. oxazepam) are inactive. This, of course, also influences the duration of action. For these reasons, it may be advisable to deviate from the three-times-per-day rhythm. For example, if sleep disorders are prominent a twice-per-day scheme should be used, with the main dose before turning in and the remainder after awakening. This scheme is also of advantage if the patient is much troubled by side effects. Another possibility is that the patient is only instructed about an upper limit and given freedom to distribute the dose as he thinks best.

When a rapid effect is required, it should be borne in mind that different benzodiazepines have different intestinal absorption times. Chlordiazepoxide is absorbed slowly (peak blood concentration only after a few hours), whereas diazepam is absorbed quickly (peak blood concentration after about an hour).

The duration of action of meprobamate is relatively short: it is eliminated fairly quickly (half-life about 10 hours) and its metabolites are pharmacologically inactive. In this respect it is superior to most of the benzodiazepines, and also to the barbiturates. Urinary excretion of 50% of a given dose of pentobarbital (one of the "short-acting" barbiturates) takes about 50 hours. The peak blood concentration of orally given meprobamate is attained after 1-2 hours.

The effect of ataractics generally becomes apparent after one to a few days. One need not wait 3-4 weeks before the effect can be evaluated, as in the case of neuroleptics and even more so with antidepressants. Combining ataractics makes no sense: the side effects are more likely to be potentiated than the therapeutic effects.

So far as we know, ataractics can be combined with other types of drugs without problems. A widely used combination is that of an antidepressant with a benzodiazepine derivative in the treatment of agitated vital depressions. There are also commercial specifics which contain amitriptyline as well as chlordiazepoxide (Limbatril, Limbritol), but personally I prefer to adjust the doses of the two compounds separately.

7. Side effects and toxic effects of benzodiazepines*

Somatic symptoms

Benzodiazepines have only slight side effects and are of low toxicity, which is a great advantage in terms of practical application. During the first few days to weeks of medication, patients not infrequently complain of fatigue, "weak legs" (possibly due to hypotonia of the muscles) and diminished powers of concentration. The lastmentioned effect can be a hazard for motorists, particularly during long, monotonous drives. They should be warned accordingly!

Larger doses can lead to a sensation which the patient describes as "dizziness." However, no revolving sensations are involved but rather a "floating" sensation which is intensified by postural changes and has proved not to be based on orthostatic hypotension. These sensations may be of central origin, and diminished tonus of the striated muscles may also play a role. Be this as it may, this phenomenon is inconvenient and, particularly for outpatients (motorists!), not without danger. In some cases it disappears spontaneously, but in others it persists until the dosage is reduced. Disorders of coordination with an atactic gait and impeded speech are likewise observed only after large doses, which in fact approximate the toxic limit.

---

*The side effects of the other ataractics are discussed in chapter XX.

As regards other side effects described (e.g. nausea, headache, diminished libido, vertigo, menstrual disorders), it is uncertain whether these are in fact side effects of benzodiazepines or features of the anxiety syndrome per se. Allergic symptoms and bone marrow inhibition can develop, but are exceedingly rare. The effect of benzodiazepines on blood pressure and cardiac function is minimal, and they can be prescribed for cardiac patients without undue risk.

Benzodiazepines potentiate the effect of other compounds with a central depressant activity. Potentiation of alcohol effects is the most important in view of its practical implications. The patient should be properly cautioned against this danger.

Habituation and addiction

Habituation and addiction are a less grave problem than might be expected in view of the activity of these compounds. Habituation (the need for larger doses in order to obtain the same effect) is uncommon, but the risk increases as the doses given and the duration of treatment increase. The same applies to addiction (dependence). Such dependence as develops is largely of a psychological nature: the patient becomes mentally unable to do without his tablets. Physical dependence—withdrawal symptoms after discontinuation of treatment—is uncommon. When a compound with active metabolites is involved, withdrawal symptoms develop not immediately after discontinuation but a few days later. Withdrawal symptoms so far described are: agitation, insomnia, vomiting, ataxia, tremors and convulsions. After protracted medication it is advisable gradually to withdraw benzodiazepines.

Psychological side effects

Two paradoxical psychological side effects have been described: increased aggressiveness and increased anxiety and agitation. I should like to make some marginal notes in this context. a) The available documentation is based on casuistry; in double-blind comparative studies these side effects have not been demonstrable (Rickels and Downing 1974); if real, therefore, they must be rare. b) It has not been established whether these are true side effects of the medication or results of failure of the medication. c) It is conceivable that, rather than true side effects, an indirect relation between psychological symptoms and medication is involved. As regards the aggression: it may be that the lowering of the anxiety level "unlocks" repressed agression, much as alcohol can do. As regards the paradoxically increased agitation: when the patient feels (over)sedated and has less grip on his defence mechanisms, secondary feelings of insecurity and anxiety could result.

Overdosage

The central symptom of overdosage with benzodiazepines is a reduced level of consciousness, ranging from somnolence to coma. Respiration, pulse and blood pressure generally are no problem unless massive doses are taken. In the case of mild intoxication there is retardation of motoricity, dysarthria, ataxia and sometimes diplopia. Treatment is symptomatic: gastric lavage is necessary, prevention of respiratory obstruction, monitoring of pulse, blood pressure and ECG, and maintenance of fluid balance. In some cases, some agitation occurs during the phase of recovery; this should not be combated with barbiturates.

Interaction with other drugs

The only dangerous combination is that with other central depressants (alcohol!) which potentiate the depressant effect. Enzyme induction in the liver does not occur in response to benzodiazepines. With barbiturates, this is a notorious problem: they stimulate in liver microsomes the activity of enzymes which degrade other agents (including anticoagulants). Patients receiving anticoagulant medication can be given benzodiazepines without undue risk.

Contraindications

Myasthenia gravis and ataxia can be regarded as the only true contraindications.

BIBLIOGRAPHY

BERGER, F. M. (1970). Anxiety and the discovery of the tranquillizers. In: *Discoveries in Biological Psychiatry*, (F. J. Ayd and B. Blockwell, Eds.) pp. 115-129, Philadelphia: Lippincott.

BERGER, F. M. (1975). Therapeutic uses of meprobamate and the propanediols. In: *Drug Treatment of Mental Disorders*, pp. 91-107. New York: Raven Press.

BOOKMAN, P. H. AND RANDALL, L. O. (1975). Therapeutic uses of the benzodiazepines. In: *Drug Treatment of Mental Disorders*, pp. 73-90. New York: Raven Press.

BROWN, J. H., D. E. MOGGEY AND F. H. SHANE (1972). Delirium tremens: A comparison of intravenous treatment with diazepam and chlordiazepoxide. *Scott. Med. J.*, 17, 9.

COSTA, E., A. GUIDOTTI, C. C. MAO AND A. SURIA (1975). New concepts on the mechanism of action of benzodiazepines. *Life Sci.* 17, 167.

DASBERG, H., E. VAN DER KLEIJN, P. J. R. GUELEN AND H. M. VAN PRAAG (1974). Plasma concentrations of diazepam and of its metabolite N-desmethyl-diazepam in relation to anxiolytic effect. *Clin. Pharmacol. Ther.* 15, 473.

DASBERG, H. AND H. M. VAN PRAAG (1974). The therapeutic effect of short-term oral diazepam treatment on acute clinical anxiety in a crisis centre. *Acta Psychiat. Scand.* 50, 326.

DIMASCIO, A. (1973). The effects of benzodiazepines on aggression: Reduced or increased? *Psychopharmacologia* 30, 95.

FISHER, C., E. KAHN, A. EDWARDS AND D. DAVIS (1973). A psychophysiological study of nightmares and night terrors. *Arch. Gen. Psychiat.* 28, 252.

GARATTINI, S., E. MUSSINI AND L. V. RANDALL (1973). *The Benzodiazepines*. New York: Raven Press.

GREENBLATT, D. J. AND R. I. SHADER (1972). The clinical choice of sedative-hypnotics. *Ann. Intern. Med.* 77, 91.

GREENBLATT, D. J. AND R. I. SHADER (1974). *Benzodiazepines in Clinical Practice*. New York: Raven Press.

JEFFERSON, J. W. (1974). Beta-adrenergic receptor blocking drugs in psychiatry. *Arch. Gen. Psychiat.* 31, 681.

KATZ, R. L. (1972). Drug therapy: Sedatives and tranquillizers. *N. Engl. J. Med.* 286, 757.

KOCH-WESER, J. AND E. M. SELLERS (1971). Drug interactions with coumarin anticoagulants. *N. Engl. J. Med.* 285, 487 and 547.

PRAAG, H. M. VAN (1975) *Research in Neurosis*. Amsterdam: Bohn, Scheltema, Holkema.

RICKELS, K. AND R. W. DOWNING (1974). Chlordiazepoxide and hostility in anxious outpatients. *Am. J. Psychiat.* 131, 442.

SCHALLEK, W., W. SCHLOSSER AND L. O. RANDALL (1972). Recent developments in the pharmacology of the benzodiazepines. *Adv. Pharmacol. Chemother.* 10, 121.

SHAND, D. F. (1975). Propranolol. *New Eng. J. Med.* 293, 280.

SMITH, R. B., L. W. DITTERT, W. O. GRIFFEN, JR. AND J. T. DOLUISIO (1973). Pharmacokinetics of pentobarbital after intravenous and oral administration. *J. Pharmacokinet. Biopharm.* 1, 5.

TICKTIN, H. E. AND N. P. TRUJILLO (1968). Further experience with diazepam for preendoscopic medication. *Gastrointest. Endosc.* 15, 91.

TORNETTA, F. J. (1965). Diazepam as preanesthetic medication. *Anesth. Analg.* (Cleve.) 44, 449.

WINSTEAD, D. K., A. ANDERSON, M. K. EILERS, B. BLACKWELL AND A. L. ZAREMBA (1974). Diazepam on demand: Drug-seeking behavior in psychiatric inpatients. *Arch. Gen. Psychiat.* 30, 349.

XX

Ataractics II: Specific Part

Effects and side effects of the ataractics as a group were discussed in the preceding chapter. This chapter deals with the individual compounds, that is to say: with some prototypes of the principal groups. It is unnecessary to describe all compounds in a given group because they differ hardly, if at all, in terms of effect. The heading "Particulars" is exclusively devoted to deviations from the general action profile discussed in the preceding chapter.

1. Benzodiazepines (Table 29)

Chlordiazepoxide (Librium)

Chemical structure. 7-chloro-2-methylamino-5-phenyl-3H-1,4-benzodiazepine-4-oxide hydrochloride.

Dosage. The daily oral dose is 10-50 mg. When used as a hypnotic, 5-20 mg is given 30 minutes before retiring. Large parenteral doses are administered in delirium tremens: 50 mg by intramuscular

Table 29. Some benzodiazepine derivatives

Chemical structure	Generic name	Trade name	Average daily oral dose in mg
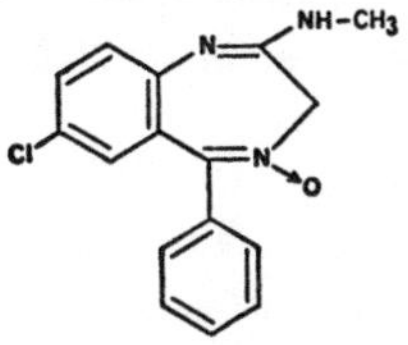	Chlordiazepoxide	Librium	10-50
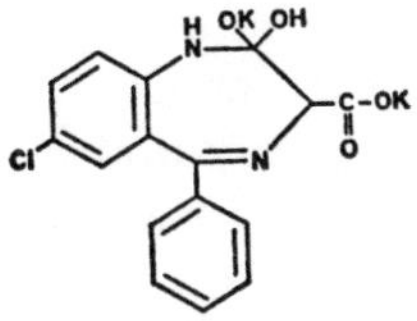	Chlorazepate	Tranxene Tranxilium	15-60
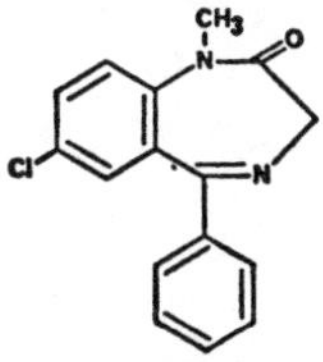	Diazepam	Levium Stesolid Valium	6-30
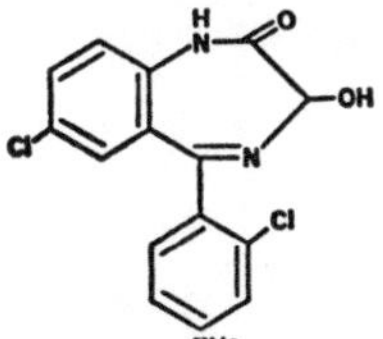	Lorazepam	Ativan Tavor Temesta	2-5
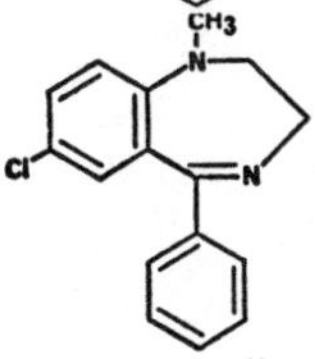	Medazepam	Nobrium	10-30
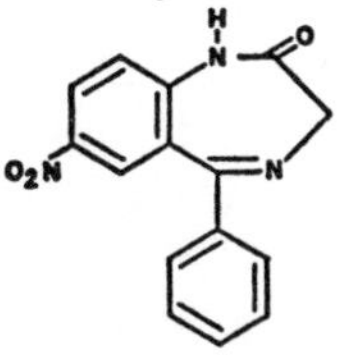	Nitrazepam	Mogadon Mogadan	5-10
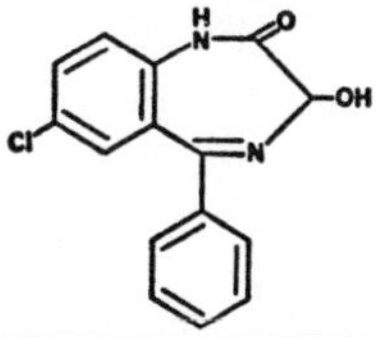	Oxazepam	Adumbran Serax Seresta	20-60

injection, to be repeated after 30-60 minutes if necessary, up to a maximum of 300 mg/24 hours. In very severe cases the first injection may be given intravenously, but only very slowly and only in a clinical setting in view of the risk of respiratory depression. Once the symptoms of the delirium abate, medication is continued by mouth, with the parenterally used doses, for a few days; the dosage is then reduced on the basis of the clinical condition.

Particulars. Chlordiazepoxide is the father of all benzodiazepines and was introduced in clinical psychiatry in 1960. Its side effects after oral administration are only slight, as described in the preceding chapter. Large parenteral doses produce more frequent and more severe side effects. One should beware in particular of muscular weakness, gastrointestinal symptoms, disturbed coordination and hypotension. This is why it is advisable to confine the patient to bed during a course of injections.

Combined preparations are *Limbritol* and *Limbatril* (chlordiazepoxide combined with amitriptyline) and *Librax* (chlordiazepoxide combined with clinidium bromide, a spasmolytic).

Diazepam (Levium, Stesolid, Valium)

Chemical structure. 7-chloro-1-methyl-5-phenyl-1,4-benzodiazepine-2(1H)-on.

Dosage. The daily oral dose is 6-30 mg. As a hypnotic, this compound is given 30 minutes before retiring in a dose of 5-10 mg. Parenteral administration (intramuscular or slow intravenous injection) is indicated in delirium tremens, acute states of anxiety or tension, and status epilepticus. In delirium tremens 10-20 mg is given intramuscularly, and the injection can be repeated after 30-60 minutes if necessary, up to a maximum of 60 mg/24 hours. It is possible to institute treatment by a slow intravenous injection (at a rate of 1 ml/minute or slower).

In acute anxiety and tension (e.g. after a "bad trip" or by way of sedation before a disagreeable medical intervention), 10 mg is given intramuscularly (this dose can be repeated twice at 30-minute intervals).

In status epilepticus, 10 mg diazepam is given by slow intravenous injection; this can be repeated at 30-minute intervals up to a maximum of 60 mg/24 hours. As soon as possible, intravenous injection is replaced by intramuscular injection, and the latter by oral administration.

Particulars. Diazepam has a more marked sedative and hypnotic effect than chlordiazepoxide. Somnolence is quite common during the first days to weeks of medication. We do not know whether diazepam or chlordiazepoxide should be preferred in the treatment of delirium tremens, or whether these compounds are therapeutic equivalents.

If large doses are given, and particularly if they are given parenterally, it is advisable to confine the patient to bed (in view of possible hypotension and disorders of coordination). With moderate oral doses this risk is very small. Parenteral administration of diazepam calls for a clinical setting in view of possible respiratory depression.

Other benzodiazepine derivatives frequently used as ataractics are the following.

Clorazepate (Tranxene, Tranxilium). In the body this compound is converted to demethyldiazepam and oxazepam. It is probably to these two metabolites that clorazepate owes its efficacy. It is given orally in a daily dose of 15-60 mg.

Lorazepam (Tavor, Temesta) is given orally in a daily dose of 2-5 mg. Used as a hypnotic, 1-2.5 mg is given 30 minutes before retiring.

Medazepam (Nobrium) is given orally in a daily dose of 10-30 mg; its sedative and muscle-relaxant effects are believed to be less pronounced than those of diazepam.

Oxazepam (Adumbran, Serax, Seresta) is an active metabolite of diazepam which is given orally in a daily dose of 20-60 mg.

The differences between the various benzodiazepines, so far as demonstrated, are small and of no therapeutic significance.

There are two benzodiazepine derivatives which are used, not as ataractics but *exclusively* as hypnotics. They are the following.

Flurazepam (Dalmadorm, Dalmane). The average oral dose is 30 mg (15-60 mg), to be taken 15 minutes before retiring. It is reported to shorten the time required to attain depth of sleep, and to lengthen the total duration of sleep.

Nitrazepam (Mogadan, Mogadon), of which 5-10 mg is given orally 30 minutes before retiring, is available in liquid and in tablet form. It has been recommended both against difficulties in going to sleep and against difficulties in continuing sleep.

Two questions are urgent: a) are these compounds, as hypnotics, really superior to the other benzodiazepines, and b) can they be used as ataractics, like the other benzodiazepines? The data required to answer these questions are not available.

2. Substituted dioles (Table 30)

Meprobamate (Equanil, Miltown, Sedapon)

Chemical structure. 2-methyl-2-propyl-1,3-propanediole dicarbamate.

Dosage. Meprobamate is given orally (tablets, powder or draught). The therapeutic range of the compound is considerable. The average daily dose is 400-1200 mg, but doses up to 2-3 g are tolerated without undue problems. The medication should be discontinued gradually because acute withdrawal may give rise to withdrawal symptoms: nausea, vomiting, convulsions, agitation or even delirious symptoms.

Particulars. Prior to the introduction of chlordiazepoxide, meprobamate was by far the most popular ataractic. It derives from mephenesin, a compound introduced as a muscle relaxant shortly after World War II. When it was found that mephenesin had sedative properties as well, efforts were made so to alter the molecule that duration and intensity of the sedative effect were enhanced. Meprobamate is a result of these efforts.

Like the benzodiazepines, meprobamate has a relaxant effect on striated muscles and also has anticonvulsant properties. However, it has not been introduced in the treatment of epilepsy.

Dizziness is a common complaint in the initial phase of medication, and usually disappears spontaneously. Hypersensitive reactions, particularly of the skin, are a common occurrence. Only large doses lead to any significant decrease in blood pressure, and atactic symptoms can also occur in those circumstances, along with hyperperistalsis of the intestine with diarrhoea. There have been no reports on liver damage, and bone marrow damage has been very rare.

Table 30. Other ataractics

Chemical structure	Generic name	Trade name	Average daily oral dose in mg
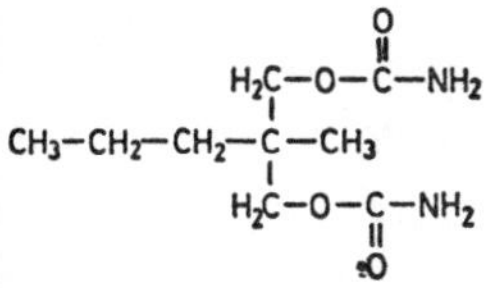	Meprobamate	Equanil Miltown Sedapon	400-1200
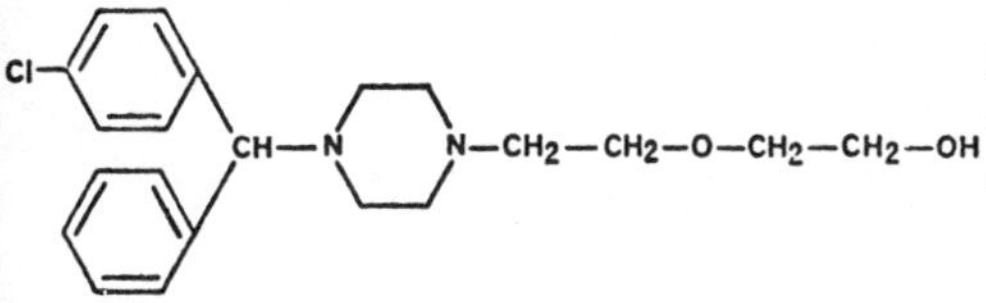	Hydroxyzine -hydrochloride -pamoate	Atarax Masmoran Vistaril	60-200
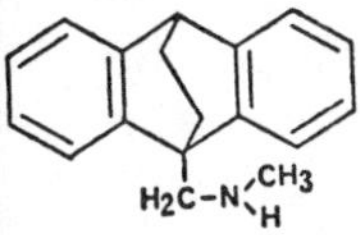	Benzoctamine	Tacitin	10-30
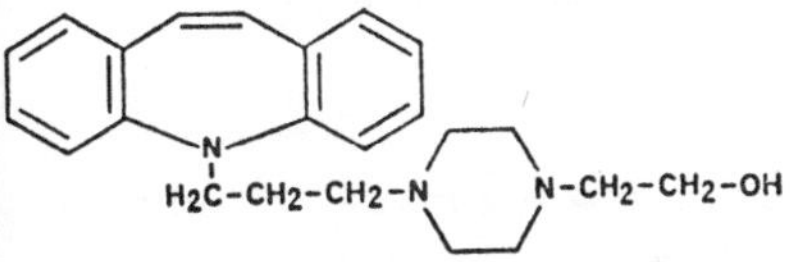	Opipramol	Ensidon Insidon	75-250
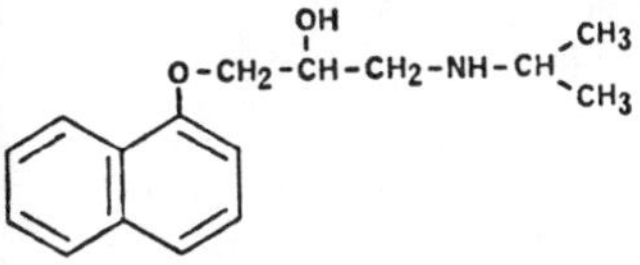	Propanolol	Inderal	40-160

Meprobamate potentiates the effects of alcohol and impairs motoring performance. The risk of addiction is believed to be greater than that with benzodiazepines.

Acute overdosage leads to loss of consciousness and hypotension. Tendon reflexes are absent, the muscles show marked hypotonia and the pupils are dilated and unresponsive to light. Convulsions are sometimes observed. Treatment is the same as that of intoxication caused by hypnotics.

Meprobamate is contained in numerous combined preparations. Chemically related compounds are *mebutamate* (Dormate) and *tyba-*

mate (Solacen, Tybatran); the former is used as a hypnotic, and the latter as an ataractic.

3. Diphenylmethane derivatives (Table 30)

The compounds of this group combine sedative with histamine-antagonistic and spasmolytic properties. The latter effects can be of advantage in the treatment of psychosomatic disorders.

Hydroxyzine hydrochloride (Atarax)

Chemical structure. 1-p-chlorobenzhydryl-4-[2-(2-hydroxyethoxy)-ethyl]piperazine dihydrochloride.

Dosage. The daily oral dose is 60-200 mg.

Particulars. Hydroxyzine is a mild sedative which, with its relatively low toxicity, can also be used in treating the emotional instability of old age. Some authors obtained good results with large doses of hydroxyzine (up to 300 mg per day) in brain-damaged children with hyperkinetic symptoms.

As pointed out, the side effects are only slight. The main side effects are dizziness and xerostomia (hydroxyzine is an anticholinergic). The former side effect usually disappears spontaneously after a few days to weeks. Overdosage can lead to hypotension and delirious symptoms.

Another hydroxyzine derivative is *hydroxyzine pamoate* (Vistaril, Masmoran), given in the same doses and with the same effects as hydroxyzine hydrochloride.

4. Tricyclic and tetracyclic ataractics (Table 30)

Benzoctamine (Tacitin)

Chemical structure. N-[(dibenzo(b,e)bicyclo-(2,2,2)octa-2,5-diene-1-yl)-methyl]-N methylamine.

Dosage. The daily oral dose is 10-30 mg.

Particulars. Benzoctamine is closely related chemically to the tetracyclic antidepressant maprotiline. Biochemically and pharmacologically, however, it clearly differs from the action profile of the antidepressants. It differs also from the benzodiazepines, e.g. in that it lacks a muscle-relaxant effect. The relation between benzoctamine and benzodiazepines in therapeutic terms has not been properly studied. Information on its addictive potency is likewise inadequate.

Side effects are mild, and usually limited to sensations of fatigue during the first few days, xerostomia and gastrointestinal symptoms.

Opipramol (Insidon)

Chemical structure. 4-[3-(5-5H-dibenz(b,f)azepinyl]-1-piperazinyl-2-ethanol.

Dosage. The daily oral dose is 75-250 mg.

Particulars. This compound is chemically related to the tricyclic antidepressants, but it is used as an ataractic. The claim that it also has antidepressant properties has not so far been adequately documented. Its side effects are mild, and usually limited to sensations of fatigue and tachycardia during the first few days, and xerostomia—a phenomenon to which the patient usually does not become accustomed. The agent has no muscle-relaxant effect.

5. Beta-blockers (Table 30)

Propranolol (Inderal)

Chemical structure. 1-isopropylamino-3-(1-naphthyloxy)-2-propanol.

Dosage. When used as an ataractic, propranolol is prescribed in a daily dose of 40-160 mg.

Particulars. This agent is particularly effective when anxiety is manifested mostly in somatic symptoms. Whether it is superior to the more conventional ataractics for this indication has not been adequately studied. If anxiety is experienced mostly in psychological terms, propranolol is probably no more effective than a placebo. Of the many somatic anxiety equivalents, functional cardiac symptoms have been most thoroughly studied. These are phenomena such as palpitations and disagreeable sensations in the cardiac region ("cardiac awareness") in the absence of organic changes. In the literature, this syndrome is found under a variety of names, e.g. hyperkinetic heart syndrome, hyperdynamic β-adrenergic circulatory state, irritable heart syndrome, neurocirculatory asthenia, Da Costa syndrome, cardiophobia, soldier's heart, effort syndrome and cardiac neurosis. This syndrome is a good indication for beta-blockers.

Propranolol has been recommended also for the treatment of withdrawal symptoms in patients addicted to alcohol, amphetamines and heroin. These claims have not been adequately substantiated.

Hypotension and bradycardia are the principal side effects. Prudence is advisable with asthmatic patients because beta-blockers can cause increased resistance in the respiratory tract. Another possibility to be taken into account is a decrease in blood sugar level as a result of inhibition of glycogenolysis in the liver. In addition there have been reports on numerous symptoms of which it is difficult to decide whether they are side effects or features of the anxiety syndrome, e.g. vivid dreams, fatigue sensations, nausea, diarrhoea, constipation, etc. They rarely necessitate discontinuation of treatment. Depressions have been described as well. In this respect the same question arises as for the abovementioned side effects. From a scientific point of view, the question of the depressogenic potency of propranolol is exceedingly relevant (chapter XVI).

In animal experiments, phenothiazines and tricyclic antidepressants potentiate the effects of propranolol because they inhibit its breakdown in the liver. Whether the same applies to the human organism has not yet been established.

Other beta-blockers have also been found effective in anxiety syndromes with a prominent somatic component, e.g. *alprenolol* (Aptine) and *oxprenolol* (Trasicor). The lastmentioned compound, when given in a single dose of 40 mg, is effective in acute, transient tension states produced by, say, speaking before an audience or having to take an examination.

BIBLIOGRAPHY

BALTER, M. B., J. LEVINE AND D. I. MANHEIMER (1974). Cross-national study of the extent of anti-anxiety/sedative drug use. *New Engl. J. Med.* 290, 769.

DUNDEE, J. W. AND W. H. K. HASLETT (1970). Benzodiazepines. A review of their ac-

tions and uses relative to anesthetic practice. *Brit. J. Anaesth.* 42, 217.
FROHLICH, E. D. (1971). Beta adrenergic blockade in the circulatory regulation of hyperkinetic states. *Am. J. Cardiol.* 27, 195.
GREENBLATT, D. J. AND R. I. SHADER (1971). Meprobamate: a study of irrational drug use. *Amer. J. Psychiat.* 127, 1297.
GREENBLATT, D. J. AND M. GREENBLATT (1972). Which drug for alcohol withdrawal? *J. Clin. Pharmacol.* 12, 429.
GREENBLATT, D. J. AND R. I. SHADER (1972). The clinical choice of sedative-hypnotics. *Ann. Intern. Med.* 77, 91.
GREENBLATT, D. J. AND R. I. SHADER (1974). Benzodiazepines. *New Engl. J. Med.* 291, 1011.
GREENBLATT, D. J. AND R. I. SHADER (1974). Benzodiazepines. *New Engl. J. Med.* 291, 1239.
HOFFBRAND, B. I., R. J. SHANKS AND I. BRICK (1976). Ten years of propranolol. *Postgrad. Med. J.* 52, Suppl. 4.
KATZ, R. L. (1972). Drug therapy: sedatives and tranquilizers. *New Engl. J. Med.* 286, 757.
KESSON, C. M., J. M. B. GRAY AND D. H. LAWSON (1976). Benzodiazepine drugs in general medical patients. *Brit. Med. J.* 1, 680.
Leading article (1975). Tranquillizers causing aggression. *Brit. Med. J.* 1, 113.
PERKINS, R. AND J. HINTON (1974). Sedative or tranquillizer? A comparison of the hypnotic effects of chlordiazepoxide and amylobarbitone sodium. *Brit. J. Psychiat.* 124, 435.
SHADER, R. I., M. I. GOOD AND D. J. GREENBLATT (1976). Anxiety states and beta-adrenergic blockade. In: *Progress in Psychiatric Drug Treatment.* Vol. 2. Ed. by D. F. Klein and R. Gittelman-Klein. New York: Brunner/Mazel.
TAGGART, P., M. CARRUTHERS AND W. SOMERVILLE (1973). Electrocardiogram, plasma catecholamines and lipids, and their modification by oxprenolol when speaking before an audience. *Lancet* 2, 341.
TYRER, P. F. AND M. H. LADER (1974). Response to propranolol and diazepam in somatic and psychic anxiety. *Brit. Med. J.* 2, 14.

XXI

Sedatives and Hypnotics

1. Definition

Sedatives are calming agents which allay anxiety and lower the level of tension, if increased. This definition also applies to the ataractics. The two groups of compounds, however, differ in one important respect: the degree of selectivity. Classical sedatives depress cortical as well as subcortical functions; the influence of the ataractics is much more limited to subcortical systems, more specifically the reticular formation and the limbic system. This difference has important practical implications. Sedatives reduce anxiety and tension less selectively than ataractics, and their influence on level of consciousness and intellectual performance is therefore more unfavourable. However, no sharp boundary can be drawn between ataractics and sedatives.

When given in larger doses, sedatives have a more hypnotic effect. The group of the sedatives imperceptibly merges with the group of the hypnotics. At any rate, some sedatives are largely used as hypnotics, while others are prescribed more as sedatives during the day. The same applies to ataractics: with increased doses they all begin to exert a hypnotic influence, and some of these compounds have exclusively been used as hypnotics. Whether this exclusiveness has a pharmacological basis or is dictated by marketing policies remains uncertain.

Sedatives have disadvantages other than the abovementioned, and these will be discussed in the relevant sections. It is my opinion that, apart from a few exceptions still to be discussed, these drugs, either used as sedatives or as hypnotics, are obsolete and should be replaced by ataractics, more specifically by benzodiazepines. These are less risky and induce fewer side effects. The benzodiazepine derivatives are more expensive, it is true, but if they are used for selective indications and during a limited period this factor need not count too much.

I nevertheless discuss the sedatives because they are still being frequently prescribed and, moreover, are present in numerous combined preparations.

There are numerous sedatives and hypnotics. They come and go, and the group is always in motion. In this chapter, therefore, I make no attempt at comprehensiveness, but merely discuss a few groups concisely, confining myself to mentioning a few examples in each group.

2. Indications

The indications for sedatives were described in chapter XIX. In this section I present some brief remarks on hypnotics and their indications, referring for a detailed discussion to studies by Kagan (1975), Kales and Kales (1974) and Williams and Karacan (1973).

1) Prescription of a hypnotic should be preceded by diagnosis of the sleep disorder involved, in *aetiological* as well as in *symptomatological* terms. Primary question: can the cause be traced? Sleep disorders can be secondary to such somatic diseases as cerebral arteriosclerosis and hyperthyroidism. Guilleminault et al. (1973) described a new "sleep disease": sleep apnoea. Whenever the patient falls asleep, respiration ceases, which means that he wakes up hundreds of times in the course of a night. There seems to be little doubt that further development of EEG studies will lead to the discovery of new "sleep diseases."

   Sleep disorders can also be secondary to (or rather: be part of) a psychiatric syndrome such as depression—which is by no means always recognized as such by the patient—or neurosis, in which sleep disorders are provoked by unresolved psychological (neurotic) conflicts. Sleep diagnosis invariably calls for a careful psychiatric examination.

The next thing to be accounted for is the exact nature of the patient's complaints: does he find it difficult to fall asleep; does he wake up early or often; is he suffering from nightmares; does he sleep during a fair number of hours but nevertheless feels that he has hardly slept at all (a syndrome which can only be identified on the basis of polygraphic findings), etc.

2) Sleep requirements show marked interindividual differences. Moreover, sleep disorders have not so far been adequately classified with the aid of sleep EEGs. For the time being, the diagnosis "disturbed sleep" is based simply on the patient's own statement: that he sleeps so poorly that his sense of well-being is affected, as well as his level of performance during the day.

3) A hypnotic is certainly not indicated in all sleep disorders. If a vital depression is involved, then antidepressants are the agents of choice; neuroleptics are to be preferred if sleep is disturbed by psychotic anxiety. Psychotherapy is indicated whenever psychological conflicts have been demonstrated which provoke and maintain the sleep disorders. In some cases simple rules of conduct can be very beneficial (e.g. do not go to bed before you are sleepy). Deconditioning (behaviour therapy) should be contemplated in all cases because sleep disorders: a) readily become an established habit; b) induce anxious tension which in turn impairs sleep.

4) Hypnotics should be used with restraint, and must not be prescribed until after careful physical and psychiatric examination; and only for a specified period of time in order to avoid habituation and dependence. On the other hand, one should not be too reluctant to prescribe them. Disturbed sleep undermines psychological (and physical) resistance. Actual problems which can in principle be resolved can in this way come to seem unsolvable. The despondency of the depressive patient can be intensified by the inability to sleep. Psychotherapy can stagnate because the patient is too preoccupied with the complaint that troubles him so much. In such cases there is no justification for persistent withholding of a hypnotic.

In all cases it should be made clear to the patient in advance that the hypnotic is prescribed for a limited period of time, in view of the risk of addiction and because the useful effect as a rule diminishes rapidly. Of course there are individuals who, for years, sleep well on the basis of a tablet, without feeling any need to increase the dose. These persons, however, probably sleep on the basis of a placebo effect, and one can only say that they are using a dangerous placebo. Benzodiazepines lead to habituation and addiction less readily than classical sedatives and hypnotics.

3. Barbiturates

Preparations

Barbiturates are still being widely used as hypnotics. They are derivatives of barbituric acid, a compound which possesses no hypnotic properties but acquires them when the two hydrogen atoms at the carbon atom in position 5 are substituted with alkyl or aryl groups (Table 31). They inhibit the activity of all stimulable tissues, but the CNS is particularly sensitive to their effect. Only after acute overdosage are other stimulable tissues such as myocardium, smooth and striated muscles influenced in this way. There are a great many

Table 31. Some barbituric acid derivatives

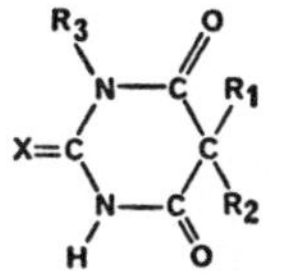

Barbiturate	Some trade names	R_1	R_2	R_3	X
Amylobarbitone sodium (U.K.) Amobarbital (USA)	Amytal	ethyl	isopentyl	H	O
Barbital	Neuronidia, Veronal	ethyl	ethyl	H	O
Butabarbital	Butisol, Soneryl	ethyl	sec-butyl	H	O
Hexobarbital	Sombulex, Evipan	methyl	1-cyclohexene-1-yl	CH_3	O
Methylphenobarbital	Prominal	ethyl	phenyl	CH_3	O
Phenobarbitone (U.K.) Phenobarbital (USA)	Luminal	ethyl	phenyl	H	O
Thiopental	Pentothal	ethyl	1-methylbutyl	H	S

barbiturates (Table 31). The choice of a particular compound is determined by the duration of its action, which ranges from 10-15 minutes to 24 hours or longer. The sedative dose is about one-third to one-fourth of the hypnotic dose.

The *short-acting barbiturates* are used as anaesthetics, for which purpose they are given intravenously. When given by mouth they are suitable as agents to induce sleep. They act quickly and relatively briefly. Examples are thiopental and hexobarbital, of which the oral dose is 250-500 mg.

Decidedly *long-acting* compounds are phenobarbital and methylphenobarbital. They are slowly absorbed, moreover, so that their optimal effect is not obtained until after a few hours. Since there is a considerable risk of a "hangover" the next morning, they are less suitable as hypnotics. Phenobarbital is mainly being used as an anti-epileptic. Its less somnifacient methyl derivative is used as a sedative, in a daily oral dose of about 60-250 mg. Barbital, the first hypnotic barbiturate, is also a long-acting compound; its daily oral dose is about 250-500 mg.

There is an *intermediate group* with a duration of action which lies between the values of the abovementioned groups. These are most widely used as sedatives and hypnotics. Well known representatives are amobarbital and butabarbital. As sedatives, both compounds are given orally in a daily dose of 2-3 × 25-50 mg. The hypnotic oral dose is 100-250 mg.

Both pentothiobarbital and amobarbital are being used in narco-analytic treatment—a method by which the patient is subanaesthetized for 15-45 minutes by intravenous administration of barbiturates in order to facilitate abreaction of conflicts and complexes and to promote psychotherapeutic contact between therapist and patient.

Injectio barbamini (Somnifene) is frequently used in prolonged sleep courses. The solution contains 100 mg barbital and 100 mg aprobarbital per ml, and 1-2 ml is given per intramuscular injection. Prolonged sleep has become obsolete as a therapeutic method, but Somnifene is still being used in status epilepticus.

Finally, barbiturates are contained in numerous *combined preparations,* together with such compounds as ataractics, other hypnotics, neuroleptics, analgesics, antihistamines, etc. A warning against these combinations is justified. Intoxications caused by them often take a much more serious course than those caused by the separate components. A notorious combination in this respect is Vesparax, which contains brallobarbital, secobarbital and hydroxyzine.

Disadvantages and dangers

The sedative effect of barbiturates is as a rule accompanied by varying degrees of dullness, reduced concentration and reduced reactivity. This is an inconvenience in certain occupations and dangerous in traffic. It is also to be borne in mind that alcohol potentiates both the sedative and the hypnotic effect of barbiturates.

When used as hypnotics, barbiturates not uncommonly produce a "hangover" the next morning: dizziness, nausea, somnolence and fatigue. The symptoms are as much more marked as the dose has been larger, the time of administration closer to the time of awakening, and the action of the compound more prolonged. It is to be noted that even short-acting compounds have a protracted "after-effect": 10-20 hours after administration, psychological functional disorders can still be demonstrated. Moreover, barbiturates disturb the normal EEG pattern of sleep. They suppress the REM phases and, after discontinuation, cause REM rebound. The exact clinical significance of these phenomena, however, is unknown. Some authors have related REM rebound to the "bad dreams" not infrequently reported after withdrawal of barbiturates.

All barbiturates increase the activity of microsomal liver enzymes which degrade other drugs, e.g. oral anticoagulants. Combination with barbiturates reduces their efficacy, and overdosage results from discontinuation of the barbiturate. By this same route, barbiturates also intensify their own degradation. This is a factor which contributes to the generally rapid habituation.

Not only does habituation to barbiturates develop readily, but the same applies to addiction. The patient develops a physical as well as psychological dependence: withdrawal, or even reduction of the dosage, is followed by a variety of somatic dysfunctions. The patient feels extremely weak and tired, but cannot sleep. He complains of nausea and abdominal cramps, and vomiting often occurs. Coarse tremors of the head and limbs are observed, and fascicular contractions in the muscles occur. The tendon reflexes are very brisk. Seizures of the grand mal type are the gravest danger; they can occur in such rapid succession that status epilepticus results. Finally, delirious symptoms may develop. What I have outlined here is the fully developed withdrawal syndrome; this, of course, occurs in various degrees of severity. For this reason discontinuation of barbiturates should always be gradual.

Overdosage of barbiturates is common—chronic in the case of addiction, and acute in attempts at suicide. In the case of *chronic overdosage* we observe a narrowing and clouding of consciousness; the gait becomes atactic and speech is thick: the patient impresses as drunk. Pains can also develop, usually headaches but also myalgia and arthralgia. Sleep is often disturbed. One should not be tempted to increase the dosage in such cases! Finally, delirious symptoms may develop, although this is relatively rare. A characteristic neurological finding in these cases is fixation nystagmus, which can be induced in all directions, while optokinetic nystagmus is abolished in all directions.

Acute intoxication with barbiturates causes reduction or loss of consciousness. The tendon reflexes are weak or absent; the pupils are usually contracted but, in contrast to morphine intoxication, they are still responsive to light. A barbiturate-induced coma is very dangerous because these compounds have a depressant effect on the respiratory centre in the medulla oblongata as well as on the vasomotor centre. This leads to respiratory insufficiency and vasodilatation with hypotension. Respiration and circulation are consequently the central concern in the treatment of these intoxications. A fatal issue is recorded in 0.5-12% of these cases, depending on the expertise of the therapeutic team.

In patients suffering from acute intermittent porphyria, barbiturates can provoke an attack. In this rare disease, therefore, these compounds are absolutely contraindicated.

It may finally be pointed out that acquired hypersensitivity to barbiturates is not rare, and that these compounds are unsuitable for aged patients and children because in these age categories they may produce paradoxical effects: instead of sedating, they induce or intensify agitation.

As already pointed out, benzodiazepines do not have these disadvantages, or at least in lesser degree, and are therefore to be preferred to barbiturates both as sedatives and as hypnotics.

4. Bromides

In the past, bromides have been widely used as sedatives and anticonvulsants, but less frequently as hypnotics. A very well-known sedative was the Charcot solution—a combination of ammonium bromide, potassium bromide and sodium bromide. For several reasons, bromides have now become obsolete. To begin with, the dosage has to be very high if a sedative effect is to be obtained (1-2 g per day); sedation is then obtained at the price of stupefaction and, moreover, the therapeutic dose approaches the toxic limit. In addition, the sedative effect develops very slowly, in the course of a few days. This slowness can be explained as follows.

After absorption, bromides rapidly distribute themselves over the extracellular space, where the bromine ion competes with the chlorine ion. With the exception of the erythrocytes, the cells of the organism are relatively inaccessible to the bromine ion. The exchange of bromine and chlorine ions is slow, and consequently an effective bromine concentration in the cells is not attained until after a few days. The often observed immediate effect of bromides (a spoonful of Charcot in all kinds of "nervousness") must therefore be based on suggestion. It follows from the above that a saltless (salt-restricted) diet should accelerate the therapeutic effect of bromides, but also the development of symptoms of intoxication.

Another disadvantage of bromides is their very slow renal excretion. The excretion of a single dose can take as long as 30 days. The risk of accumulation is therefore considerable. When the blood bromine level exceeds 50 mg/100 ml, symptoms of intoxication develop: the patient becomes dull, slow and often irritable and recalcitrant. Appetite is decreased, and sleep disturbed. Regular bromide use can also give rise to skin lesions, which can be of a maculopapular or of a more acne-like nature. In serious cases (blood levels exceeding 100 mg/100 ml) the patient becomes dysarthric and atactic; the Babinski reflex becomes positive and tremors develop. Finally, delirious symptoms may occur. A bromide delirium can show a striking resemblance to the delirium tremens of the alcoholic.

Since the kidney virtually does not discriminate between the bromine ion and the chlorine ion, bromide intoxication is treated by administration of chloride (as NaCl or NH_4Cl), water and a chloruretic. The excess chloride is excreted and "takes the bromide with it." Haemodialysis may be indicated.

Bromides are still contained in some "nerve tablets" available without prescription, fortunately in such minute quantities that, when used in the normal way, they are harmless (as well as probably ineffective).

5. Mono-ureids

Although several compounds in this group contain a bromine atom, their activity is probably not based on this atom but determined by the molecule per se. However, the bromine atom is released, and can come to play a role in intoxications. These compounds are mild, short-acting sedatives which are widely used, even without prescription; habituation and addiction therefore are regularly seen.

The group of the mono-ureids includes *carbromal* and *bromisoval*, which are given by mouth in a daily dose of 3 × 300-500 mg (Fig. 35).

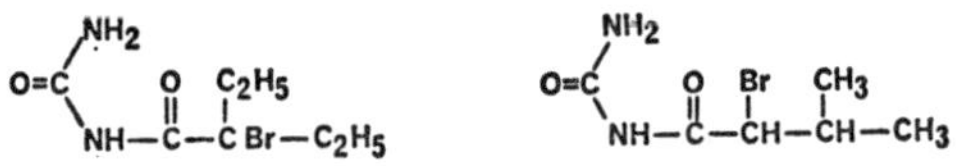

Figure 35. Some mono-ureids. Left: carbromal (Adalin, Carbrital, Diacid). Right: bromisoval (Bromural).

6. Aldehydes and halogenated alcohols

The principal representatives of these two groups are paraldehyde and chloral hydrate, respectively (Fig. 36). Of the "classical" sedatives, these are the only two compounds for which I would go to bat. They are good and relatively harmless sedatives with a quickly established effect (after 15-30 minutes) which, in therapeutic doses, exert little influence on blood pressure, respiration and cardiac function. Particularly in dealing with confused, agitated elderly patients, they can be very useful. In these patients barbiturates often have a

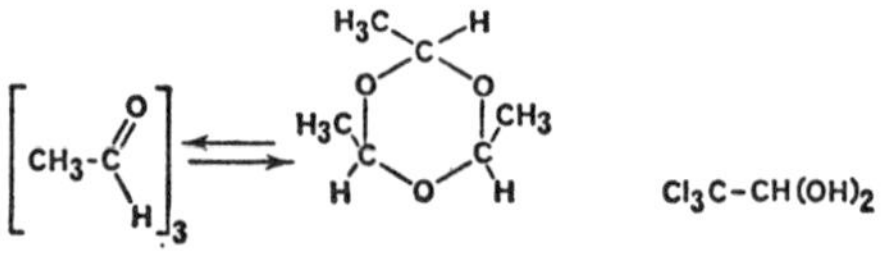

Figure 36. Paraldehyde (left) and chloral hydrate (right).

paradoxical effect, neuroleptics entail a risk of hypotension, and ataractics are often insufficiently effective.

For regular use, paraldehyde is preferable to chloral hydrate because its toxicity is low and it has a wide therapeutic range, whereas the therapeutic and toxic doses of chloral hydrate are fairly close together. Protracted use of the latter, moreover, can give rise to lesions of the kidneys and liver.

Both agents have a very disagreeable taste (although this does not seem to prevent addiction to them). The bad taste can be fairly effectively corrected as follows.

R. Paraldehyde	30 g
Compound gum powder	6 g
Althaea syrup	75 ml
Orange oil	6-9 dr
Methyloxybenzoate solution up to	300 ml
(1 tablespoonful = 1.5 g paraldehyde)	

R. Chloral hydrate	30 g
Water	30 ml
Chloroform	300 mg
Peppermint oil	6 dr
Althaea syrup up to	300 ml
(1 tablespoonful = 1.5 g chloral hydrate)	

Paraldehyde is a polymer of acetaldehyde. Some 70% of it is metabolized in the liver, and the remainder disappears via the lungs. This is why the patient's exhaled breath assumes a disagreeable odour within a few minutes of ingestion. Renal excretion is negligible. Little is known about the toxicology of the substance.

Paraldehyde can be administered by mouth, rectally (suppositories or enema) and by intramuscular injection; the dose per administration is 2-3 g (maximum 5 g) up to a maximum of 15 g (10 g if given intramuscularly) per 24 hours.

Chloral hydrate is a derivative of ethylalcohol. It can irritate the gastric wall and should therefore not be given to gastric patients. It is also to be borne in mind that the excretory products can cause positive reduction of urine. Allergic skin reactions are not uncommon. Prudence should be observed in dealing with patients who are receiving anticoagulants. Like the barbiturates, chloral hydrate can accelerate the metabolism of these substances by activation of microsomal liver enzymes. Acute chloral hydrate intoxication causes a syndrome resembling that of acute barbiturate intoxication, and is treated in the same way.

The agent can be given orally or rectally (suppositories or enema); the dose per administration is 1-1.5 g (maximum 3 g), to a maximum of 6 g per 24 hours.

A tasteless compound is *dichloralphenazone* (Duodorm, Welldorm), a molecular compound which consists of two chloral hydrate molecules and one antipyrine molecule. The daily dose recommended for sedative purposes is 3 × 250 mg.

7. Piperidine derivatives

Two compounds of this group are in use as hypnotics: *glutethimide* and *methyprylone* (Fig. 37). The usual dose prescribed of either compound is 200-400 mg. These are mild hypnotics with a rapidly established effect which lasts about 5-8 hours. Contrary to what was initially believed, habituation and addiction to both compounds are possible.

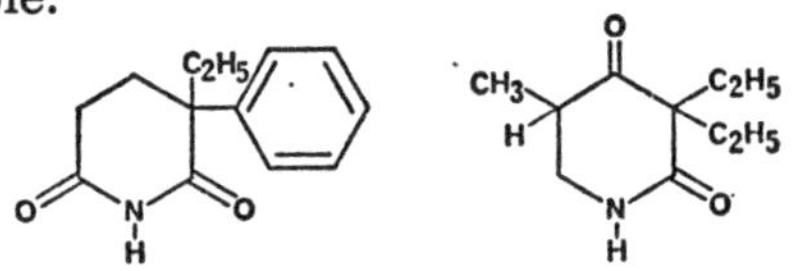

Figure 37. Some piperidine derivatives. Left: glutethimide (Doriden). Right: methyprylone (Nodular, Noctan, Dimerin).

8. Some other compounds

Probably the most harmless of all sedatives is *tinctura valerianae*, of which 3 × 20 drops per day is usually prescribed.

Methaqualone (Revonal, Quaalude) is used as a sedative (daily oral dose 3 × 75 mg) and as a hypnotic (dose 150-300 mg). As usual, habituation and addiction are a problem. Protracted use of this compound can lead to polyneuritis. Intoxications with this drug are serious. *Mandrax* is a compound which combines methaqualone with the sedative antihistamine diphenhydramine.

Opiates (morphine subcutaneously or pantopon subcutaneously or orally) were widely used as sedatives in the past, particularly in agitated depressions. Although they are certainly effective within this range of indications, these compounds must now be regarded as obsolete. There are several reasons for this. There is a grave risk of addiction; also, for the protection of staff members, opiates should not be available in a psychiatric ward. In addition, they have a marked depressant effect on respiration; elderly patients and those with a decreased metabolism (hypothyroidism, Addison's disease) are particularly susceptible to this effect. Opiates are absolutely contraindicated in the case of poor pulmonary function and disturbed liver functions (risk of accumulation) as well as after head injuries. In the latter case, their miotic effect and influence on the sensorium can interfere with neurological diagnosis. Moreover, hypoventilation is highly undesirable in these circumstances.

BIBLIOGRAPHY

Greenblatt, D. J. and R. I. Shader (1972). The clinical choice of sedative hypnotics. *Ann. Intern. Med.* 77, 91.

Guilleminault, C., F. L. Eldridge and W. C. Dement (1973). Insomnia with sleep apnea: a new syndrome. *Science* 181, 856.

Kagan, F. (Ed.) (1975). *Hypnotics, Methods of Development and Evaluation.* New York: Spectum Publications.

Kales, A. and J. D. Kales (1974). Sleep disorders—recent findings in the diagnosis and treatment of disturbed sleep. *N. Eng. J. Med.* 290, 487.

Kales, A., E. O. Bixler, T. L. Tan, M. B. Scharf and J. Kales (1974). Chronic hypnotic use: ineffectiveness, drug withdrawal insomnia, and hypnotic drug dependence. *J. Am. Med. Ass.* 227, 513.

Kales, A., J. Kales and E. Bixler (1974). Insomnia: an approach to management and treatment. *Psychiatric Annals*, 4, 28.

Koch-Weser, J. and D. J. Greenblatt (1974). The archaic barbiturate hypnotics. *N. Eng. J. Med.* 291, 790.

Koch-Weser, J. and E. M. Sellers (1971). Drug interactions with coumarin anticoagulants. *N. Engl. J. Med.* 28, 487 and 547.

Kuntzman, R. (1969). Drugs and enzyme induction. *Ann. Rev. Pharmacol.* 9, 21.

Leading Article (1976). Glutethimide, an unsafe alternative to barbiturate hypnotics. *Brit. Med. J.* 1, 1424.

McKenzie, R. E. and L. L. Elliot (1965). Effects of secobarbital and d-amphetamine on performance during a simulated air mission. *Aerospace Med.* 36, 774.

Praag, H. M. van and H. Meinardi (Eds.) (1974). *Brain and Sleep.* Amsterdam: Erven Bohn.

Regestein, Q. R. (1976). Treating insomnia: a practical guide for managing chronic sleeplessness circa 1975. *Compr. Psychiat.* 17, 517.

Smith, R. B., L. W. Dittert, W. O. Griffen et al. (1973). Pharmacokinetics of pentobarbital after intravenous and oral administration. *J. Pharmacokinet. Biopharma.* 1, 5.

Wikler, A. (1968). Diagnosis and treatment of drug dependence of the barbiturate type. *Am. J. Psychiat.* 125, 758.

Williams, R. L. and I. Karacan (1973). Clinical disorders of sleep. In: *Sleep Research and Clinical Practice*, ed. by G. Usdin, New York: Brunner/Mazel. pp. 23-57.

Wong, R. T. H. and M. Wiener (1973). Approach to the management of insomnia. *Drug Ther.* 3, 77.

XXII

Psychodysleptics

1. Some notes on natural psychodysleptics

Psychodysleptics—otherwise known as psychotomimetics, psycholytics, eidetics, hallucinogens or psychotogenics—are compounds which so disorganize mental life that severe psychopathological disorders result. By this definition, the group of the psychodysleptics would encompass a not unimportant part of the pharmacopoeia, for many drugs fulfil this criterion if they are given in sufficiently large doses. The definition given, therefore, requires the following qualification: psychodysleptics produce the abovementioned effect when given in doses which cause no significant symptoms of physical intoxication.

Undoubtedly the most widely known compound in this group is LSD (lysergic acid diethylamide), a semi-synthetic product. However, there are also numerous natural psychodysleptics. They are found, for example, in the venom of certain reptiles and amphibians. An example is *bufotenin*, a compound closely related to serotonin which is found in the skin of some toad species (Fig. 38). Psychodysleptics

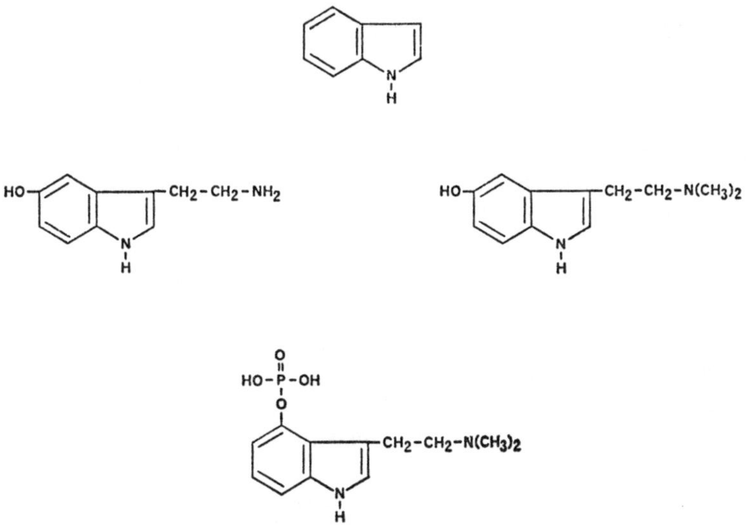

Figure 38. Indole ring and some indole derivatives.
Top: indole.
Left: 5-hydroxytryptamine (serotonin)
Right: 5-hydroxy-N-dimethyltryptamine (bufotenin)
Bottom: O-phosphoryl-4-hydroxy-N-dimethyltryptamine (psilocybine)

of vegetable origin are more numerous and have been known much longer, in fact since time immemorial. Because of their intoxicating, euphorizing or hallucinogenic potency, they were used to obtain pleasure, as medicinal agents, and for mystical-religious purposes. Some illustrative examples follow.

In the Middle Ages, an extract from the herb Corydalis cava was used as medicine against certain forms of insanity. The psychotoxic principle from this herb has been identified as *bulbocapnine.* In the thirties of this century, the Frenchman Baruk and the Dutchman De Jong have made extensive experiments with this alkaloid. They corroborated the observation of Peters that bulbocapnine induces a cataleptic syndrome in test animals, and from this fact they drew various far-reaching conclusions concerning the origin of schizophrenia, more specifically of the catatonic types. Their conclusions went too far, but this does not alter the fact that these investigators were among the pioneers of experimental psychopharmacology.

The leaves of the coca shrub (Erythroxylon coca) have a central stimulant and, in large doses, also an intoxicating and hallucinogenic effect; this was why they were used in the ritual ceremonies of certain South American Indian tribes. In the middle of the 19th century, Albert Niemann succeeded in isolating the active principle from these leaves, which was called *cocaine*. Freud is known to have experimented with this compound in his early years, and he devoted a detailed study to its psychological effects. Surprisingly, he did notice that his tongue and oropharyngeal cavity became "furry" but failed to recognize the significance of this phenomenon. It was not Freud but his fellow-townsman the ophthalmologist Koller who introduced cocaine as a local anaesthetic in medicine.

In this context I also mention *hashish*—called marihuana in South America—as an intoxicant with a disinhibiting, euphorizing effect, prepared from the hemp plant (Cannabis sativa var. indica). The psychotoxic principle from hemp is among the cannabinol derivatives. It has been said of the great 19th-century French psychiatrist Morel that he made his pupils use hashish in order to give them some understanding of the world in which a mental patient lives. The use of hashish originates from Central Asia but spread over large parts of the Orient and the New World. Until recently, Europe remained relatively immune, despite the impassioned descriptions by such lions of literature as Moreau de Tours ("Du hachich et de l'aliénation mentale," 1845) and Baudelaire ("Les paradis artificiels, 1860). In the course of the past decade, however, the use of hemp—in the form of marihuana cigarettes—has increased tremendously.

As a final example I mention *mescaline*, a compound chemically related to adrenaline and with effects resembling those of LSD: taken in doses of 0.5-1.5 g, it alters the world of perception and experience without drastically lowering the level of consciousness (Fig. 39). Mescaline is the psychotoxically active principle from Anhalonium lewinii, a Mexican cactus species which the local Indians call peyotl. During their religious ceremonies, priests chew dried slices of this plant in order to enter a state of ecstacy. In 1888, Lewin published a detailed description of this plant and its use by

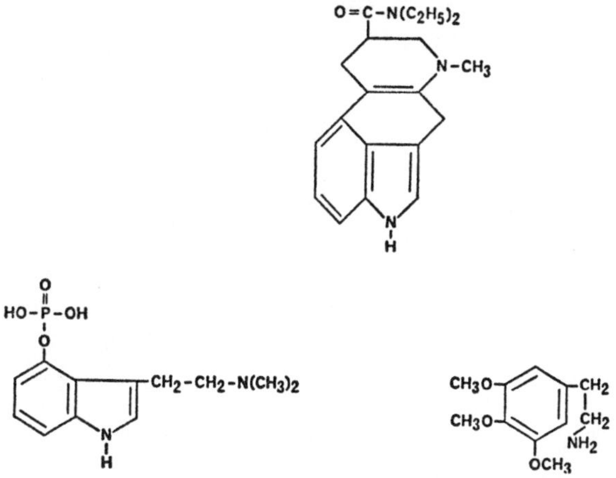

Figure 39. Three hallucinogenic compounds with similar effects.
Top: LSD (lysergic acid diethylamide)
Left: psilocybine
Right: mescaline

the local population. The active principle was isolated by Heffter in 1898; twenty years later, in 1919, Spaeth succeeded in elucidating its structure.

A few years after Lewin's publications, Prentiss and Morgan (1895) and, independently, Mitchell (1896) made investigations into the effect of mescaline on the human psyche. Their experiments have since been repeated and extended in numerous countries. Mescaline was in fact the first compound which, because of its psychodysleptic properties, attracted the attention of the world of science and was studied systematically instead of only incidentally. After the discovery of LSD is was relegated to obscurity. For therapeutic purposes it has rarely been used. As a drug of pleasure it has not become very popular, in spite of the glowing words which Aldous Huxley found to describe the world of bliss and torment which, he maintained, could be entered by using this agent ("The doors of perception"; "Heaven and hell").

2. Scientific and practical aspects of psychodysleptics

Prior to World War II, the world of psychiatry took little notice of the group of psychodysleptics. In fact it was only mescaline that was studied more or less systematically. This situation was drastically changed in the fifties. The sensational discovery of LSD has certainly played a role in this respect but, viewed in larger focus, this interest is really understandable only in the context of the rapid rise of biological-psychiatric research in that period (chapter V). It was gradually understood that, with the psychodysleptics, one had received tools of great *scientific* value, above all with regard to psychopathological research. These drugs make it possible to imitate psychiatric states, so to speak. Such "model psychoses" (actually disease models) provide an opportunity for systematic study of certain psychopathological symptoms, at least in principle. Many investigators hold that deliberate disturbance of psychological balance is ethically unacceptable. I may mention in passing that chemical means are not necessary per se to induce model psychoses. It has been established that marked limitation of sensory impressions (so-called sensory deprivation) can also induce psychotic syndromes.

Secondly, psychodysleptics owe their scientific significance to their catalysing effect on research into the biological determinants of psychotic behaviour. Much research has been done into their mechanisms of action. This nourished the hope of gaining some insight, through this approach, into the pathogenesis of certain psychotic symptoms or syndromes. A second line of research focused on the question whether the organism itself could be considered capable of producing hallucinogenic substances under certain conditions. The question is less far-fetched than it may seem to be at first sight. As already discussed in chapter IV, the brain contains monoamines which locally act as neurotransmitters. At their inactivation they are methylated. If a methyl group attaches itself to the monoamine molecule at an abnormal site, then substances with a hallucinogenic potency can result. Mescaline, for example, is a trimethylated dopamine derivative, and bufotenin is a dimethyl derivative of serotonin. The questions are: does the brain contain the enzymes required for such abnormal methylations and, if so, when do these become active? These questions are much less ephemeral than, say, a wild-goose chase after toxins which the liver is believed to produce in schizophrenia, as has taken place in the past.

Finally, the question of the *practical* value of psychodysleptics arose. Are they of importance as adjuvants in "uncovering" types of psychotherapy? Is the "material" which emerges in the pharmacogenic state of disintegration of diagnostic value? It is these questions that will be discussed in the following sections—not the biochemical aspects, which I have discussed in my book *Depression and Schizophrenia* (1977). Nor will psychopathological research be discussed; this is not so much because I regard it as exceeding the scope of this book, but because this research has so far been too sporadic to lend itself to a summary.

It is no longer a matter of course that psychodysleptics, and more specifically LSD, are discussed in a practical book on psychotropic drugs. Arguments against including them, however, are in my opinion not convincing; and I shall begin by explaining why.

3. LSD use, LSD abuse, LSD research

LSD discredited

In the fifties, LSD received ample attention in medicine and pharmacology. Over 1000 publications were devoted to this compound between 1951 and 1962. LSD raised great expectations as an adjuvant to psychotherapy and, even more so, as a possible key to the enigma of the biochemical roots of "schizophrenia." The turn of the tide was heralded by problems which arose at Harvard University, when it was found that undergraduates were using LSD without medical supervision, as part of a mystical cult.

Human research waned and, in the course of the sixties, practically ceased altogether. Psychiatrists who continued to make use of this agent were regarded as irresponsible charlatans or, at best, viewed with suspicion. Animal experiments were not at all encouraged, for fear of illegal distribution of LSD. Research stagnated, but not because the compound has been fully investigated. On the contrary, its mechanism of action is still largely unexplained, and we have no conclusive data on the practical value of this agent in psychiatry. There were other reasons to discredit LSD and thwart its further investigations. These were not of a primarily medical nature.

The most important of these factors was the rise of the drug culture and drug cult in the course of the sixties. Drugs became features of a way of life. They were glorified as keys to a new world with unlimited (transcendent) possibilities. These so-called subcultures generated fear and anger among the established citizens. Moreover, drugs can be dangerous, and this applies in particular to the "star-drug" LSD. Unsupervised use of this drug, often in large doses, inevitably led to accidents: protracted psychotic states, suicides, residual psychopathological symptoms, e.g. depersonalization syndromes. LSD, the darling of the nonconformist "left," also enjoyed the active, but unpublicized attention of the "right." The military significance of LSD was studied; human individuals served as test subjects, sometimes unknowingly. And this did not exactly improve the image of LSD.

A third factor: the new mystics began to describe the bliss of the LSD intoxication in glowing terms. Their pleas resembled a confession of faith more than a scientific argumentation. Two examples, which come from the medical profession and are in a relatively austere key: "... Intense states of belief may be created in some of those who go through the hallucinated confused state, which is afterwards felt to have been of tremendous emotional significance" (Sargant and Slater 1963). And Savage et al. (1962) wrote: "Our own conception is that people live an inauthentic existential modality (i.e. alienation), and that illness arises from an inability to see meaning in life. LSD provides an encounter which brings a sudden liberation from ignorance and illusion, enlarges the spiritual horizon and gives a new meaning to life." These are only two examples among many. In 1966, in an earlier work, I wrote: "Statements of this kind, in which incidental individual experiences are generalized in an unacceptable way, hold little power of conviction. In fact they are more likely to raise suspicion concerning the soundness of this method of treatment. This is why in my opinion they are to be regretted because, as a result, LSD could be prematurely discredited." This prediction has proved to be correct. The new mystics began to advocate "psychedelic therapy," which involves administration of LSD in relatively very large doses—up to 1500 mg per administration. They rejected psychiatric supervision, and again accidents happened.

Finally, psychiatrists themselves are to be blamed. They, too, published reports on miraculous cures obtained with LSD, for example in chronic alcoholism, after only one or a few LSD sessions. And no attempts were made to counterbalance private enthusiasm by introducing suitable control measures.

Dangers of LSD

I wish to make it very clear that this chapter does not mean to advocate the use of LSD. It is merely a plea for LSD research. To me, the balance between benefit (i.e. possible importance of this research) and risk is in favour of the former. But I do not in any way wish to underestimate the potential dangers, which can be summarized as follows.

1) The use of LSD in a medical setting entails a risk of illegal distribution.
2) Imminent and manifest psychoses can exacerbate in response to LSD, although there is no convincing evidence that LSD as such is capable of producing protracted psychosis.
3) A "bad trip" can reinforce (latent) suicidal tendencies.
4) Chronic symptoms of depersonalization have been described, but it is difficult to evaluate the role of LSD in their pathogenesis. Was LSD resorted to precisely because of experiential deficiency, or was this deficiency caused by LSD? At any rate, this (alleged) complication has been observed mainly after LSD abuse (use without psychiatric supervision), often in combination with other agents.
5) LSD is believed to damage chromosomes and to have a teratogenic effect. The books on this subject have not yet been closed but, quite apart from this, would any sensible psychiatrist venture to treat a pregnant woman with LSD?
6) Addiction has been mentioned as a potential risk of LSD use, but probably without justification. True addiction to LSD as such has not been described. It is possible that rapid habituation to the LSD effect plays a role in this context: if LSD is used more frequently than once a week, then its effect diminishes quickly. This entails the risk that, precisely because LSD becomes less effective, one resorts to a substitute which does cause addiction.

LSD research

I am fully aware of these dangers, but do not regard them as decisive arguments against LSD research as long as a number of requirements are met.

1) LSD therapy is provided in a psychotherapeutic context, by a psychotherapist who maintains a therapeutic relationship with the patient.

2) LSD therapy is given in a clinical setting so that its results can be studied in detail and untoward (side) effects combated immediately.

3) For LSD therapy, a separate unit should be available, with a specialized psychotherapeutic and nursing staff because: a) the personnel involved need experience, b) LSD therapy and LSD research entail a great deal of work, and c) concentration of this work enhances its efficiency, and also reduces the risk of illegal drug traffic.

4) Therapy starts with small doses (25 μg); these are increased if necessary, but a dose of 150 μg per administration must not be exceeded.

My statement that the risks are not a decisive argument against the use of LSD should be understood in a relative sense—in relation to the yield to be expected from LSD research. This yield is a dual one. To begin with, an answer can be expected to the question whether LSD can really accelerate psychotherapy and, if so, in which groups of patients this is most likely to occur. In view of the long duration of many courses of psychotherapy and the great expenses involved, the answer to this question is of the greatest practical importance. Secondly, there is the question of the diagnostic importance of LSD. Can the "material" brought forth in an LSD session elucidate the diagnosis and give a more precise indication for the type of therapy to be used? In view of the lack of reliable criteria in determining indications for various psychiatric therapies, this question is likewise of considerable importance.

Subjects of LSD research

Given the many problems with LSD and the delicate, sensation-prone character of its use, I would limit research for the time being to groups of patients who pose serious diagnostic and therapeutic problems. One might object that in this way LSD is not given a fair chance; but on the other hand there is the argument that (within certain limits) more risks can be accepted as fewer therapeutic alternatives are available.

I would first of all test the therapeutic potency of LSD in neurotic patients who make little progress under analytically-oriented therapy. I would test the diagnostic value of LSD in that group of (generally youthful) patients who consult a psychiatrist because they feel "empty"—deficient in establishing adequate contacts with others; whose spiritual development stagnates and who are often bogged down at school or in the work situation, but who show no psychotic symptoms. In such cases the problem of differential diagnosis is whether we are dealing with a neurosis with severe repression or with a deficiency of the "instrument" due to a (schizophrenic?) process. During the period 1958-1962, when I was regularly making use of LSD, I gained the impression that in the former cases LSD brings forth a considerable amount of "material" and breaks the vacuum, whereas in the latter category the vacuum persists and LSD produces not much more than vegetative symptoms.

These would be my research subjects, but others may have better suggestions. The only point I wish to make is that it would be regrettable if LSD research were relegated to oblivion on the basis of considerations and arguments which chiefly pertain to LSD abuse. The questions which are still moot are of too great practical importance to let this happen. This is also why I thought it justifiable to include a chapter on LSD and related compounds in a practical book on psychotropic drugs in 1977.

4. The history of LSD

LSD is a semi-synthetic alkaloid which consists of lysergic acid—a natural compound which is found in all ergot alkaloids—and a diethylamide group which is synthetically attached to it. The natural psychodysleptics also include compounds closely related to LSD. For example, the psychotoxic substance in the seeds of the Mexican plant Rivea corymbosa proved to consist of a mixture of d-lysergic acid, d-isolysergic acid amide, and lysergol. The native population calls these seeds ololiuqui and uses them for magic purposes.

Although it was synthesized as early as 1938, the hallucinogenic potency of LSD was not discovered until 1943, on April 16th of that year, and by accident. Hofmann, a Swiss chemist, wrote the following in his laboratory report on that day.

> Last Friday I had to stop work in the middle of the afternoon and go home to rest, because I was overcome by a remarkable restiveness, associated with a slight sensation of vertigo. At home I lay down and sank into a state resembling intoxication which was not unpleasant and characterized by an exceedingly activated imagination. In a twilight state with my eyes closed (I found the daylight disagreeably harsh), I found a continuous stream of fantastic images of extraordinary vividness and in intensive, kaleidoscopic colours to come to my mind.

Hofmann at first thought of an intoxication caused by some solvent, but later remembered that in the course of that afternoon he had been working with LSD, be it only with a few milligrammes. He decided to ingest 250 μg of that substance, and this proved to be sufficient to confirm his suspicion. Possibly as a result of war conditions, this discovery initially caused little commotion. Only four years later, when Stoll had published the first psychiatric report on LSD, did the psychiatric world begin to realize the significance of this compound.

LSD is indeed a very unusual substance, for two reasons. First of all because its hallucinogenic effect usually becomes manifest in response to *minimal quantities:* 250-50 μg. For comparison, I present the following list of approximate minimal doses required to produce a psychological effect with some other psychotropic drugs (in gamma = μg = 0.000001 g).

ethylalcohol	by mouth	7000000 - 20000000
chloral hydrate	by mouth	1000000 - 2000000
cocaine	subcutaneously	80000 - 300000
mescaline	by mouth	10000 - 20000
morphine	subcutaneously	5000 - 10000
atropine	subcutaneously	3000 - 10000
methamphetamine	by mouth	1500 - 3000
LSD	by mouth	30 - 50

That traces of a compound were able to influence the course of certain mental processes in an approximately constant and reproducible way was unheard of and surprising. It raised the suspicion that LSD probably exerted an influence on a very circumscribed series of cerebral metabolic processes.

Another unusual feature of LSD is that it produces psychopathological disturbances while leaving *consciousness* practically *unclouded*. This is a unique property. In toxic psychoses—and as such the LSD psychosis must be regarded—there is always some degree of clouding of consciousness. Hallucinatory sensations and experiences of a delusion-like nature which occur at an undisturbed level of consciousness are considered to be much more suggestive of schizophrenic psychoses. It was, therefore, not surprising that many investigators, in high optimism, initially believed that LSD could really be used to imitate a schizophrenic psychosis, and that elucidation of the mechanism of action of LSD could provide the (biochemical) key to the "schizophrenia" problem. Such optimism was anything but justifiable, if only because it makes no sense to equate a transient state of disintegration with a few schizophrenic features but with largely intact disease insight to the psychopathologically very polymorphous, chronic, disabling disease process which is called schizophrenia.

The introduction of LSD in psychiatry coincided with a second important discovery. In the early fifties, a new hormone-like substance was discovered: 5-hydroxytryptamine (5-HT; serotonin). This compound was found in high concentrations in blood platelets, in the yellow cells of the intestinal wall, and in the brain. Woolley and Shaw (1954) placed a hyphen between LSD and serotonin. They established that LSD antagonizes certain serotonin effects in the periphery. Peripherally, LSD and serotonin proved to behave as competitive antagonists. On this finding they based their famed hypothesis on the mechanism of central LSD actions. They postulated that the antagonism between LSD and serotonin manifests itself not only peripherally but also centrally, and that the LSD psychosis could result from a relative serotonin deficiency in the brain. This hypothesis soon proved to be untenable in this simple form, but its great merit was that it was the first hypothesis in the field of biological psychiatry to be based on experimental findings, and one which, in principle, could be clinically tested. In two different ways, therefore, this hypothesis is a classical one.

5. The course of the LSD syndrome

LSD syndrome and LSD psychosis

The LSD syndrome is preceded, and sometimes also accompanied, by symptoms of a vegetative type, e.g. accelerated pulse, mydriasis and more or less pronounced acrocyanosis. Salivation can either increase or decrease; the facial complexion becomes either ruddy or pale. The blood pressure usually increases slightly. Some patients in addition complain of nausea, dizziness or headache. The literature mentions numerous other prodromal signs, but it is questionable whether these are indeed related to the LSD intoxication per se. No correlation has been established between the severity of the vegetative symptoms and the intensity of the psychopathological disturbances. I worked frequently with LSD during the period 1958-1962. At that time abuse of this compound was unknown (in The Netherlands), and laymen hardly knew of its existence. Mysterious expectations could not yet play a role in the causation of LSD symptoms. Some 50% of the test subjects observed during this period showed only a vegetative reaction. In subsequent years, when the magic of LSD was widely glorified, this percentage diminished substantially. It seems evident that the LSD syndrome can comprise strong placebo elements.

LSD is usually taken by mouth. Some 30-60 minutes later the first signs of mental disorganization can manifest themselves: the true LSD syndrome develops. I deliberately use the word syndrome, not psychosis. Only a minority of cases involve true psychosis. The manifestations of the LSD syndrome gradually increase in intensity over a period of 2-3 hours and then attain a plateau of varying duration before they gradually abate. The state of intoxication usually ends some 6-8 hours after administration of LSD.

Manifestations of the LSD syndrome

Disorders of *visual perception* are among the first and also among the most constant manifestations. The duration of after-images increases. In a later stage, moreover, visual hallucinations develop, particularly when the subject closes the eyes. These hallucinations are often of an elementary nature (e.g. geometric figures such as points, lines, circles), but sometimes they are of a really scenic character. The objects perceived are often in movement and have a strikingly bright colour. It is a general rule that colours are perceived as harsher and more vivid during LSD intoxication. Yet the hallucinations are rarely "real": as a rule the patient retains a degree of critical distance and disease insight, and the term pseudo-hallucinations therefore seems more appropriate. Illusionary falsifications, too, are not uncommon.

Not only the optic but also the acoustic excitability increases, and as a result the patients are often hypersensitive to sounds. Auditory hallucinations, however, are rare.

In addition a degree of *alienation*, from self and from the environment, develops. These sensations can be very concrete and so assume a bizarre character. For example, certain parts of the body such as an arm or a foot are experienced as spurious, as not really belonging to the body. Sometimes the patient reports that his body feels literally strange, e.g. "soft," "cold," "soap-like." The environment, too, can be perceived as unreal, as some sort of stage setting. In terms of time perception, too, derealization can occur. The patient experiences some sort of timelessness—a sensation as if time has ceased to pass. In other cases, however, fragmentation of time is experienced: every moment is experienced as if it were isolated, and unrelated to the preceding or the following moment.

Disorders of visual perception and symptoms of depersonalization are nearly always features of the LSD syndrome, although their intensity varies widely. While they may be abundant and overwhelming in one patient, they may be traceable in the other patient only by questioning. And the same applies to healthy test subjects. It has so far been impossible to correlate these differences with structural features of the premorbid personality. The significance, if any, of pharmacokinetic factors (LSD absorption, turnover rate, etc.) has not been studied.

A variety of *other symptoms* can develop in response to LSD, although less regularly than the above discussed. Mention may be made of synaesthetic disorders: stimulation of a given sensory area leads to homologous as well as heterologous perceptions; e.g. hearing a sound also produces a visual image, and vice versa. In addition, unusual distortions of perspective and spatial relations may occur. Distances are estimated quite wrong. The room in which the patient is assumes different dimensions—it becomes shorter or on the contrary very narrow and long. Objects and persons can also be perceived distorted, as if seen in a curved mirror. Sometimes the patient identifies the distorted face of his therapist or nurse with persons of his home environment: father, mother, friends, etc. "The patient," says Baker (1964), "may be said to perceptualize the transference." Although the ability to concentrate is as a rule somewhat affected, the level of consciousness is not usually lowered by LSD. Orientation as to places and persons always remains intact. In fact, lucidity may increase so that all sensory stimuli are perceived with unusual sharpness, and sometimes as fraught with unusual significances. In these cases the term "mind expansion" seems appropriate.

The mood changes markedly even in the same patient within one session. There may be "elation" or on the contrary some depression. Fluctuations are at any rate characteristic of the LSD syndrome in general. A patient can give a fairly stabilized impression at a given moment, and show unmistakable regression a moment later.

As already pointed out, the manifestations discussed usually disappear 6-8 hours after administration of LSD. Mild residual symptoms such as a degree of disinhibition (which often facilitates contact with the patient), reduced ability to concentrate, mild depressiveness and sleep disorders, however, can persist 24 hours or longer.

Manifestations of the LSD syndrome can suddenly return although no additional LSD has been used. Such sensations are probably provoked by internal or external situations comparable to those which prevail during an LSD session. These so-called flashbacks are generally of short duration.

LSD psychoses

In some cases (we do not know exactly how many) the LSD syndrome assumes psychotic features. Insight into the cause of the manifestations disappears. Real hallucinations and delusions (e.g. paranoid delusions) occur; the patient can become very anxious and acutely suicidal. On the other hand, ecstatically blissful experiences are also possible, but these are rare. The development of psychotic symptoms is sufficient reason to discontinue the session. To do this, a neuroleptic is administered (e.g. 50-75 mg chlorpromazine by intramuscular injection, to be repeated after 60 minutes if necessary). This is usually sufficient to cause the psychosis to disappear. However, there are reports on cases in which the psychosis persisted even after LSD could be assumed to have been eliminated from the organism. Do these cases involve a release of endogenous (e.g. schizophrenic) psychosis, or disintegration due to emotional tension provoked during the LSD session (psychogenic psychosis), or a truly pharmacogenic psychosis, directly resulting from an influence of LSD on the brain? We cannot be sure. In many cases the plausibility of one of the first two possibilities can be demonstrated. The lastmentioned possibility cannot be excluded, but no positive indications in either direction are available.

Psychoses have been described mostly in cases of unsupervised LSD use. This risk is small, however, in non-depressive patients with no history of psychosis who receive LSD therapy from a trained therapist. In view of the possibility of the abovementioned complications, the therapist should not leave the patient alone during the LSD session. Another reason is that the solitary patient often very actively and successfully resists disintegration and regression. It is only when he is aware of being more or less under protection that he dares "let go."

6. Rationale and application of LSD

Rationale

LSD produces a degree of disintegration. Disintegration implies loosening or possibly disruption of the ego structure. The inevitable consequence is attenuation of inhibitions and disappearance of censoring resistances. In the most general terms, it can be said that disintegration always entails regression; regression to a more primitive level of emotional and intellectual development. This regression is often readily observable in response to LSD. The patient becomes more or less infantile and develops a child-like, dependent reaction pattern. Logical thinking with its intellectual-rational overtones recedes, in favour of a more magical, prelogical form of image-thinking.

As a result of this regressive movement (or so, at least, can the course of events be presented in more or less understandable terms), all sorts of events of the past are revived in memory; but not only are they revived in memory, they are often re-lived, re-experienced as intense realities. This often happens with emotion-laden experiences which have remained un-assimilated. In addition, unfulfilled wishes can be experienced as fulfilled. Occasionally a patient mentions religious-cosmic experiences, in which he can enter an ecstatic state of bliss. Such contents are often quite striking in their differentiated substance and poetic expression. In substance and expression, they can far exceed the level which could be expected of the patient in view of his formal education and past history of development.

It is for the abovementioned reasons that LSD has been applied in psychotherapy—not because of its disintegrating effect as such, but with a view to its result: the release of unconscious and conflict-laden experiential material. LSD has been described as an "abreactive agent." As such it has even acquired the predicate "deep," which is to say that it can reactivate very early or very thoroughly repressed experiences. In this respect it differs from carbon dioxide inhalation and narcoanalysis (pentothal treatment) with which one generally reaches only rather "superficial" layers.

Even more important is the following difference: LSD does alter consciousness but scarcely lowers the level of consciousness. The phase of disintegration is generally experienced consciously, and remembered. The experiences undergone under carbon dioxide or pentothal, however, are usually subject to total or partial amnesia; consequently it is difficult to utilize them for psychotherapeutic purposes.

Applications

In psychotherapy, LSD has been utilized for two different purposes, which differ gradually rather than essentially.

1) As adjuvant to psychoanalytic therapy. During phases of stagnation in the therapeutic process, LSD can be useful: it

causes the emergence of new "material" and often also intensifies dream life.

2) As an aid in psychocathartic therapy. In such therapy the accent is on having the patient re-experience traumatizing situations of the past, which have remained unassimilated and were repressed. An essential feature of this method lies in repetition, for in the long run the emotional charge of such experiences can substantially diminish, and evident relaxation can ensue. Of course, in most cases the process of abreaction as such is not sufficient. The patient must be helped to re-accept the actualized experiences, but in a more mature manner. An LSD course, therefore, is never an isolated therapy, but is always embedded in a broader psychotherapeutic context.

In psychocathartic therapy with LSD, large doses have been used (>150 μg per session). As already pointed out, however, the risk of (psychotic) complications increases as the dosage increases.

To summarize: LSD has been used in the treatment of a wide variety of neurosis, and this use is known as *psycholysis*. The rationale of this method seems acceptable, but reliable data on its efficacy are not yet available. Determination of indications, too, has remained a moot point. Which types of neuroses are and which are not (or less) suitable for this type of treatment; what is the significance of the premorbid structure in this respect; what is the significance of the duration of symptoms—these have been and continue to be controversial questions. For example, compulsive neuroses are regarded by some as an indication par excellence, whereas others consider them to be contraindications. The same applies to states of depersonalization; some have reported beneficial effects from the intensification of various modalities of experience in response to LSD, but others observed aggravation after termination of the LSD intoxication. Even the boundaries of the range of indications are still controversial. The current view is that LSD is particularly well-suited to the treatment of neurotics; but some investigators have reported their best results in "psychopathic personalities." Nor is there any certainty about the relative value of LSD therapy, i.e. its value as compared with that of other cathartic methods such as narcoanalysis, carbon dioxide inhalation and hypnosis.

Therefore, those who consider LSD to be ready for introduction in psychotherapy are as much in the wrong as those who regard it as a diabolical invention. What is really needed is systematic LSD research.

7. Short-acting compounds

There are compounds which produce an effect similar to that of LSD but short-lived (3-4 hours). In this context I mention the synthetic compound dipropyltryptamine and the natural compound psilocybine. The latter is the psychotoxically active principle of Psilocybe mexicana Heim—a mushroom used even in pre-columbic times by Mexican priests in ritual ceremonies. It was isolated in 1958 by Hofmann (the same chemist who discovered the hallucinogenic effect of LSD), and identified as O-phosphoryl-4-hydroxy-N-dimethyltryptamine. Both compounds have an indole ring and are related to serotonin (Fig. 37).

A strong interest is taken in these compounds in particular by psychiatrists who use psycholysis in outpatient treatment. As I explained in section 3 above, it is my view that application of these agents should be confined to a clinical setting for the time being.

BIBLIOGRAPHY

Baker, E. F. W. (1964). The use of lysergic acid diethylamide (LSD) in psychotherapy. *Canad. Med. Ass. J.* 91, 1200.

Berg, J. H. van den (1951). Ein Beitrag zur Psychopathologie des Meskalinrausches. *Folia Psychiat.* (Amst) 54, 385.

Beringer, K. (1927). *Der Meskalinrausch. Seine Geschichte und Erscheinungsweise.* Monographien d. Neurol. u. Psychiat. H. 49, Berlin: Springer Verlag.

Braude, M. C. and S. Szara (Eds.) (1976). *Pharmacology of Marihuana.* New York: Raven Press.

Dahlberg, C. C., R. Mechaneck and S. Feldstein (1968). LSD research: The impact of publicity. *Amer. J. Psychiat.* 125, 685.

Efron, D. (Ed.) (1970). *Psychotomimetic Drugs.* New York: Raven Press.

Freedman, D. X. (1968). On the use and abuse of LSD. *Arch. Gen. Psychiatry* 18, 330.

Freud, S. (1884). Über coca. *Centralbl. f.d. ges. Therapie* 2, 289.

Glass, G. S. (1973). Psychedelic drugs, stress and the ego. The differential diagnosis of psychosis associated with psychotomimetic drug use. *J. Nerv. Ment. Dis.* 156, 232.

Hofmann, A., A. Frey, H. Ott, Th. Petrzilka (1958). Konstitutionsaufklärung und Synthese von Psilocybin. *Experientia* 14, 397.

Jong, H. de and E. H. Baruk (1930). *La catatonie expérimentale par la bulbocapnine,*: Paris: Masson.

Jong, H. H. de (1945). *Experimental Catatonia.* Baltimore: Williams and Wilkins.

Lewin, L. (1888). Ueber Anhalonium Lewinii, Naunyn-Schmiedebergs *Arch. exp. Pathol. u. Pharmakol.* 24, 401.

MAIER, H. W. (1926). *Der Kokainismus*. Stuttgart: Thieme-Verlag.
Marihuana. New Support for immune and reproductive hazards. Research News. (1975). *Science* 190, 865.
MCGLOTHLIN, W. H. AND D. O. ARNOLD. (1971). LSD revisited. *Arch. Gen. Psychiat.* 24, 35.
MITCHELL, S. W. (1896). The effects of Anhalonium Lewinii (the Mescal button) *Brit. Med. J.* 2, 1625.
PRAAG, H. M. VAN (1966). *Psychopharmaca. Een leidraad voor de praktiserende medicus*. Assen: Van Gorcum.
PRAAG, H. M. VAN (1968). Hallucinogens, a Trojan horse? *Ned. T.v. Geneesk.* 112, 1985.
PRAAG, H. M. VAN (1971). Marihuana. Folklore and Science? *Ned. T. v. Geneesk.* 115, 270.
PRENTISS, D. W. AND A. M. MORGAN (1895). Anhalonium Lewinii (mescal button) *Ther. Gaz.* 9, 577.
SARGANT, W. AND E. SLATER (1963). *An Introduction to Physical Methods of Treatment in Psychiatry*. Edinburgh and London: E. and S. Livingstone Ltd.
SAVAGE, C., J. TERRILL AND D. D. JACKSON (1962). LSD, transcendence and new beginning. *J. Nerv. Ment. Dis.* 135, 425.
SIVA SANKAR, D. V. (1975). *LSD—a total study*. PJD Publi. Ltd. Westbury New York.
STOLL, W. A. (1947). Jysergsäure-diäthylamid, ein Phantastikum aus der Mutterkorngruppe. *Schweiz. Arch. Neurol. Psychiat.* 60/61, 279.
TINKLENBERG, J. R. (Ed.) (1975). *Marihuana and Health Hazards*. New York: Academic Press.
WOOLLEY, D. W. AND E. SHAW (1954). A biochemical and pharmacological suggestion about certain mental disorders. *Proc. Nat. Acad. Sci.* 40, 228.

XXIII

Pharmacotherapy of Addictions

1. Opiates, narcotic analgesics, opioids

Opiates are alkaloids prepared from the seed-pod of Papaver somniferum. On the basis of their chemical structure, they are divided into two groups: phenanthrene derivatives, e.g. morphine and codeine, and benzyl quinolines, which include the vasodilator papaverine. Crude opium contains 10% morphine. The latter is its principal active constituent, and the pharmacology of opium is roughly that of morphine. Opium itself is used as a drug of pleasure (it is mostly smoked, snuffed or taken by mouth), as is morphine (which is usually injected).

Until recently, the terms opiates and *narcotic analgesics* were used as synonyms because opium itself and the phenanthrene derivatives combine psychotropic with analgesic properties. In actual fact, they are the strongest pain-killers available to medicine. The other major group of analgesics—the antipyretic analgesics such as acetosal (acetylsalicylic acid)—are less effective but also less dangerous. Be this as it may, at present the group of narcotic analgesics comprises not only opiates but also a series of (semi-)synthetic compounds which are or are not related to morphine in terms of chemical structure but in any case share a number of pharmacological characteristics with it. So instead of narcotic analgesics, this group of compounds could better be called *opioids*.

The notorious addictive drug *heroin* is a semi-synthetic opioid (Fig. 40). It was marketed in 1898 by the German firm of Bayer as a non-addictive substitute for morphine! It is obtained by attaching two acetyl groups to morphine. In the brain, heroin is hydrolysed to monoacetylmorphine and morphine. These are probably the active products, not heroin itself. That heroin is more potent than morphine on a mg basis, and is experienced as stronger by the user, is due to the fact that it is more readily fat-soluble and passes the blood-CSF barrier more quickly than morphine. The central morphine concentration therefore rises more rapidly than after morphine. It is precisely the quick, strong (but brief) effect that the heroin mainliner values.

A completely synthetic compound is *methadone* (Fig. 40), evolved by German chemists and introduced as an analgesic towards the end of World War II. Its chemical structure shows only some

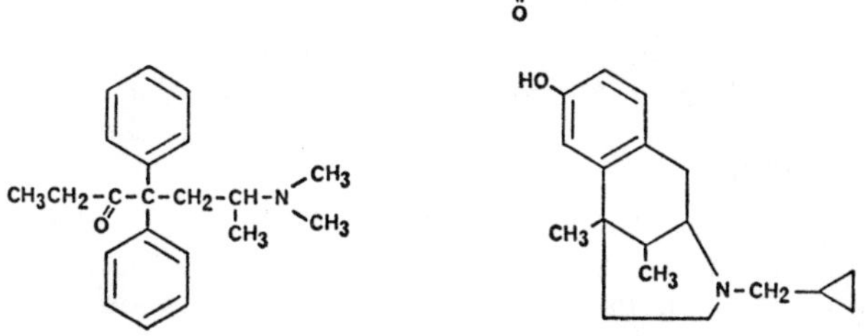

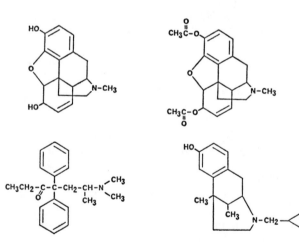

Figure 40. Some opiates and opioids.
Top left: morphine
Bottom left: methadone
Top right: heroin
Bottom right: cyclazocine

superficial resemblance to that of morphine, but in terms of pharmacological properties the two compounds are qualitatively identical.

2. Methadone: a form of substitution therapy

The treatment of addiction to opioids will not be discussed in detail because it calls for methods which can only be used in specialized (outpatient) clinics. In the treatment of this type of addiction, drugs can be used along with individual and group psychotherapy and social intervention. One strategy in this context is substituting a less dangerous drug for a dangerous addictive drug. This method is used in heroin addiction. The "therapeutic" agent is usually methadone which, for several reasons, is a lesser evil than heroin. These reasons can be summarized as follows.

1) It acts longer than heroin, and the addict can do with a single administration per day.
2) The compound can be given by mouth. Parenterally, methadone is not much more effective than orally, and the urge to start "shooting" is therefore less strong. From a hygienic point of view, oral administration is preferable to injection.
3) Methadone, too, causes physical dependence: when it is withdrawn or when an opiate antagonist is given, withdrawal symptoms develop. These, however, are less severe than those after withdrawal of heroin, and the craving for resumption is therefore less overwhelming.
4) The addictive potency of methadone is less marked than that of heroin, although it does exist. The so-called overall abuse potential is considered to be about the same as that of morphine.
5) Habituation to the sedative effect of methadone develops rapidly, and the side effects are unimportant. Once a user is stabilized on methadone, it is almost impossible for an outsider to perceive any evidence of its use.

Methadone therapy is usually instituted in a clinical setting, starting with a daily dose of 2 × 5 mg. This dose is slightly increased every 3-4 days until, after 4-6 weeks, a daily dosage of 50-100 mg is attained which can be given in a single dose. If the dosage is increased too quickly, then the patient becomes dull, somnolent and apathic. After discharge, the patient initially reports daily at the outpatient clinic to take his (now legally available) drug. Later, he reports less frequently (e.g. 2-3 times per week) and is given methadone to take home for the days in between. This approach has led to illicit trafficking and abuse of methadone. This is why a strong interest is taken in longer-acting compounds. One such compound is acetylmethadol (acetyldimepheptanol), which is effective for 72 hours and is now being tested in patients but has not yet been released for non-experimental use.

A patient on a so-called methadone maintenance programme is still addicted, but nevertheless a substantial number of these patients are able to lead fairly normal and productive lives. A critical analysis of methadone programmes has been published by Lennard et al. (1972). Methadone is used, not only in substitution therapy but also as a bridging agent in therapeutic programs aimed at total abstinence.

3. Narcotic antagonists

Another possibility of pharmacotherapy of opioid addiction lies in the use of so-called narcotic antagonists. Such compounds antagonize some or all of the effects of narcotic analgesics, by occupying the receptors to which the narcotics usually attach themselves. They occupy the place of the narcotic but are unable to activate the receptors. The antagonism is of a competitive nature, and the affinity of the conventional antagonists for the receptor exceeds that of morphine, so that they supersede this compound. Narcotic antagonists are structurally related to morphine, and many have a morphine-like activity as well as a morphine-antagonizing activity. Compounds of this type are known as partial antagonists or agonists-antagonists.

Narcotic antagonists attenuate or even abolish the effects of opioids. Moreover, physical dependence cannot develop because the receptors in question are occupied. This determines their usefulness in the treatment of addicts: the absence of a) psychotropic effects and b) withdrawal symptoms eliminates two reinforcers of drug-seeking behaviour. An important disadvantage of the currently available antagonists is that they are (too) short-acting compounds. If he wishes, the patient can leave the tablets alone and, shortly after, enjoy the full "benefit" of his shot. This is why antagonists can hardly be effectively used without intensive psychotherapeutic and social guidance. Although the objectives are relatively modest, the results of methadone programmes have so far been more favourable than those obtained with narcotic antagonists.

A pure antagonist, already clinically tested, is *naloxone*. It has no morphine-like properties and produces no effects in normal test subjects. Its therapeutic usefulness, however, is limited because it is short-acting (4-6 hours), and the efficiency of an oral dose is much more limited than that of an intravenous injection. Consequently this compound is not very suitable for use in actual practice. Another pure antagonist which acts a little longer and is efficient when given orally is *naltrexone;* with this antagonist, however, little experience has so far been gained.

A more promising compound is *cyclazocine*. An oral dose of 4-6 mg causes a block which persists for 24 hours. This is a partial antagonist which has retained a slight analgesic, respiratory depressant and euphorizing effect. Habituation to this effect develops quickly, however, while the narcotic-antagonistic effect persists. As a result of the remaining morphine-like properties, abrupt discontinuation of treatment is followed by withdrawal symptoms. These, however, are mild as compared with the syndrome which develops after withdrawal of true narcotics, and they are of a different nature. Typical withdrawal symptoms are a tendency to scratch and a sensation of electric shocks passing through the head. Subsequently there may be diarrhoea, lacrimation, rhinorrhoea, anorexia and other symptoms. No craving for this compound develops. A much more disagreeable consequence is that many partial antagonists, including cyclazocine, can induce anxiety and restlessness, and may even have hallucinogenic effects. In that case the patient is subject to fearsome (pseudo)hallucinations and nightmares, often accompanied by parasympathicomimetic manifestations such as hyperhidrosis. The patient experiences this as highly disagreeable, and the risk of abuse of these antagonists is therefore small. This is an advantage over methadone.

Before narcotic antagonists are administered, the patient must be weaned from the opioids because, in the case of physical dependence, antagonists can provoke severe withdrawal symptoms.

4. Disulfiram in chronic alcoholism

Mechanism of action

The principle of pharmacotherapeutic deconditioning is used not only in opioid addiction but also in addiction to alcohol. With anti-alcoholic agents, in fact, one goes even further. The subjectively agreeable effect of alcohol is not extinguished (as narcotic antagonists extinguish the pleasurable effect of opioids), but turned into its opposite: the patient is made to feel very bad indeed.

The most widely used anti-alcoholic agent is disulfiram (Antabuse; Refusal) (Fig. 41). Its effect is based on interference with alcohol metabolism (Fig. 42). In the liver, alcohol is converted to acetaldehyde by the enzyme alcohol dehydrogenase. Normally,

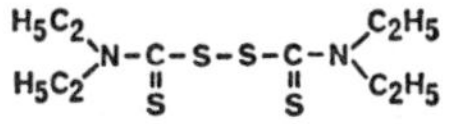

Figure 41. Disulfiram (Antabuse; Refusal)

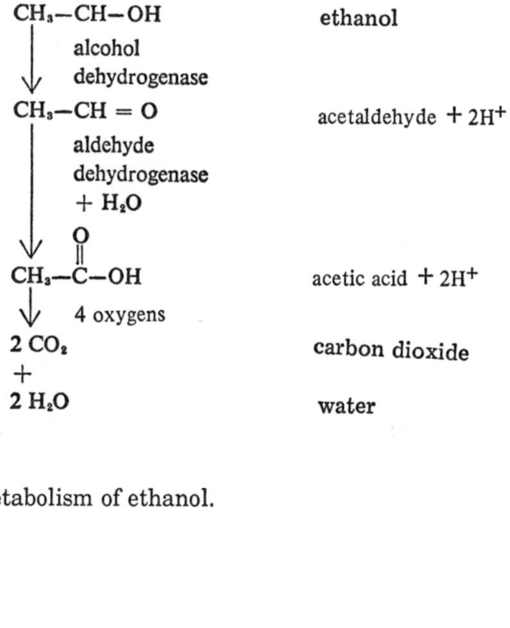

Figure 42. Metabolism of ethanol.

acetaldehyde is further oxidized to acetic acid with the aid of the enzyme aldehyde dehydrogenase. It is the lastmentioned reaction that is blocked by disulfiram, which thus leads to acetaldehyde accumulation. Whenever a person who has used disulfiram drinks an alcoholic beverage, symptoms of acetaldehyde poisoning develop. In volunteers, the alcohol/disulfiram reaction has been imitated by infusion of acetaldehyde. Not all the symptoms produced by the combination disulfiram/alcohol can be ascribed to acetaldehyde. This combination decreases blood pressure, whereas acetaldehyde causes increased blood pressure. The hypotension is explained by the fact that disulfiram inhibits dopamine-ß-hydroxylase—the enzyme which converts dopamine to noradrenaline. Consequently noradrenaline synthesis diminishes, sympathetic activity is suppressed, and the blood pressure falls.

Application

Disulfiram therapy begins with a test drink—a procedure not entirely without risk, for which the patient should be hospitalized. In my opinion it is incorrect to prescribe disulfiram without test drink, because in this way one bypasses the cardinal point of deconditioning: to associate the use of alcohol with exceedingly unpleasant sensations.

Once hospitalized, the patient receives 2 × 0.5 g disulfiram daily during 4 days, and on the fourth day is given a small amount of alcohol (the so-called test drink), e.g. 10-20 ml hard liquor (40% alcohol) or 50-100 ml wine or 100-200 ml beer. The disulfiram dose is then reduced to 0.25-0.5 g per day, depending on the side effects. The dose is given in the morning and medication is continued for an indefinite time. During the hospital period, the test drink can be repeated several times. The following symptoms develop after the test drink.

1) After about 5 minutes the skin of the face, neck and chest becomes red and the patient reports a sensation of heat. He feels pulsations in the head, and a headache can develop. Vasodilatation in the sclerae can also occur. The pulse rate increases while the blood pressure shows a slight decrease.
2) After 30-60 minutes the patient becomes nauseated and sometimes has to vomit. The erythema disappears, to be re-

placed by quite marked pallor. The patient complains of headache, palpitations, thirst and dizziness, and marked hyperhidrosis is noted. There is an unmistakable feeling of illness and the blood pressure can show a marked decrease at this stage. The syndrome gradually abates within 1-2 hours, whereupon the patient, very tired, often falls asleep.

The test drink is taken while the patient is in a quiet room. He should not be left alone, and pulse and blood pressure should be regularly checked because complications may occur, especially from the cardiovascular system, e.g. cardiovascular shock, arrhythmias and cardiac decompensation. Respiratory depression is also possible, and convulsions may occur. Disulfiram is therefore contraindicated in the presence of cardiac and pulmonary disease, and in epilepsy. Evidently, these patients should not be given a test drink. Disulfiram is largely metabolized in the liver and is therefore contraindicated also in patients with poor liver functions.

According to Benkert and Hippius (1974), an excessive disulfiram/alcohol reaction can be arrested by intravenous injection of 1 g ascorbic acid (vitamin C) or 40 mg of the antihistamine promethazine (Phernergan).

Disulfiram itself usually causes little trouble. Possible side effects are skin changes (acne, urticarial eruptions), disorders of potency, headache, dizziness and gastrointestinal disorders. Psychological side effects have also been described (e.g. restiveness and fatigue), but in the actual case it is difficult to decide whether these manifestations represent pharmacological effects or are determined by the enforced abstinence. Psychotic reactions can occur but are rare. It is generally possible to control the side effects by reducing the dosage. They are seldom a reason to discontinue medication.

The effect of disulfiram begins after 12-18 hours and continues for 4-6 days after discontinuation of medication. This compound is fat-soluble, and accumulates in the fat stores, from which it is only slowly released. Moreover, disulfiram elimination is slow.

Like all addiction, alcoholism poses a biological as well as a sociological and psychological problem. Disulfiram medication is therefore meaningful only if the patient at the same time receives psychotherapeutic and sociotherapeutic guidance. The medication may be helpful to the patient when the temptation to drink is very strong.

Implantations

Disulfiram can be implanted and, in principle, the patient can thus be protected from himself; he cannot give in at moments of weakness and interrupt the medication. I wrote "in principle" because so far there have been no indications that currently available compounds do achieve the objective and can be used to maintain an effective blood disulfiram concentration over longer periods. As a rule, 1 g disulfiram in the form of a number of compressed tablets is implanted into a muscle of the abdominal wall under general anaesthesia. Blood disulfiram concentrations exceeding 0.1 mg/100 ml (regarded as the minimal effective concentration in oral therapy) are found only during the first week following implantation. It is therefore likely that the favourable effects described after disulfiram implantation have been psychologically, not pharmacologically determined. Proof could be obtained by comparing the effect of disulfiram with that of placebo implantation. I have no knowledge of any such comparative study.

5. Other (potential) anti-alcoholic agents

An agent with a mechanism of action similar to that of disulfiram, but shorter-acting, is *calcium carbimide* (Dispan), which is believed to exert less influence on the cardiovascular system. The daily dose is 2 × 50-100 mg, to be taken at an interval of 12 hours.

When combined with alcohol, the hypoglycaemic *sulphonyl urea derivatives* produce symptoms comparable to those of a (mild) disulfiram/alcohol reaction. The blood acetaldehyde concentration rises, probably via inhibition of the enzyme aldehyde dehydrogenase as in the case of disulfiram.

The antiprotozoal *metronidazole* (Flagyl) has been reported to reduce both the effect of and the craving for alcohol, and as such to be of value in the treatment of alcoholics. These reports are not well-documented and the underlying mechanism is obscure.

Finally, a new line of biochemical research is of interest although it has not yet yielded results of practical value. Investigations have indicated as plausible that the euphorizing and stimulant effects of some addictive compounds are related to activation of catecholaminergic systems in the brain. This applies specifically to alcohol and amphetamines. Alcohol increases the rate of catecholamine (CA) synthesis in the brain but does not influence the rate of serotonin synthesis. On the behavioural level, ethanol increases motor activity in rodents. This stimulant effect remains absent after premedication with *α-methyl-p-tyrosine* (α-MT), an inhibitor of tyrosine hydroxylase and therefore of dopamine and noradrenaline synthesis. This suggests that CA are of importance in the stimulant effect of ethanol.

These data stimulated an effort by Ahlenius et al. (1973) to study the interaction of α-MT and ethanol in human individuals. Ten normal subjects (social drinkers) were premedicated with α-MT and were then given 50 ml aquavit every 10 minutes for 40 minutes (i.e. a total of 200 ml). Use was made of a so-called double-blind/cross-over arrangement. This means that: a) the test subject receives either a placebo or α-MT while he himself and the observer are unaware of the choice, and b) the experiment is repeated in such a manner that on the second occasion the placebo group receives α-MT and the α-MT group is given a placebo. In this setup, each test subject serves as his own control.

The drinking situation was made as natural as possible, and approximated a party situation. The test subjects knew each other and were seated at a round table, with appetizers available ad libitum. Behaviour rating was done by three sober observers who were thoroughly familiar with all the test subjects. In all test subjects, α-MT proved to reduce the stimulant and euphorizing effects of ethanol. Whether habituation to this α-MT effect develops is unknown.

Comparable experience has been gained with amphetamines (Jönsson et al. 1971). These compounds increase motor activity in all test animals studied. They enhance CA-ergic activity in the brain, partly by facilitating release of CA into the synapse and partly by blocking their re-uptake into the neuron. It was found that α-MT antagonized both the biochemical and the behavioural effect, and interaction is therefore suspected in this case also. It seems likely that this also applies to human individuals, because in amphetamine addicts α-MT vigorously suppresses the stimulant and euphorizing effects of amphetamines. However, habituation to this effect develops quickly, and the practical importance of a α-MT in this context therefore seems small.

6. Chlormethiazole in alcoholic delirium

Indications

Chlormethiazole (clomethiazole edisylate; Hemineurine; Distraneurine) is a synthetic product, chemically related to the thiazole part of the thiamine (Aneurine; vitamin B_1) molecule (Fig. 43).

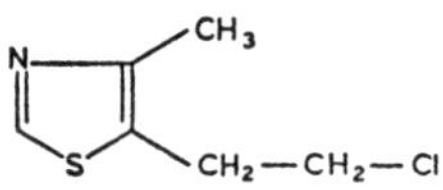

Figure 43. Chlormethiazole (clomethiazole edisylate; Hemineurine; Distraneurine).

Pharmacologically it has sedative and anticonvulsant properties. Particularly in Germany and in the Scandinavian countries it has been successfully used in the treatment of addicts, and more specifically:

1) in the treatment of delirious states caused by abuse of alcohol or drugs (especially sedatives and ataractics);
2) in the prevention of these syndromes after abrupt discontinuation of excessive use of alcohol or sedatives/ataractics;
3) in the treatment of other withdrawal symptoms which can occur following withdrawal of alcohol, sedatives/ataractics or opioids.

These indications are largely based on uncontrolled studies. In controlled studies, chlormethiazole was found to be more effective than a placebo; and with regard to alcohol withdrawal symptoms it was of the same therapeutic efficacy as the neuroleptic trifluoperazine (Madden et al. 1969). Its effect has not been compared with that of benzodiazepine derivatives, particularly chlordiazepoxide. This would be important because many psychiatrists regard these agents as first-choice compounds in the treatment of alcohol withdrawal symptoms.

The use of chlormethiazole as a hypnotic is not advisable because dependence develops quickly. In the treatment of addicts, therefore, its use should be restricted to a short period, not exceeding a few weeks.

Chlormethiazole, administered intravenously, is also used in the treatment of status epilepticus. Some authors regard it as a first-choice agent for this purpose, preferable to parenteral administration of diazepam or hydantoin derivatives. The mechanism of action of this compound is unknown.

Dosage

Patients with not-too-severe symptoms are first given an oral booster dose of 600-1200 mg. During the subsequent 24 hours, the dosage is adjusted to the clinical condition. Doses should not exceed 600 mg per 90 minutes or 8 g per day. In most cases 3 g, in fractional doses distributed over 24 hours, is sufficient.

In severe delirium, 40-100 ml of an 0.8% solution for infusion can be given by intravenous injection in 3-5 minutes (100 ml of the solution contains 0.8 g of the active substance). A more customary procedure is to administer this solution by slow intravenous drip. In this case the drip rate should be 60-150/minute, to be continued until sleep ensues. The drip rate is then so adjusted that (superficial) sleep continues (arousal should remain possible). The dose given by drip should not exceed 8 g/24 hours. As a rule, the switch to oral administration can be made after 1-3 days. In view of the risk of addiction, this treatment should not be continued longer than about 2 weeks for alcoholics. Unlike alcohol withdrawal, that of sedatives and ataractics is more gradual so that in these cases treatment should be continued somewhat longer.

Side effects

During parenteral treatment respiration, pulse and depth of sleep should be carefully monitored because with this mode of administration the blood pressure can fall, respiration can be depressed, and the patient can enter a coma. In oral medication the side effects are only slight: exanthema, increased tendency to sneeze and cough, and gastric symptoms. Hypotension is rare. The risk of addiction has already been stressed.

7. The rationale of multi-vitamin preparations in chronic alcoholism

Alcohol and avitaminoses

The psychiatric consequences of chronic alcohol abuse are numerous. The most widely known consequence is delirium tremens, which can be a phenomenon of intoxication as well as of acute withdrawal. Chronic abuse can also lead to deterioration of the ability to memorize and to retain memories. Two syndromes can develop more or less acutely: the Korsakow syndrome and the Wernicke syndrome. The former is characterized by disorientation, particularly in time, confusion and amnesia; the amnesia and disorientation are "compensated" by various confabulations. The Wernicke syndrome comprises acute neurological symptoms such as ataxia and paresis of the ocular muscles, but in addition the patient is confused and disoriented. The boundary between the two syndromes is therefore ill-defined.

These psychiatric consequences of chronic alcohol abuse are believed to have two causes: 1) a direct toxic effect of alcohol on the CNS; 2) malnutrition, and particularly deficiency in vitamins, especially water-soluble vitamins such as those of the B-group, which the organism cannot retain for any long period. The malnutrition results from two circumstances: a) nutrition largely consists of "empty" (alcohol) calories, without proteins, minerals and vitamins; b) the gastric mucosa is often chronically inflamed so that digestion and absorption are reduced.

Multi-vitamin preparations

This is why multi-vitamin preparations are prescribed to chronic alcoholics. In acute complications (delirium tremens, Korsakow and Wernicke syndromes), they are initially given parenterally (for a few weeks) to ensure rapid substitution and to short-circuit the intestinal tract. Vitamins are *supplements* to, *not substitutes* for the compounds used to control with withdrawal symptoms.

A multi-vitamin preparation of this type is Parentrovite, which can be given by intramuscular or intravenous injection but also by mouth (in which case it is called Oralvite). It is available in ampoules of 10 ml which contain high concentrations of thiamine, riboflavin, pyridoxine, nicotinamide and ascorbic acid. One ampoule daily is given during one week; this dosage is then reduced to 3 ampoules per week for two weeks, whereupon treatment is continued by oral administration (1-3 dragées per day).

This preparation has also been recommended for use in the treatment of mentally disturbed elderly patients with a history of chronic nutritional neglect.

BIBLIOGRAPHY

AHLENIUS, S., A. CARLSSON, J. ENGEL, H. SVENSSON AND P. SÖDERSTEN (1973). Antagonism by alpha methyltyrosine of the ethanol-induced stimulation and euphoria in man. *Clin. Pharmacol. Ther.* 14, 586.

BENKERT, V. AND H. HIPPIUS (1974). *Psychiatrische Pharmakotherapie.* Berlin, Heidelberg, New York: Springer Verlag.

BRAUDE, M. C., L. S. HARRIS, E. L. MAY, J. P. SMITH AND J. E. VILLARREAL (Eds.) (1974). *Narcotic Antagonist.* New York: Raven Press.

CARLSSON, A. AND M. LUNDQVIST (1973). Effect of ethanol on the hydroxylation of tyrosine and tryptophan in rat brain in vivo. *J. Pharm. Pharmacol.* 25, 437.

DOLE, V. P., M. E. NYSWANDER AND M. J. KREEK (1966). Narcotic blockade. *Arch. Intern. Med.* 118, 304.

DOLE, V. P., M. E. NYSWANDER AND A. WARNER (1968) Successful treatment of 750 clinical addicts. *J. Am. Med. Assn.* 206, 2708.

FINK, M. (1972). Opiate dependence. Treatment and prophylaxis. In: *Biochemical and Pharmacological Aspects of Dependence and Reports on Marihuana Research,* Ed. H. M. van Praag. Haarlem: Erven Bohn.

FRISCH, E. P. (Ed.) (1966). *Chlormethiazole (Heminevrin, Distraneurin)* Copenhagen: Munksgaard.

GLATT, M. M., H. R. GEORGE AND E. P. FRISCH (1965). Controlled trial of chlormethiazole in treatment of the alcohol withdrawal phase. *Brit. Med. J.* 2, 401.

HOLLISTER, L. E., J. J. PRUSMACK AND W. LIPSCOME (1972). Treatment of acute alcohol withdrawal with chlormethiazole (Heminevrin). *Dis. Nerv. Syst.* 33, 247.

JÖNSSON, L. E., E. ÄNGGARD AND L. M. GUNNE (1971). Blockade of intravenous amphetamine euphoria in man. *Clin. Pharmacol. Ther.* 12, 889.

KINGSTONE E. AND S. A. KLINE (1975). Disulfiram implants in the treatment of alcoholism. Some mechanisms of action. *Int. Pharmacopsychiat.* 10, 183.

Leading Article (1976) Alcohol and the brain. *Brit. Med. J.* 1, 1168.

LENNARD, H. L., L. J. EPSTEIN AND M. S. ROZENTHAL (1972). The methadone illusion. *Science* 176, 881.

LUNDWALL, L. AND F. BAEKELAND (1971). Disulfiram treatment of alcoholism: a re-

view. *J. Nerv. Ment. Dis.* 158, 381.
Madden, J. S., D. Jones and E. P. Frisch (1969). Chlormethiazole and trifluoperazine in alcohol withdrawal. *Brit. J. Psychiat.* 115, 1191.
Malcolm, M. T., J. S. Madden and A. E. Williams (1974). Disulfiram implantation critically evaluated. *Brit. J. Psychiat.* 125, 485.
Martin, W. R. (1973). Opioid antagonists. *Pharmacol. Rev.* 19, 463.
Martin, W. R., D. Z. Jasinski and P. A. Mansky (1973). Naltrexone, an antagonist for the treatment of heroin dependence. *Arch. Gen. Psychiat.* 28, 789.
Whyte, C. R. and P. M. J. O'Brien (1974). Disulfiram implant: a controlled trial. *Brit. J. Psychiat.* 124, 42.
Wilmarth, S. S. and A. Goldstein. (1974). *Therapeutic Effectiveness of Methadone Maintenance Program in the U.S.A.* Publication no. 3. World Health Organization, Geneva.

XXIV

Pharmacotherapy of Sexual Disorders

1. Suppression of sexual behaviour

Hypersexuality, be it directed normally or abnormally, is often a source of delinquent behaviour, particularly if the sexual impulses have a strong aggressive charge. Abnormally directed sexual impulses need not be abnormally strong to bring the individual in question into a court of law. For this reason, these individuals require treatment, quite apart from the question whether they themselves experience these impulses as morbid or rather as a variety of the normal. We are dealing here with typically masculine "diseases." Women rarely face criminal charges because of sexual aberrations.

The treatment of sexual delinquents is difficult, and usually involves diverse methods: psychotherapy, behaviour therapy, pharmacotherapy, and possibly even psychosurgery (although the value of this type of treatment is still controversial). In pharmacotherapy, two types of compounds have been used: neuroleptics and hormones. Diminished libido and impotence are side effects of neuroleptics but they are (fortunately) not common occurrences, and their development cannot be predicted. This is why neuroleptics are hardly suitable for the treatment of sexual deviations. An exception is the butyrophenone derivative benperidol. This is the only neuroleptic demonstrated to have probably a *specific* libido-inhibiting effect. According to Bancroft et al. (1974), it is not inferior to cyproterone acetate in this respect, although it produces more disturbing side effects.

Of the hormonal therapies, oestrogen administration is the most widely used. Although it is effective, its practicability is very limited because of the side effects: nausea, vomiting, and particularly feminization. An unusual but very serious complication can be mammary carcinoma. Progesterone-like substances are likewise believed to have a desexualizing effect, but practical experience with these products has been limited. The latest hormonal strategy is the use of anti-androgens. These are synthetic compounds which inhibit the effect of natural and synthetic androgens on peripheral and central (the so-called mating centres in the hypothalamus) effector cells. Probably they competitively oust androgens from the receptors. Substances which inhibit androgen synthesis, such as oestrogens, are not regarded as belonging to this group. Anti-androgens have been under investigation some 40 years. Since 1973, one representative of this group has been used in male hypersexuality: the competitive androgen antagonist cyproterone acetate (Androcur) (Fig. 44).

Few controlled studies have so far been made, and these few have covered only brief periods (1-2 months). With this restriction in mind, it can be stated that the results have so far been encouraging. The compound produces *physiological* effects: 1) reduced ability to have an erection; 2) delayed or absent ejaculation; 3) inhibition of

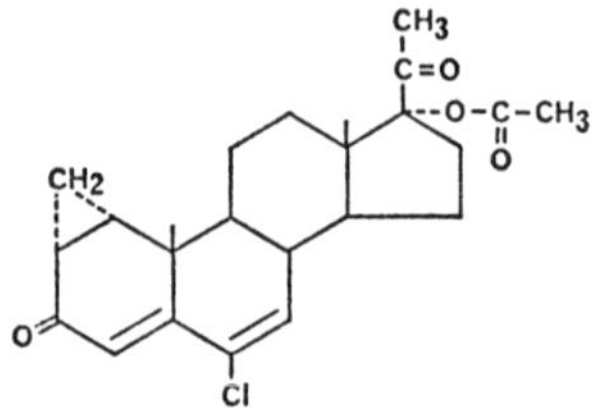

Figure 44. Cyprosterone acetate (Androcur), a substance with an anti-androgenic effect.

spermatogenesis. In addition it has *psychological* effects: 1) sexual impulses become less strong; 2) the sexual fantasies become less powerful. The direction of sexual impulses and the contents of sexual fantasies are not influenced. So far as we know, the effects of cyproterone acetate are reversible.

The psychological and physiological effects of cyproterone acetate do not always run parallel, and this entails a risk. When potency diminishes more markedly than desire, a severe degree of frustration can result. This is one of the reasons for using this type of pharmacotherapy only in combination with psychotherapy.

Suppression of sexuality is a very serious intervention, which can only be considered indicated in sexual delinquents and/or in those who suffer seriously as a result of their sexual aberration.

Dosage

The usual daily dose of cyproterone acetate is 2 × 50 mg, to be taken in the morning and in the evening. If no changes have occurred after 4-6 weeks, then the dosage can be increased to 200 mg per day and, briefly, to 300 mg per day, in three fractional doses. Once the desired effect is obtained, the minimal effective dose should be determined. This is usually about 2 × 25-50 mg per day. If the dosage is adequate, then suppression of sexuality as a rule becomes apparent after 2-4 weeks.

Side effects

In the initial phase of treatment the patient may complain of fatigue, apathy and despondency. Often, however, it is difficult to establish whether these symptoms are pharmacogenic or psychogenic, induced by what in actual fact is a mutilating intervention.

In the presence of endocrine or metabolic disorders, the internist should be consulted before this compound is prescribed. Since it can influence longitudinal growth, it should not be given to growing boys (should a convincing psychiatric indication to do so ever exist). The same applies to sexually mature women: cyproterone acetate is contraindicated, but women do not develop psychiatric symptoms for which this medication could be contemplated.

2. Stimulation of sexual behaviour

On this subject I can be brief: There are no known agents which have been demonstrated to intensify the libido or enhance potency via a pharmacological route. The only exception is amphetamines, which can stimulate sexual desire and intensify orgasm as well as prolong the pleasure. For this purpose, however, large (parenteral) doses are required which entail grave risks and are never medically justifiable. Oestrogens and androgens, which are occasionally prescribed to middle-aged or elderly women and men, respectively, have not been demonstrated to enhance diminished sexual activity. For a review of (alleged) aphrodisiacs, I refer to a publication by Hollister (1975).

BIBLIOGRAPHY

BANCROFT, J. (1974). *Deviant Sexual Behaviour, Modification and Assessment.* Oxford: Clarendon Press.

BANCROFT, J., G. TENNANT, K. LOUCAS AND J. CASS (1974). The control of deviant sexual behaviour by drugs. *Brit. J. Psychiat.* 125, 310.

BANCROFT, J. H. J. (1971). The application of psychophysiological measures to the assessment and modification of sexual behaviour. *Behav. Res. Ther.* 9, 119.

COOPER, A. J., A. A. A. ISMAIL, A. L. PHANJOO AND D. L. LOVE (1972). Anti-androgen (cyproterone acetate) therapy in deviant hypersexuality. *Brit. J. Psychiat.* 120, 59.

EDITORIAL (1976). Cyprosterone acetate. *Lancet* 1, 1003.

FIELD, L. H. (1973). Benperidol in the treatment of sex offenders. *Med. Sci. Law* 13, 195.

HOLLISTER, L. E. (1975). Drugs and sexual behavior in man. *Life Sci.* 17, 661.

NEUMANN, F. (1974). *Androgens and Antiandrogens.* Berlin, Heidelberg, New York: Springer Verlag.

SANDLER, M. AND G. L. GESSA (Eds.) (1975). *Sexual Behavior: Pharmacology and Biochemistry.* New York: Raven Press.

PART FIVE

Special Topics

Special effort to promote the interest of students in science is needed in face of the demand for clinical relevance. I believe the best hope lies not in a return to the traditional methods of instruction in basic science courses but in the personal example of the scientists both 'basic' and 'clinical' who should insist that an appreciation of science must be an objective for all students. There are many ways in which this objective may be achieved; but I am sure that, just as it is essential for the students to meet doctors behaving as doctors, so it is essential for them to meet scientists behaving as scientists. The student and the scientist must be brought together for a grander purpose than the passive transfer of acceptable stories.

E. J. Moran Campbell
Lancet, 17 January 1976.

XXV

Psychotropic Drugs in Children

1. Structure of this chapter

Of the psychotropic drugs discussed in this chapter, the central stimulants receive most attention because, of all psychotropic drugs, they have been most thoroughly studied in children and because they have specific indications in children. Moreover, there is no evidence that the therapeutic action profile and the pattern of side effects of the other psychotropic drugs in children differ essentially from those in adults. The remarks I shall make in this respect are merely supplements to what has already been pointed out in the relevant specific chapters. These chapters are therefore indispensable for a good understanding of paediatric psychopharmacology.

The discussions of the various groups of psychotropic drugs will be preceded by a general discussion of the use of these agents in children.

2. Delayed evolution of paediatric psychopharmacology

Paediatric psychopharmacology is an underdeveloped area as compared with psychotropic drugs research in adults. Development and evaluation of methods of registration; differentiation of related syndromes and studies of possible differences in response to psychotropic drugs; application of suitable control measures—all these procedures are more or less taken for granted in adults but have been used only sparingly in children. Consequently, much research in this field is not very reliable. While diagnostic criteria have often been inadequately defined, their communicative value is also limited. The delayed evolution is strikingly expressed in the limited number of publications on paediatric psychopharmacology in relation to the totality of the psychopharmacological literature. And their number is small also in the absolute sense.

To explain the situation, two factors are of importance. The first lies in the methodological problems. The second is to be found in the fact that many child psychiatrists are reluctant a priori to prescribe psychotropic drugs. Both factors will be discussed in some detail.

3. Causes of delayed evolution

Abundance of methodological problems

Research into the effects of drugs in human individuals is no longer what it used to be for many years: a pastime of clinicians. It has become a separate discipline: human pharmacology. This is a difficult discipline, particularly if it concerns itself with the influence of drugs on psychological functions, and even more so if children are the objects of study. These additional problems are traceable to the simple fact that a child is a growing organism.

Psychopharmacological research always requires the use of (at least) two groups—test group and control group—which (at least) should tend to be diagnostically homogeneous. In the diagnosis of disorders in children, age is an important variable. Behaviour which is quite normal at a given age—e.g. distractibility, hyperactivity, dependency—becomes abnormal when it persists at a later age. In children more than in adults, moreover, the nature of psychopathological manifestations differs with age. A single year's difference in early childhood can be diagnostically much more important than a difference of decades in adult life. This implies that the groups studied should be matched not only according to diagnosis, duration of symptoms, and preferably sex and IQ as well (as in adults), but also according to age. This makes it difficult to compose groups of sufficient size to give results which can be statistically analysed.

There is something else. Adult psychiatric syndromes are made up of symptoms which can usually be differentiated without too much difficulty. In early childhood, however, psychiatric reactions are more amorphous and less differentiated; this of course impedes their classification and categorization. The amorphousness, by the way, might well be spurious; it might be a result of the fact that, in psychiatric diagnosis, greater emphasis is usually placed on the patient's verbal introspective expressions than on his visually observable behaviour. A delusion is generally diagnosed on the basis of what the patient says rather than on the basis of what he does. Young children, however, still verbalize imperfectly, and consequently psychiatric disorders are expressed more directly in their behaviour and relations to others. In a more "ethologically" oriented diagnostic approach, the lack of differentiation might well prove to be non-existent.

Evaluation of therapeutic results also poses an abundance of problems in children, for one has to determine changes (if any) in an individual who is, as such, constantly changing. The younger the child, the higher the growth rate and the more difficult the evaluation.

Finally, the fact has to be taken into account that, more than the adult organism, the developing organism is susceptible to exogenous (somatic and psychological) influences. This applies to regressive influences which impede recovery, as well as to regenerative influences. Children are more vulnerable than adults, but also more resilient. Evaluation of the effect of a therapy demands that all other variables which might influence the syndrome be kept constant so far as possible. This requirement, standardization of the test situation, is even more difficult to fulfil in children than in adults. This may explain the fact that pharmacotherapy regularly produces surprises in children: results which are inconsistent with earlier, parallel or somebody else's observations. The predictability of therapeutic results is certainly less than that in adults.

Reluctance of child psychiatrists

Many child psychiatrists show a certain reluctance to prescribe psychotropic drugs, particularly in less serious cases (outpatients) and/or cases accessible to psychotherapy. What are the potential risks that cause this reluctance?

1) Psychotropic drugs could readily provide *parents* with an alibi for minimizing the emotional problems with which the child struggles; on the other hand, their use could unnecessarily alarm parents and make them exaggerate the severity of the disturbances.
2) *Children*, particularly so-called problem children, might experience the psychopharmacotherapy as a panacea or, on the other hand, see it as a punishment or as a means of coercion by which authorities impose their will and try to force them to cooperate.
3) Psychotropic drugs could be a temptation to the *therapist* to avoid confrontation with his patient's vital problems, and could thus undermine the doctor-patient relationship.
4) Finally, mention is made in this context of the possibility of side effects which outweigh the therapeutic effects. Psychotropic drugs interfere with perceptive and cognitive functions and can thus reduce scholastic performance. By reducing emotional susceptibility, moreover, they may disturb the psychotherapeutic relation.

These considerations are undoubtedly valid but, as such, are not sufficient to explain the reluctance completely. After all, it can be explained to all persons involved what can and what cannot be expected of a drug. Of course, drugs influence the subtle lines of communication between child, parents and psychotherapist, but the possible dangers can be discussed with child and parents and thus avoided (provided, always, that the physician has a sensible attitude towards drugs). As regards the balance between desired and undesired effects: this is a delicate one, certainly in children, and requires highly individualized attention. But the same applies equally to adults. In principle, however, an acceptable balance can be achieved in most cases.

I therefore believe that, in addition to a rational ground, the reluctance also has an irrational ground, namely the tendency to classify methods of psychiatric treatment vertically rather than horizontally. In this vision, pharmacotherapy is not merely a different mode of treatment as compared with verbal types of therapy but an inferior method, a second choice, an approach not to be seriously considered until verbal psychotherapy has failed. In this vision, psychotropic drugs are degraded to a rather irritating interference with the therapist's desire for psychotherapeutic omnipotence.

Regardless of whether the reluctance is essentially rational or irrational, it is a fact that it has assumed a rationale in the course of time: sparing use of a method causes knowledge of the method to remain fragmentary, and this in turn is a valid argument in favour of continuing to use the method only sparingly.

4. Central stimulants

The so-called hyperkinetic (or hyperactivity) syndrome

Central stimulants have a specific range of indications in child psychiatry. These indications are found within the group of hyperkinetic children. This statement requires elucidation, because hyperkinetic children have become subject to many myths, and stimulants have been abused in their treatment.

Hyperkinesia is a syndrome of varying aetiology, which occurs in all degrees of severity and is four times as frequent in boys as in girls. Its principal symptoms are the following.

a. *Hyperactivity*, almost incessant or at least occurring in situations in which children of comparable age are as a rule quiet. The motor activity is not very orderly and hardly purposeful. The child starts all sorts of things but does not finish them. Coordination of motor activities as such may be disturbed. Activity readily increases in response to exogenous stimuli.
b. *Impulsiveness*. Impulses are readily responded to, and there is little room for "either/or" considerations. The parents

complain that the child does such dangerous things, or makes such tactless remarks.

c. *Increased distractiveness*, as a result of which the child is unable to focus his attention on a particular subject for any length of time. For this reason, scholastic performance is often substandard.

d. *Decreased frustration tolerance* is often (but by no means always) observed, the children showing unusually explosive responses to frustrations.

In early childhood, manifestations of the hyperkinetic syndrome develop physiologically when the child tires. When tired, adults become inactive but young children as a rule become animated, overly active and "difficult." When this behaviour pattern is more or less habitual, the child is called hyperkinetic.

Some hyperkinetic children show psychological and neurological signs of slightly disturbed cerebral functions (partial learning problems; slightly disturbed coordination; chorea-like "jerkiness," etc.), but others show no such signs. Inversely, numerous children with cerebral lesions show no hyperkinetic symptoms. Some hyperkinetic children show disturbances in personality development, e.g. fear of failure, uncertainty, poorly controlled aggressiveness, reduced frustration tolerance, emotional explosiveness, etc. Others who are equally hyperkinetic show a normal personality development. The hyperkinetic syndrome can also be encountered in deeply disturbed children suffering from psychosis or from the consequences of anatomical brain lesions. Finally, the results of family studies indicate the likelihood that genetic factors may be of importance also in the aetiology of this syndrome.

The hyperkinesia concept, therefore, must not be used as a diagnosis. It denotes a *syndrome* which can be caused by a variety of factors: organic cerebral, psychogenic and hereditary. And in many cases there are no demonstrable aetiological factors at all. In its *aetiological non-specificity*, the hyperkinetic syndrome in children can be compared with the vital depressive syndrome and the anxiety syndrome in adults.

Hyperkinetic syndrome and "minimal brain dysfunction"

The terms hyperkinetic syndrome and minimal brain dysfunction (MBD) are not synonyms. MBD is a vaguely defined concept which covers a whole range of more or less mild neurological (e.g. slight disorders of coordination) and psychological (e.g. partial learning problems) functional disorders. It has not been established with certainty in which cases it is justifiable to ascribe such changes to not further specified functional disorders of the brain. One might expect that criteria would have been formulated, e.g. certain EEG changes, diseases during pregnancy, incidents at parturition, etc. Nothing of the sort has been done, and for this reason the term MBD is not much more than a smoke screen to conceal diagnostic ignorance.

Be this as it may, MBD is certainly not identical to the hyperkinetic syndrome. As already pointed out, this syndrome *can* be accompanied by circumscribed psychological or neurological disorders, but these may equally well be absent.

Therapeutic range of action of stimulants

Stimulants are *not* the agents of choice in the treatment of *all* children with manifestations of the hyperkinetic syndrome. Neuroleptics are decidedly to be preferred in cases involving manifest psychosis or a borderline state. In these cases, stimulants may have an adverse effect: aggravate unrest or cause psychosis to become manifest. In the presence of severe anatomical brain lesions, stimulants are usually inadequate. In the remaining cases, the chance of a favourable effect is 60%. The others show no response, or an insufficient response, or evidently respond much better to other psychotropic drugs. We do not know the factors which determine success, nor do we have any predictors. The only possible strategy is that of trial-and-error. In this context it is fortunate that the therapeutic effect of stimulants, if it occurs at all, comes quickly. Within a day or a few days behaviour becomes less chaotic, more purposeful; restiveness diminishes and concentration improves. In many cases, performance at school is the best yardstick. Be this as it may, a therapeutic attempt with stimulants takes but little time.

Is the effect of stimulants in hyperkinesia really paradoxical?

The term paradoxical has been used because it had been expected that, in hyperkinetic children, stimulants were more likely to make behaviour more chaotic than to give it structure. Although nothing is known with certainty about the mechanism of action of stimulants used for these indications, it is an attractive hypothesis that, in these cases too, their therapeutic effect is based on central activation. Young children become disinhibited and hypermotile when tired. They cannot "shift back to a lower gear," as adults do. Yet we must assume that in these circumstances their CNS is not overaroused but underaroused. This would explain the fact that barbiturates, which further depress the CNS, often have an adverse effect if used to sedate hyperactive children, aggravating the restiveness instead of arresting it. If in hyperkinetic children the CNS is habitually "underaroused," then the therapeutic efficacy of stimulants would be explained. If this theory is correct, then the effect of stimulants in these cases is a traditional, not a paradoxical one. And physiological studies have shown that this theory is not entirely untenable (e.g. Knopp et al. 1973; Satterfield et al. 1974).

Are stimulants effective only in hyperkinesia?

This question has been studied in particular by Fish (1968), and she answers it in the negative. She found that stimulants also produced good results in insecure, inhibited, anxious children with fear of failure, and more specifically in those with school phobias. These children became less shy and reticent, and gained self-confidence. In these children it seems that the conventional stimulant effect develops, similar to that in adults. The therapeutic effect of stimulants in hyperkinetic children has been properly documented in controlled studies, but the effect for the forementioned indication has not. There is something else. So far as we know, hyperkinetic children have never become addicted to amphetamines. It seems to me, however, that this risk does exist in anxious, insecure children, although I must add immediately that no instances of addiction have so far been described.

Dosage

In the treatment of hyperkinetic children, most experience has been gained with two stimulants: dextro-amphetamine and methylphenidate. We do not know which of the two give the best results. I regard methylphenidate as the first choice because it exerts less influence on appetite than d-amphetamine and because the sympathicomimetic activity in the periphery is less pronounced. Its side effects are on the whole less marked.

The initial daily dose of d-amphetamine as well as of methylphenidate is 0.25 mg/kg body weight. The dose is doubled every week to an average of 2 mg/kg for methylphenidate and 1 mg/kg for d-amphetamine (always assuming that no severe side effects occur). If methylphenidate is ineffective, then an amphetamine derivative (usually d-amphetamine, which is more potent per mg than laevo-amphetamine or dl-amphetamine) can be tried. If the one stimulant causes an increase in hyperactivity, then the other is likely to do the same. In such cases a neuroleptic or ataractic is to be preferred.

Stimulants are usually given three times per day, every 4 hours, because they are quickly metabolized and their therapeutic effect diminishes after 3-4 hours. The last dose is given at 1600 hrs so as not to disturb sleep too much.

Duration of treatment

This depends on the results. Every 3-6 months there should be a period during which dosage is reduced or even discontinued under strict supervision. If the condition deteriorates, the medication has to be resumed. This therapy is as a rule discontinued as adolescence starts, but some authors (e.g. Renshaw 1975) continue longer, even up to age 19.

Habituation to the therapeutic effect has not been described, and this raises doubt about the theory which postulates that the effect is based on the traditional arousing effect of stimulants, for habituation to this effect is the rule.

Side effects

The principal side effects are disturbed sleep and reduced appetite. The former is minimized by giving the last fractional dose no later than 1600 hrs; the latter is minimized by having the doses ingested immediately *after* meals (even though this does reduce intestinal absorption). Nevertheless, "amphetamine children" often show some degree of growth retardation.

Abdominal pain and nausea frequently occur in cases in which the dosage is increased too quickly. Addiction to amphetamines prior to adolescence has never been described.

Stimulants have some epileptogenic activity. This is why they should be combined with anticonvulsants when used in the treatment of children with clinical or EEG evidence of epilepsy. One should start with a few days of anticonvulsant medication only, to ensure that an optimal concentration in the brain is attained before stimulant medication is started.

Stimulants and other therapies

Even if it is effective, stimulant medication alone is often not enough. A search should be made for, and attention given to, psychological and social problems which impede the child's growth and development. Experience has shown that, in most cases, indications are found for psychotherapeutic and/or paedagogic measures, or for remedial teaching. As a component in a more comprehensive therapeutic programme, however, stimulant medication can be very useful.

5. Ataractics, sedatives, hypnotics

Ataractics are sedative compounds which differ from neuroleptics in that they lack de-emotioning (antipsychotic) activity, and from sedatives (barbiturates, bromides, etc.) in that their hypnotic effect is less and their anxiolytic (anxiety-reducing) effect more pronounced. They make the patient much less dull, and hardly affect intellectual performance.

Sedatives and ataractics are certainly effective in cases of anxiety and/or motor unrest of non-psychotic origin. Whether they should be prescribed to children is another question. For sedatives, and particularly for barbiturates, the answer is no. As discussed in chapter XXI, they produce too many side effects; and young children not infrequently show a "paradoxical" response: instead of calming down, they become restive. As anticonvulsants, however, barbiturates can still be indicated in the treatment of children.

The position of ataractics in child psychiatry is uncertain. Research has focused mainly on chlordiazepoxide, diazepam and hydroxyzine, and undoubtedly their effect is superior to that of a placebo. But when are they indicated? In the hyperkinetic syndrome they are not first choice, because stimulants are therapeutically more effective (Zrull et al. 1963). In psychoses, neuroleptics are far preferable. Ataractics can be prescribed in the case of marked anxiety of neurotic origin if psychotherapeutic intervention fails, but only for a brief period. It does not seem to be a very wise therapeutic policy to teach a young child to suppress feelings of dysphoria and tension by means of drugs. Moreover, a substance such as chlordiazepoxide is suspected of being able to produce a "paradoxical" effect: to reduce impulse control and intensify aggressiveness. As in the case of adults, however, this suspicion is based on incidental observations rather than on systematic research.

Particularly the Bellevue group (Fish and her co-workers) has recommended the antihistamine diphenhydramine as an effective and harmless sedative for children under 12, with an IQ exceeding 70. It is reported to lose some of its efficacy as adolescence begins. It is uncertain whether diphenhydramine is to be regarded as an ataractic or rather as a conventional sedative. Because of its antiallergic and anti-emetic effect, the compound is useful in the treatment of neurotic children who vomit much or show asthmatic symptoms. Such somatic symptoms can sometimes be interpreted as anxiety equivalents. Diphenhydramine is used also to control acute dystonic reactions caused by neuroleptics. And finally it is used as a hypnotic for children. Another hypnotic which can be prescribed to children, if necessary, is chloral hydrate. It is an old agent which, as in adults, is often overlooked.

6. Neuroleptics

Indications

There are strong indications that pre-adolescent psychoses are favourably influenced by neuroleptics, much as psychoses at a later age are. This applies to psychoses of the schizophrenic type, to those associated with anatomical brain lesions, and to disintegration states of largely psychogenic origin. They can also be indicated in the treatment of children suffering from overwhelming anxiety and those who show uncontrollable aggressive or destructive behaviour towards self, others, or objects.

Of the phenothiazines, chlorpromazine and thioridazine have been best studied. Both are superior to a placebo when used for the indications under discussion. In severely disturbed children, chlorpromazine had a favourable effect in 80% of cases, whereas none improved in response to a placebo (Korein et al. 1971). Chlorpromazine has a stronger sedative effect than thioridazine, and thus has an unfavourable effect on scholastic performance. Moreover, it exerts a more marked influence on the extrapyramidal system. For these reasons, thioridazine is to be preferred. If the latter gives unsatisfactory results, then chlorpromazine should be tried because its antipsychotic effect is probably more pronounced than that of thioridazine.

Of the phenothiazines which increase rather than depress motor activity, trifluoperazine and fluphenazine have been studied. Both are active neuroleptics, indicated in particular if the child is reticent and hypoactive, and shows little response to the environment. Both compounds have a strong affinity for the extrapyramidal system and can provoke parkinson-like as well as hyper(dys)kinetic symptoms. The same applies to trifluperidol, a neuroleptic of the butyrophenone type, with an activating effect. According to Campbell et al. (1972), it is superior to trifluoperazine in the treatment of young autistic children. Its therapeutic range is narrow, however, and it readily provokes extrapyramidal symptoms.

Haloperidol is another butyrophenone derivative which has been studied in children. It is of value in particular when hyperactivity and aggressiveness are prominent features. It is one of the strongest sedatives available to cope with psychotic unrest. It has also been used, with varying success, in the treatment of the Gilles de la Tourette syndrome.

In the group of the thioxanthene derivatives, experience has been gained mostly with thiothixene. According to Campbell et al. (1972), it is therapeutically superior to chlorpromazine and less sedative, which is a great practical advantage.

Pimozide, a representative of the diphenylbutylpiperidine derivatives (the latest group of neuroleptics), has so far only occasionally been used in child psychiatry. The results have been encouraging, particularly in children with autistic symptoms.

Side effects

The principal side effects of neuroleptics are the extrapyramidal symptoms. Hypokinetic-rigid symptoms seem to be less frequent in children than in adults, but hyperkinetic and dyskinetic symptoms are more frequent. Inactivating neuroleptics induce largely manifestations of the former type, while activating neuroleptics are more likely to induce those of the latter type. The extrapyramidal symptoms are rarely dangerous, but always alarming. With the conventional anti-parkinson drugs (e.g. orphenadrine; Disipal), however, hypokinetic and dyskinetic symptoms can be adequately controlled, or even prevented. Large doses of phenothiazines over longer periods are to be avoided. As in adults, this approach can lead to irreversible lesions of the extrapyramidal system. Efforts to determine the minimal effective dose should always be made.

Phenothiazines are epileptogenic compounds. In children with clinical or EEG evidence of epilepsy, administration of anticonvulsants (or increase of their dosage) is to be considered.

In some cases, very inconvenient weight gains may make it necessary to reduce caloric intake.

Neuroleptics often improve the child's contact with the environment and enhance the child's communicativeness also about pathological thoughts and experiences. As a result, the condition of inhibited, negativistic or autistically preoccupied children may initially *seem* to deteriorate.

Other applications

Chlorpromazine and thioridazine have been tested in children with hyperkinetic symptoms. They had a beneficial effect, which is not surprising in view of their sedative action. Nevertheless I regard stimulants as first choice when the hyperkinetic child is not psychotic, because stimulant medication is less drastic than neuroleptic medication. Stimulants do not have the de-emotioning effect which, in non-psychotic children, is undesirable. Moreover, they do not sedate and scholastic performance is therefore not negatively affected.

7. Dosage of neuroleptics and ataractics

In the discussion of neuroleptics and ataractics I have not mentioned doses. The reason is that susceptibility of neuroleptics and ataractics is individually widely variable. Conversion of adult doses to children's doses by the usual conversion formulae will often given faulty results. Little is known about the pharmacokinetics of psychotropic drugs in children.

The best strategy is: start with a small dose and increase gradually on the basis of clinical findings and side effects, if any. One should not be reluctant to increase to a high level (as long as intensive supervision is possible). Children often show a higher tolerance to these drugs than adults, and require a larger dose than might be expected in view of age and body weight. Since neuroleptics as well as ataractics have a wide therapeutic range (i.e. an ample margin between therapeutic and toxic doses), a flexible dosage policy is acceptable. A frequent cause of failure of medication with these agents is underdosage or premature discontinuation of treatment.

In spite of these reservations, I have listed some dosages in Table 32. These are explicitly meant to serve general orientations, and should be utilized with the necessary flexibility.

It is advisable to continue psychotropic medication for at least

Table 32. General orientation on the dosage of some psychotropic drugs in the treatment of children.

Drug	Dosage (in mg/kg/day) Range	Average
chlorpromazine (Largactil)	1.0 - 5.0	2.0
trifluoperazine (Terfluzine)	0.01 - 0.4	0.1
fluphenazine (Moditen)	0.01 - 0.1	0.05
thioridazine (Mellaril)	0.5 - 4.0	2.0
haloperidol (Serenase, Haldol)	0.02 - 0.1	0.07
chlordiazepoxide (Librium)	0.25 - 1.5	1.0
diazepam (Valium)	0.1 - 0.5	0.3
hydroxyzine (Atarax)	0.5 - 2.0	1.0
diphenhydramine (Benadryl)	2.0 - 10.0	4.0
phenobarbital (Luminal)	1.0 - 3.0	2.0
chloral hydrate	30 - 70	50
orphenadrine (Disipal)	1.5 - 4.0	2.0

six weeks before it is definitely regarded as ineffective. Failure of a neuroleptic (or ataractic) does not mean that another agent of this category would necessarily also be ineffective. Only if at least two compounds have proved to be ineffective can a therapy be considered to have failed.

8. Lithium

Nothing is known with certainty about the usefulness of lithium in the treatment of pre-adolescents. If one believes that vital depressions can occur in childhood also, then it would be rational in view of experience gained in adults to consider lithium prophylaxis in cases showing a substantial relapse rate. On the other hand, I have some reservations: little research has so far been carried out to provide a basis for such a decision; some side effects which seem acceptable in adults are very undesirable in children (e.g. diminished thyroid function); finally, chronic medication of young children is a serious intervention. All in all, I am not sure whether the benefit/risk balance will always be in favour of the former. Any practitioner who prescribes lithium in an effort to cope with mood fluctuations in a young child should regard this as an experiment which requires a very careful follow-up.

Intriguing observations were reported by Gram and Rafaelsen (1972), who pointed out that lithium may have a more or less specific anti-aggressive effect and reduces explosiveness, destructiveness and irritability; but these observations are still to be corroborated. Sheard (personal communication) observed a similar effect in adults sentenced for aggressive crimes.

9. Antidepressants

Views on the incidence of vital depressions in pre-adolescence are controversial. Fish (1968) regards it as rare in children, but Frommer (1967, 1968) describes the syndrome as regularly observed. Retrospective studies of adult patients with unipolar or bipolar depressions indicate that vital depression is indeed not rare in children but manifests itself in a different way from that in adults. Children retire, become taciturn, spend wakeful nights, eat less, may show a tendency to run away, and may perform less well at school and so develop a school phobia. They may express various somatic complaints. The mood is depressed. The lastmentioned symptom probably precedes the other manifestations instead of resulting from them, as is often believed. However, a vicious circle can of course readily develop: depressiveness, reduced scholastic performance, depressed mood, etc. Another argument which indicates that we are really dealing with types of (vital) depressiveness is that antidepressants have a therapeutic effect (or at least tricyclic compounds have; MAO inhibitors have hardly been tested in children). In adults, the rate of success with tricyclic antidepressants in vital depressions is about 65%. According to Renshaw (1975) this rate is lower in preadolescents, but no exact data are available.

Most experience has been gained with imipramine and amitriptyline, and practitioners are therefore well-advised to confine themselves to these two compounds for the time being. Amitriptyline is a sedative antidepressant and therefore indicated whenever the depressive syndrome is associated with manifest anxiety, marked tension or motor hyperactivity. Imipramine, on the contrary, is (slightly) activating rather than sedative, and is therefore the compound of choice whenever apathy rather than unrest is the dominant feature.

Side effects produced by these agents can include xerostomia, blurred vision, difficult micturition (anticholinergic effects), and sleep disorders (particularly with imipramine and especially if the last dose is given shortly before retiring). A substantial weight gain may be observed. Hypotension is rarely a problem. In some cases the daily dose of amitriptyline is given in a single dose shortly before retiring. Its sedative effect promotes sleep, and the side effects are less of a problem because they mostly develop during sleep. Whether the blood concentration does not diminish too much in the course of the 24-hour interval between the doses remains unknown. Little is in fact known about the pharmacokinetics of psychotropic drugs in children, and this also applies to antidepressants.

As regards dosage, the policy is again: start low (1 mg/kg) and increase slowly under strict supervision; there should be no reluctance to attain relatively high levels (3-4 mg/kg), but high-dosage medication should be as brief as possible. Above all: the dosage is to be individualized, for there are no extensive clinical data and/or pharmacokinetic data to guide the therapist.

Imipramine was found to be effective also in hyperkinetic children, although less so than methylphenidate (Rapoport et al. 1974). Why it should be effective is unknown. Imipramine has been successfully used also in the treatment of school phobias (Gittelman-Klein and Klein 1973), but the children involved may have been suffering from disguised depressions. The compound has also been used in enuresis nocturna (25-50 mg before retiring) (Sprague and Werry 1971). The therapeutic effect is possibly based on relaxation of the bladder musculature in combination with reduced depth of sleep.

10. Anticonvulsants

In 1938, hydantoin derivatives were introduced as anticonvulsants and found to be effective in grand mal as well as in psychomotor epilepsy. Subsequently published reports indicated that these compounds could also be useful in psychological disorders not associated with epilepsy. When it was established, moreover, that a large percentage of children with behaviour disorders show (non-specific) EEG changes, these compounds began to be used in child psychiatry for a variety of indications—with greatly varying results. There is no convincing evidence that these compounds merit a place in child psychiatry.

Of the anti-epileptic carbamazepine (Tegretol), it has been stated by many investigators that, in addition to an anticonvulsant effect, it exerts a favourable influence on behaviour disorders and character problems in epileptic patients, regardless of age. This compound, too, has been recommended for children with behaviour disorders whose EEG is not optimal (but not necessarily epileptic). The anti-epileptic primidone (Mysoline) has also been used for this indication. The underlying studies are methodologically questionable; the diagnostic criteria applied, moreover, are too vague and too heterogeneous to be conclusive of any more or less circumscribed range of indications. The subject requires further investigation. Specifically, the abovementioned anti-epileptics should be compared with neuroleptics and ataractics in diagnostically well-defined groups.

11. Conclusions

I must end as I began, with the observation that our knowledge of paediatric psychopharmacology is still fragmentary. Even more urgently than in dealing with adults, we need an accepted system of diagnoses and diagnostic criteria. Properly validated and age-standardized rating instruments are scarce. Methodological requirements are not infrequently disregarded. Nevertheless, it seems justifiable to present at least one general conclusion: that psychotropic drugs can substantially improve social adjustment and accessibility to psychotherapy in particular in psychotic children (with delusions and/or hallucinations), in hypermotile children, and in anxious children. If they are effective, moreover, then they are usually quickly effective; and this is a considerable advantage, e.g. in cases which readily tend towards chronicity. The conclusion cannot be more detailed. Further definition of the range of action of these compounds is impossible and awaits further investigations.

A second conclusion concerns the relation between pharmacotherapy and psychotherapy. As we have seen, psychotropic drugs are given for syndromally determined indications, regardless of the aetiology of the syndrome and regardless of its nosological categorization. To give an example: they are given, not because a child is considered to be suffering from schizophrenia but because delusions, hallucinations, restiveness or anxiety are observed.

In principle it can be stated that the susceptibility of symptoms to psychotropic drugs is unrelated to their severity. This means that psychotropic medication is to be considered not only for patients who show a very severe drug-susceptible syndrome but also for those who show this syndrome in a milder form, and also if the syndrome seems to be largely psychogenic and accessible to psychotherapy. To phrase it in somewhat more popular terms: psychotherapy and pharmacotherapy are not enemies. It is logically justifiable and therefore sensible to make an attempt at controlling a given morbid condition by simultaneous efforts via different routes (chapter V).

For the same reason I consider a division of competencies—in the sense of assigning psychotherapy to one therapist, and medication to another—to have more disadvantages than advantages, particularly in the treatment of outpatients. Psychotropic drugs readily become involved in the neurotic interaction between child and parents. In my opinion, the psychotherapist is the right person to prevent such complications, or to identify and discuss them.

BIBLIOGRAPHY

ANNELL, A. L. (Ed.) (1972). *Depressive States in Childhood and Adolescence*. Stockholm: Almquist & Wiksell.

CAMPBELL, M., B. FISH, T. SHAPIRO AND A. FLOYD, JR. (1972). Acute responses of schizophrenic children to a sedative and stimulating neuroleptic: A pharmacologic yardstick. *Curr. Ther. Res.* 14, 759.

CANTWELL, D. P. (Ed.) (1975). *The Hyperactive Child. Diagnosis, Management, Current Research*. New York: Spectrum Publications.

CLAGHORN, J. L. (1972). A double-blind comparison of haloperidol (Haldol) and thioridazine (Mellaril) in outpatient children. *Curr. Ther. Res.* 14, 785.

CONNORS, C. K. (1972). Pharmacotherapy of psychopathology in children. In: *Psychopathological disorders of childhood*, Ed. by H. C. Quay and J. S. Werry. New York: Wiley.

CRUZ, F. F. DE LA, B. H. FOX AND R. H. ROBERTS (Eds.) (1973). Minimal brain dysfunction. *Ann. New York Acad. Sc.* 205.

DIMASCIO, A., J. J. SOLTYS AND R. I. SHADER (1970). Psychotropic drug side effects in children. In: *Psychotropic drug side effects*, Ed. by R. I. Shader and A. DiMascio. Baltimore: William & Wilkins.

EISENBERG, L. (1968). Psychopharmacology in childhood: a critique. In: *Foundations in child psychiatry*, Ed. by E. Miller. Pergamon Press, Oxford.

EVELOFF, H. H. (1970). Pediatric psychopharmacology. In: *Principles in Psychopharmacology*, Ed. by W. G. Clark and J. del Guidice. New York: Academic Press.

FISH, B. (1971). The "one chiild, one drug" myth of stimulants in hyperkinesis. *Arch. Gen. Psychiat.* 25, 193.

FISH, B. (1968). Drug use in psychiatric disorders of children. *Am. J. Psychiat.* 124, 31.

FISH, B., M. CAMPBELL, T. SHAPIRO AND A. FLOYD JR. (1969). Comparison of trifluperidol, trifluoperazine and chlorpromazine in preschool schizophrenic children: The value of less sedative antipsychotic agents. *Curr. Ther. Res.* 11, 589.

FROMMER, E. A. (1967). Treatment in childhood depression with antidepressant drugs. *Brit. Med. J.* 1, 729.

FROMMER, E. A. (1968). Depressive illness in childhood. *Brit. J. Psychiat.* (special Publication no. 2): *Recent Developments in Affective Disorders: A Symposium*, Ed. by A. Coppen and A. Walk.

GITTELMAN-KLEIN, R. (1975). Review of clinical psychopharmacological treatment of hyperkinesis. In: *Progress in Psychiatric Drug Treatment*, Ed. by D. F. Klein and R. Gittelman-Klein. New York: Brunner/Mazel.

GITTELMAN-KLEIN, R. AND D. F. KLEIN (1973). School phobia: diagnostic considerations in the light of imipramine effects. *J. Nerv. Men. Dis.* 156, 199.

GITTELMAN-KLEIN, R. AND D. F. KLEIN (1976). Methylphenedate effects in learning disabilities. *Arch. Gen. Psychiatry* 33, 665.

GRAHAM, P. (1974). Depression in pre-pubertal children. *Dev. Med. Child. Neurol.* 16, 340.

GRAM, L. F. AND O. J. RAFAELSEN (1972). Lithium treatment of psychotic children and adolescents: a controlled clinical trial. *Acta Psychiatr. Scand.* 48, 253.

GROSS, M. B. AND W. C. WILSON (1974). *Minimal Brain Dysfunction*. New York: Brunner/Mazel.

HOLLISTER, L. E. (1973). *Clinical Use of Psychotherapeutic Drugs*. Springfield, Ill.: Charles C Thomas.

KALVERBOER, A. F., H. M. VAN PRAGG AND J. MENDELWICZ (Eds.) (1977). *Minimal Brain Dysfunction. Fact and Fiction*. Basel: Karger.

KNOPP, W., L. E. ARNOLD, R. L. ANDRAS AND D. SMELZER (1973). Predicting amphetamine response in hyperkinetic children by electronic pupillography. *Pharmakopsychiat. Neuro-Psychopharmak*. 6, 158.

KOREIN, J., B. FISH, T. SHAPIRO, E. W. GERNER AND L. LEVIDOW (1971). EEG and behavioral effects on drug therapy in children: Chlorpromazine and diphenhydramine. *Arch. Gen. Psychiatry* 24, 552.

LUCAS, A. R., H. J. LOCKETT AND F. GRIMM (1965). Amitriptyline in childhood depressions. *Dis. Nerv. Syst*. 26, 105.

MCANDREW, J. B., Q. CASE AND D. TREFFERT (1972). Effects of prolonged phenothiazine intake on psychotic and other hospitalized children. *J. Autism. Child. Schizo*. 2, 75.

MORRISON, J. AND M. STEWART (1973). The psychiatric status of the legal families of adopted hyperactive children. *Arch. Gen. Psychiat*. 28, 888.

O'MALLEY, J. AND L. EISENBERG (1973). The hyperkinetic syndrome. *Seminars in Psychiatry* 5, 95.

OMENN, G. (1973). Genetic issues in the syndrome of minimal brain dysfunction. *Seminars in Psychiatry* 5, 5.

POUSSAINT, A. F. AND K. S. DITMAN (1965). A controlled study of imipramine (Tofranil) in the treatment of childhood enuresis. *J. Pediatr*. 67, 283.

PRAAG, H. M. VAN (Ed.) (1978). *Minimal Brain Dysfunction. Fact and Fiction*. Karger, Basel.

Psychopharmacological Bulletin, Special Issue: *Pharmacotherapy of Children*, NIMH, 1973.

RAPOPORT, J. L., P. O. QUINN, G. BRADBARD, D. RIDDLE AND E. BROOKS (1974). Imipramine and methylphenidate treatments of hyperactive boys. *Arch. Gen. Psychiatry* 30, 789.

RENSHAW, D. C. (1975). Psychopharmacotherapy in children. In: Ayd, F. L. (Ed.) *Rational Psychopharmacotherapy and the Right to Treatment*. New York: Ayd Medical Communications.

SATTERFIELD, J. H., D. P. CANTWELL AND B. T. SATTERFIELD (1974). Pathophysiology of the hyperactive child syndrome. *Arch. Gen. Psychiat*. 31, 839.

SPRAGUE, H. L. AND J. S. WERRY (1971). Methodology of psychopharmacological studies with the retarded. In: N. R. Ellis (Ed.) *International Review of Research in Mental Retardation*. New York: Academic Press.

UCER, E. AND K. C. KREGER (1969). A double-blind study comparing haloperidol with thioridazine in emotionally disturbed, mentally retarded children. *Curr. Ther. Res*. 11, 278.

WOLPERT, A., M. B. HAGAMEN AND S. MERLIS (1967). A comparative study of thiothixene and trifluoperazine in childhood schizophrenia. *Curr. Ther. Res*. 9, 482.

ZRULL, J. P., J. C. WESTMAN, B. ARTHUR AND W. A. BELL (1963). A comparison of chlordiazepoxide, D-amphetamine, and placebo in the treatment of the hyperkinetic syndrome in children. *Am. J. Psychiat*. 120, 590.

XXVI

Psychotropic Drugs in the Aged

1. Functional and organic disorders in the aged

Psychological disorders in the aged are commonly ascribed to anatomical brain lesions, more specifically to (pre)senile and arteriosclerotic processes or a combination of these. This is why therapeutic pessimism is so often shown with regard to elderly patients with psychological disorders. This attitude is not justified. The automatic association of "old and disturbed" with "irreversible degeneration of brain tissue" is inappropriate, for two reasons: a) elderly patients may suffer from "functional" psychological disorders, i.e. disorders in the aetiology of which degeneration of cerebral tissue is not an important factor or seems to have acted merely as a trigger; b) organic cerebral damage in advanced age is not necessarily based on senile or arteriosclerotic processes and, moreover, can be reversible.

The above implies that psychological disorders in the aged call for careful psychiatric and physical diagnosis and that, in therapeutic terms, courage should not be too readily lost. The next two sections present some notes on psychogeriatric diagnosis, succinctly and therefore without any claim to comprehensiveness.

2. Psychopathological disorders in the aged as a result of anatomical brain lesions

Psychiatric symptoms

A number of psychiatric disorders in the aged are generally regarded as direct consequences of anatomical brain lesions.

1) Cognitive disorders. Particularly functions of memory begin to fail. Many things are no longer remembered very clearly, and this applies in particular to the more recent past. Subsequently, memories of early experiences also fade. New events are less well-memorized and less readily remembered. Also, it takes more time to learn something new.
2) Personality changes with, as points of crystallization, diminished impulse control and decreased emotional stability. On the one hand the patient is irritable and aggressive; on the other hand he is quickly moved to the point of tears. Moreover, less agreeable personality traits, successfully concealed or masked in the past, can become more overt.
3) Disorders of orientation, too, are typical. Temporal orientation is often first disturbed, followed by spatial and personal orientation. As a result, the patient's conversation can be rather incoherent.
4) Delirious syndromes. The patient is or becomes confused; the level of consciousness is lowered; anxious visual and sometimes also auditory hallucinations occur, and incoherent "ragged" delusions develop. Delirious syndromes in the aged develop mainly at night and are usually self-limiting, i.e. they tend towards spontaneous recovery or improvement within a few hours.

Transient brain lesions

The symptoms listed under 1 through 3 above can be permanent or transient. In the latter case their origin is almost certainly vascular: intermittent deficiency of the cerebral circulation which has not yet caused permanent damage. In many cases there are not only psychiatric symptoms but also transient neurological focal symptoms which may have the features of stimulation (epileptic manifestations) or loss of function (pareses).

Permanent brain lesions

If the psychiatric symptoms persist, then it must be assumed that permanent brain lesions have occurred, due to either senile degeneration or insufficient circulation. In the former case, senile plaques are found in the brain and Alzheimer's so-called neurofibrillar tangles. The plaques consist of masses of swollen nerve fibres and nerve endings filled with degenerated mitochondria and lysosomes. Amyloid is contained in the centre. Neurofibrillar tangles contain masses of tangled intraneuronal fibrillae. These pathological changes are found in particular in the frontal and temporal areas, and in the hippocampus. There density correlates closely with the degree of psychological deterioration during life, but the reverse does not apply. Psychological deterioration may have been substantial, whereas the anatomical situation in the brain "is not all that bad."

The anatomical changes produced in the brain by cerebral arteriosclerosis consist of smaller and larger infarcts. In some cases, what might be described as cicatricial tissue occurs through glia proliferation; in other cases, complete tissue degeneration occurs and pseudocysts are formed. The degree of arteriosclerosis can show marked local variations, within the brain as well as outside. For example, cerebral arteriosclerosis can be very pronounced, whereas peripheral arteriosclerotic changes (in heart, kidney, etc.) are only slight. The reverse situation is equally common.

Non-senile, non-vascular lesions

Anatomical lesions in the brain in elderly patients need not necessarily be due to senile degeneration or vascular disorders. I shall list a few other processes: subdural haematoma due to use of anticoagulants or caused by a fall due to dizziness or orthostatic hypotension (drugs!); brain tumour, the incidence of which increases with increasing age; low-pressure hydrocephalus—a condition amenable to surgery and therefore one of the few examples of a process which leads to reversible dementia. Chronic (ab)use of alcohol can be an important factor in (early) mental deterioration. A possible cause of dementia which for the time being is regarded as rare is encephalitis caused by a slow-growing virus.

If anatomical changes in the brain are irreversible, then two things may be expected of therapy: a) prevention of additional damage, and b) the taking over of functions by undamaged parts of the CNS via adequate techniques of rehabilitation.

Pseudo-dementia

An elderly individual may seem demented although in fact he (she) is not, e.g. as a result of drug intoxication. Digitalis preparations, for example, can provoke confusion and restiveness, and so can sedatives and hypnotic agents. l-DOPA can be responsible for a whole range of psychopathological symptoms, from confusion to "schizophreniform" syndromes. Unidentified or inadequately treated non-neurological diseases (e.g. cardiac decompensation, respiratory insufficiency, hypertrophy of the prostate, diabetes mellitus) can likewise seriously affect psychological vigour, flexibility and achievements, and may be the cause of *pseudo*-dementia: symptoms of deterioration not based on anatomical brain lesions and, in principle, reversible.

3. Functional psychological disorders in the aged

In this context the word "functional" indicates three characteristics.

a. It is uncertain whether the psychological symptoms in question are causally related to anatomical deterioration of the brain.

b. If such a relation is plausible, then its nature is uncertain: Did the anatomical damage merely act as trigger, or are the psychological symptoms completely determined by it.

c. The only certainty is that these psychological symptoms can develop also when the brain shows *no* anatomical lesions.

In this context I should first of all mention *depressive syndromes*. Depressions, both of the vital and of the personal type, are quite common in the aged. When a patient has a history of (vital or personal) depressive phases earlier in life, alone or in combination with (hypo)manic periods, he himself or the physician will probably recognize the situation. When a first depressive phase is involved, it will probably be identified as such if it is of the personal type; it will rightly be ascribed to the problems of old age: loneliness, mandatory retirement, financial worries, physical ailments, etc. Treatment will accordingly consist of psychotherapeutic and sociotherapeutic measures, focused on acceptance of the situation, activation, and improvement of the circumstances.

A first vital depressive phase, however, is often not recognized as such, for several reasons: the depression is mistaken for dementia; it can be masked by a complex of physical complaints (masked depressions); it can be mistaken for a personal depression caused by psychological and social factors. In addition to hereditary and exogenous-somatic factors, psychosocial factors can also play an important role in the aetiology of vital depressions. The differential diagnosis between vital and personal depressions, therefore, is based exclusively on symptom differentiation. The importance of proper differentiation between these syndromes is evident, for personal depressions are generally not amenable to antidepressant medication, whereas vital depressions are. Of course pharmacotherapy is not a substitute for psycho- and sociotherapeutic measures; but it is an important supplement to these measures.

Recognition and adequate treatment of depressions are of great importance. Depressive symptoms can make the aged patient look much more demented than he is, and can totally obscure the mild light of his final years.

Paranoid syndromes are quite common at an advanced age, although less common than depressions. Their relation to the anatomical integrity of the CNS is likewise uncertain. On the one hand we see cases in which suspicion is a characteristic feature of the premorbid personality structure, and in which deterioration is not a prominent feature. In such cases the organic factor is probably at best a secondary feature: a "trigger" (e.g. a mild defect of memory as a stepping stone to the delusion of being the victim of thefts), or a flexibility-reducing factor which makes it more difficult to find a socially acceptable form of adjustment. On the other hand, in cases with no history of pronounced suspicion but with evident current mental deterioration, there is some justification for a diagnosis of organically-determined paranoid psychosis. Of course there are numerous transitions, and in these cases the diagnosis is a rather arbitrary one.

Treatment of these syndromes is difficult. The results of psychotherapy are generally poor. Neuroleptics should always be tried in cautiously increasing doses, while monitoring the blood pressure. This approach is sometimes, but by no means always, successful. We know of no factors which in this respect have any predictive value. In some cases elderly patients have to be admitted to a mental hospital because they cannot be socially managed due to their delusions, although the remaining personality is still quite intact.

In addition, there are the *neuroses*. If we look at the list of patients of the majority of psychotherapists, we may gain the impression that neuroses are disorders of the young. This is a false impression, arising from the preconceived idea of many psychotherapists that only individuals on the ascending line of life need be considered for psychotherapy.

Neuroses are quite common also in the aged. This is a matter of course. The young neurotic grows old; not every young neurotic receives treatment; not every treatment of a young neurotic is successful; and, finally, there are no indications that neuroses tend to disappear spontaneously with increasing age.

There are also patients whose neurotic disorders—depressive syndromes, anxiety states, compulsive symptoms, periods of apathy etc.—do not become manifest until later in life. This, too, is not surprising. Old age carries its inevitable frustrations. In old age an essentially vulnerable personality who has lived under favourable conditions (good marriage, satisfactory work, etc.) and has managed to avoid disabling psychological disorders, can be severely tested. Loss of marital partner, work and prestige; financial restrictions; disappointment about an insufficient interest shown by the children; loneliness, disabling diseases and fear of death—to mention only a few factors—can exceed a (weak) level of integration and provoke symptoms of neurotic decompensation.

The tenet that neurotic disorders primarily call for psychotherapy applies without restriction to the aged neurotic also. A statement such as "too old for psychotherapy" is scientifically untenable and ethically unjustifiable. Of course the specific qualities of the patient will be taken into account in determining the type and purpose of therapy; but this applies to any patient who presents for treatment, and the elderly patient is no exception to this rule.

Finally it may be mentioned here that *chronic* and *chronic recurrent (schizophrenic) psychoses* can also become manifest in old age, either in a "pure" form or mixed with so-called organic symptoms. In the former case, neuroleptic medication is the treatment of choice. In the latter case, neuroleptic agents are certainly to be tried, but there is a considerable chance that their therapeutic effect will be meagre.

4. Problems of psychopharmacotherapy in the aged

Treatment of elderly patients with (psychotropic) drugs poses its peculiar problems for several reasons. The most important of these reasons follow:

1) Pharmacokinetic factors are of paramount importance. The pharmacokinetics of a drug are a function of its absorption, distribution, metabolism and excretion, and of the level of activity of the corresponding receptors.

   It is assumed on clinical grounds (little pharmacokinetic research has been done) that absorption of drugs can diminish in old age. In such cases, efforts can be made to establish whether the drug does produce its effect if administered in liquid form or parenterally. Much more important, in practical terms, are the processes which cause the reverse effect: abnormally high blood levels over abnormally long periods. These processes are reduced degradation (due to delayed enzyme induction, among other things) and diminished excretion (diminished renal function) of the drug. Because the lean body mass diminshes and is replaced by fat, moreover, retention of fat-soluble substances is promoted.

   Receptor sensitivity can diminish in the course of the years, as Belville et al. (1971) demonstrated for analgesic drugs. Sensitivity to these compounds changes with increasing age, even though blood and tissue concentrations remain unchanged. Receptor sensitivity to various drugs can either decrease or increase, but information on these processes is still scanty.

2) Many elderly patients suffer from somatic illnesses, either already diagnosed or, worse, as yet unrecognized. The most common conditions are: cardiac decompensation, respiratory infection, carcinomas, cirrhosis of the liver, diabetes mellitus, malnutrition and peripheral neuritis. In the presence of such conditions prescription of psychotropic drugs is more hazardous. Such drugs, for example, can reduce the blood pressure (e.g. neuroleptics), depress respiration (e.g. barbiturates) or increase glucose tolerance (e.g. MAO inhibitors). In this context, it is to be noted that in the case of severely demented elderly patients the morbid history, as an important source of information, may be absent or unreliable.

3) Many elderly patients are receiving medication for somatic illnesses, and these may potentiate or reduce the (side) effects of psychotropic drugs. Thiazide diuretics, prescribed for hypertension, can provoke an acute hypotensive crisis if combined with phenothiazines or tricyclic antidepressants. Barbiturates can enhance the degradation of coumarin-type anticoagulants in the liver, thus reducing their effect. MAO inhibitors of the hydrazine type potentiate the effect of antidiabetics. These are merely a few examples. For a more comprehensive review of negative drug interactions, I refer to Salzman et al. (1970) and Keyes (1965).

4) Paradoxical reactions are more frequently observed in the aged than in younger patients, e.g. insomnia and agitation caused by barbiturates; increased aggressivity caused by ataractics of the benzodiazepine type; delirious symptoms caused by a phenothiazine-type neuroleptic (due to decreased blood pressure with diminished cerebral circulation?).

In view of all these factors, more side effects of (psychotropic) drugs can be expected with increasing age. This expectation has proved to be correct. Hurwitz (1969) studied a large group of psychiatric and other patients (internal diseases) and found side effects in 21.3% of those aged 70-79, 7.5% of those aged 40-49, and 3% of those aged 20-29. In a study described by Learoyd (1972), no less than 16% of patients admitted to a psychogeriatric ward showed more or less serious side effects of psychotropic drugs which they had previously received.

The elderly patient is particularly susceptible to cardiovascular (hypotension) and extrapyramidal side effects (of neuroleptics for example), to paradoxical effects of sedative and ataractics, to urinary retention (caused by neuroleptics and tricyclic antidepressants) and to depression of respiration (due to central depressant compounds). Side effects are not only more frequent but also more intensive. Drugs which provoke hypotension or constipation in younger patients can lead to a cerebrovascular accident or acute intestinal obstruction due to paralytic ileus in geriatric patients.

For these reasons it is of importance to observe the following rules when dealing with elderly patients.

1) The initial dose should be small, and increased gradually on the basis of the ratio between therapeutic and side effects.
2) The minimum effective dose should be established, and regular efforts should be made to establish whether one could do with less, or even without.
3) Regular monitoring is imperative.
4) Combined pharmacotherapy is to be avoided if at all possible in view of possible untoward interactions and in order to prevent the patient from confusing the various dosage schemes (defects of memory!). Cases in which dramatic improvement is observed after reduction or discontinuation of (psychotropic) medication are by no means rare!

5. Psycholeptics

Neuroleptics

As much as in younger patients, neuroleptics are indicated in elderly patients who show psychotic symptoms, regardless of whether these are of a schizophrenic, delirious, paranoid or other nature. One does gain the impression from the literature that neuroleptics are slightly less effective in the aged than in younger patients, but it is not clear whether this is definitely related to more advanced age or rather to the fact that (to avoid possible side effects) smaller and therefore possibly suboptimal doses are generally prescribed for elderly patients. Clinical manifestations of dementia per se (e.g. defects of memory, memorizing and other intellectual functions) do not improve in response to neuroleptics.

The choice of a neuroleptic is free in the sense that there are no indications that particular neuroleptics are particularly effective in elderly patients. The guideline in selecting a neuroleptic should therefore be the patient's clinical condition and the risk of side effects. The widest experience has so far been gained with a few phenothiazines, the thioxanthene derivative chlorprothixene and the butyrophenone derivative haloperidol. The practitioner is well-advised to confine himself to these compounds and may take advantage of the following guidelines.

If a *neuroleptic with a sedative component* is to be prescribed, then suitable possibilities are in particular: thioridazine (Mellaril), chlorpromazine (Largactil, Thorazine), alimemazine (Nedeltran), chlorprothixene (Taractan) (initial dose of these four: 50 mg per day), or haloperidol (Haldol) (initial dose 0.5 mg per day).

An advantage of thioridazine is that it exerts but little influence on the extrapyramidal system; a disadvantage is that its antipsychotic effect is not very pronounced, and generally less marked than that of chlorpromazine.

An advantage of chlorpromazine is that it is a relatively strong antipsychotic; a disadvantage is that it relatively often provokes extrapyramidal (especially parkinson-like) symptoms.

It is also to be borne in mind that all phenothiazines, including the two mentioned above, can reduce the blood pressure, and that both thioridazine and chlorpromazine (given in large doses) can influence the function of the heart. Conduction disorders as well as arrhythmias (ventricular and supraventricular) have been described. Cardiac patients should therefore be approached with caution.

An advantage of alimemazine is that it has relatively little effect on cardiac function, blood pressure and motor activity. A disadvantage is that its antipsychotic effect is inferior to that of the other phenothiazines mentioned here. The same applies to the thioxanthene derivative chlorproxithene.

The advantages of haloperidol are its intensive sedative effect on (psychotic) restiveness and its only slight effect on blood pressure. Moreover, the epileptogenic action of this agent is less pronounced than that of phenothiazine derivatives. A disadvantage is its relatively pronounced influence on the extrapyramidal system.

It can be said of all neuroleptics, but more of phenothiazines than of butyrophenones, that they are central and peripheral anticholinergic agents. A study by El-Yousef et al. (1973) has shown that reduction of central cholinergic activity is a psychosis (confusion)-inducing factor—all the more reason to be prudent with neuroleptics and careful with anticholinergic antiparkinson agents (in extrapyramidal reactions) in the treatment of elderly patients, who in any case have a certain susceptibility to psychotic reactions. As a result of peripheral anticholinergic activity, urinary retention, constipation and glaucoma can develop or exacerbate. Xerostomia is a more inconvenient than harmful side effect. The new anti-parkinson agent amantadine (Symmetrel: 200-400 mg per day) is to be preferred because it does not produce these anticholinergic effects.

As *neuroleptics with an effect tending more towards motor activation*, perphenazine (Trilafon) or trifluoperazine (Stelazine) can be considered (initial dose in both cases 2 mg per day). Like all phenothiazines of the piperazine series, they are very active extrapyramidally, and can provoke hypokinetic as well as hyperkinetic (and dyskinetic) symptoms.

Ataractics and sedatives

These drugs, and more specifically the benzodiazepines and meprobamate, can be very useful when anxiety, tension and motor unrest are dominant features but not manifestly nourished by psychotic disorders of thinking (delusions) and experiencing (hallucinations). Time-tested agents are chlordiazepoxide (Librium, initial dose 5 mg per day), diazepam (Valium, initial dose 2 mg per day) and meprobamate (Miltown, initial dose 200 mg per day).

Ataractics have many advantages over the classical sedatives, and in particular the barbiturates: an overdose is less toxic; habituation and addiction develop less readily; their action focuses more selectively on anxiety and tension—level of consciousness and therefore intellectual performance are less markedly influenced.

The side effects of ataractics, moreover, are mild: muscular weakness, fatigability (muscular hypotonia!) and a sensation of lightness in the head are the principal side effects. It is of importance for their use in the treatment of elderly patients that they exert no or hardly any influence on blood pressure, and that paradoxical reactions are less common than after barbiturates.

I would advise against the use of barbiturates as daytime sedatives. I have already outlined the principal disadvantages, and now add that they can enhance the activity of drug-degrading enzymes in the liver. This applies, for example, to the enzymes involved in the degradation of coumarin-type anticoagulants. As a result, underdosage of these anticoagulants and, after discontinuation of the barbiturate, overdosage threaten.

Hypnotic agents

Sleep can pose a grave problem in old age. Moreover, periods of restiveness and disorientation are more frequent during the night than during the day.

For the above discussed reasons, barbiturates are not the first choice. One should first try hypnotics of the benzodiazepine series, e.g. nitrazepam (Mogadon, 5-10 mg per night) or flurazepam (Dalmane, 15-30 mg per night). If a barbiturate is nevertheless desired, then butabarbital (50-100 mg per night) or pentobarbital (50-100 mg per night) are acceptable because Stotsky and Borozne (1972) and Pattison and Allen (1972) have demonstrated that these compounds are effective and produce relatively few side effects.

Good hypnotics of the classical type are also paraldehyde and chloral hydrate. They merit consideration in particular in the case of nocturnal restiveness and confusion. Paraldehyde can be given orally, rectally (suppository or enema) and also by intramuscular injection: 2-3 g (maximum 5 g) per dose to a maximum of 15 g (10 g when injected intramuscularly) per 24 hours. Chloral hydrate can be orally or rectally (suppository or enema) administered: 1-1.5 g (maximum 3 g) per dose to a maximum of 6 g per 24 hours. It can irritate the gastric wall and should therefore not be given to gastric patients. It should also be borne in mind that the excretory products can cause positive reduction in urine. Caution is also to be observed with patients receiving anticoagulants: like the barbiturates, chloral hydrate can accelerate the metabolism of these compounds by activation of microsomal liver enzymes.

With all hypnotic agents there is a risk of habituation and addiction. They should be prescribed for a limited time, and this should be discussed in advance with the patient. Some patients derive more benefit from an antidepressant than from a hypnotic (in vital depressions); others are better off with psychotherapy (neurotic conflicts or existential crises) or with a regimen (do not go to bed until you feel tired): insomnia is a behaviour pattern which establishes itself very rapidly and can provoke anxiety, even though the real need for sleep actually diminishes in old age.

Lithium

The two principal indications for lithium—as a therapeutic agent in mania and as a prophylactic agent in recurrent vital depressions (unipolar depressions) and manic-depressive conditions (bipolar depressions)—are valid also for the aged patient. The risks of lithium medication, however, are graver than at an earlier age, for reasons which can be briefly discussed as follows.

1) Toxic symptoms originating from the CNS and neuromuscular apparatus (e.g. tremors) develop at lower serum levels.

2) The half-life of lithium increases. It is 24 hours in middle age and 36-48 hours in old age, possibly as a result of decreased glomerular filtration in the kidney. Lithium should therefore be prescribed in smaller doses than for younger patients: no more than 600-900 mg per day.

3) As a result of dietary sodium restriction, the kidney retains more lithium and the serum level can quickly rise to a dangerous level.

4) Thiazide diuretics increase the lithium uptake by the proximal renal tubules. In patients well-stabilized on lithium, such a drug can cause lithium intoxication within 1-2 days. Spironolacton (Aldactone) is probably the safest diuretic for a patient receiving lithium. It is an aldosterone antagonist which influences mainly the distal renal tubules and consequently less rapidly leads to lithium retention.

5) Lithium reduces the release of T3 (tri-iodothyronine) and T4 (thyroxine) in the thyroid gland. It can cause enlargement of this organ and hypothyroidism—a syndrome which can imitate the symptoms of depression and dementia. With increasing age, the serum T3 concentration in particular diminishes. Aged patients are consequently extra-sensitive to these lithium effects.

To be brief: the aged lithium patient should be monitored even more carefully than the younger lithium patient.

6. Psychoanaleptics

Tricyclic antidepressants

These are indicated in the treatment of vital depression, regardless of the age at which it becomes manifest. Imipramine (Tofranil), amitriptyline (Elavil) and doxepine (Sinequan) have been most thoroughly tested in aged patients. The therapeutic results obtained with amitriptyline and doxepine are superior to those of imipramine, possibly because they have a more marked sedative effect than the latter (in old age the vital depressive syndrome is more likely to be of an agitated than of a retarded character). According to Grof et al. (1974), amitriptyline and doxepine are therapeutically equivalent, but doxepine has fewer anticholinergic and cardiovascular side effects.

As with neuroleptics, one should beware of side effects in the aged. One of the principal side effects is orthostatic hypotension. The patient should be instructed to avoid coming abruptly upright from a recumbent or sitting position, and to be cautious when stooping.

In toxic doses, any tricyclic antidepressant acts like a cardiac toxin. Conduction disorders and marked arrhythmias can occur. Is an already injured heart in danger with therapeutic doses? There is no certainty about this, but there are indications that it is indeed. In a retrospective study, acute death was found to be more frequent in a group of cardiacs who had been treated with amitriptyline than in a matched group of cardiacs who had not received this compound (Moir 1973). Even though the results of a retrospective study are not conclusive, one is nevertheless well-advised to consult a cardiologist before prescribing a tricyclic antidepressant to an elderly patient. However, the maxim "abstain when in doubt" does not apply here. Heart diseases are serious, but so is a vital depression, which not infrequently takes a fatal course (suicide) and in any case is a markedly disabling condition. Some risk, therefore, seems acceptable.

Like neuroleptics, tricyclic antidepressants exert a peripheral and central anticholinergic influence. The former complex of actions can lead to states of confusion. The latter is likewise of great importance because it impedes micturition, delays defecation and increases intraocular pressure. Xerostomia is a more inconvenient than serious consequence.

It should finally be pointed out that tricyclic antidepressants can block the activity of guanethidine (Ismelin), an antihypertensive widely used by elderly patients. Blood dyscrasia, to conclude, is rarely observed but nevertheless a possibility to be taken into account.

As initial dose of imipramine, as well as of amitriptyline and doxepine, I advise 25-50 mg per day, to be increased by 25 mg per week under guidance of the blood pressure, to a maximum which generally should not exceed 150 mg per day. In the case of manifest cardiac abnormalities, ECG monitoring is indicated, at least during the first six weeks. A medication should not be considered ineffective until improvement has failed to occur four weeks after attaining the maximum dosage.

In the treatment of agitated depressions, tricyclic antidepressants are often combined with phenothiazine-type neuroleptics. So far as we know, this combination causes no serious problems. There are indications, however, that the neuroleptics delay the degradation of the antidepressants so that potentiation of their (side) effects is a possibility to be borne in mind.

There are no indications that tricyclic antidepressants of the monomethyl series—nortriptyline (Aventyl), protriptyline (Vivactyl) and desipramine (Pertofrane)—have advantages over the dimethyl derivatives in elderly patients. Moreover, nortriptyline increases the half-life of antipyrine and coumarin-type anticoagulants because it inhibits the activity of the degrading enzymes in the liver.

MAO inhibitors

Monoamine oxidase (MAO) inhibitors are better not prescribed for elderly (out)patients. Their marked hypotensive effect, the difficulty of combining them with many other agents, and the dietary restrictions which they impose on the patient (no tyramine-containing products) are inconveniences for patient and therapist alike.

Oestrogens

Anecdotal data have given oestrogens the reputation of valuable mood-improvers in depressions of the menopause and climacteric.

There are no hard facts to confirm these clinical impressions. Until more data are available, I would therefore advise against the use of oestrogens for this indication, partly also because of our ignorance of the possible side effects (thrombosis?, carcinoma?).

7. Drugs which possibly influence intellectual functions

The focal psychiatric symptom of senescence is deterioration of intellectual functions. In geriatric psychopharmacology, the accent is therefore on compounds which might delay, arrest, or even reverse this process. The results of efforts to find or evolve such compounds have so far been poor.

Vasodilators

These have been most widely used, including papaverine, nicotinic acid and cyclandelate (Cyclospasmol). The rationale of this strategy is the notion that ischaemic lesions of the brain caused by cerebral arteriosclerosis could be prevented by vasodilation, which increases circulation and oxygen supply. The question is whether this goal is in fact achieved. The abovementioned compounds are not selective: they dilate the vessels throughout the organism, and most markedly so in the skin. It is quite conceivable that the net supply to the brain in fact decreases as a result of their administration. Moreover, arteriosclerosis decreases the dilatability of the cerebral vessels, and it may therefore well be that the increased blood supply concerns sites where such an increase is least necessary. Finally, an improved blood supply need not necessarily mean an improved energy supply in the area in question. It has been said of cyclandelate that it not only improves the blood supply but also directly stimulates oxidation of glucose.

Unfortunately we still lack the techniques of investigation required to find satisfactory answers to questions of this kind; an evaluation of vasodilators, therefore, has to be based exclusively on the clinical results obtained with them. There are no convincing arguments that nicotinic acid and papaverine are effective in arteriosclerotic dementia. I do note in this context that this result can have been influenced by the difficulty of diagnosing cerebral arteriosclerosis—especially in its milder forms—and by the lack of psychological instruments to diagnose and monitor this condition in a reliable way. A few double-blind studies have shown the likelihood that cyclandelate (400-1600 mg per day) exerts a more favourable influence on certain intellectual functions than a placebo (Ball and Taylor 1967; Fine 1971; Smith et al. 1968). The duration of this effect is unknown. In some patients, moreover, the therapeutic effect was demonstrable at psychological examination but of little practical significance.

Hydergine

This combination of three hydrogenated ergot alkaloids is believed to have a dual effect: vasodilation and a direct stimulating effect on the retarded energy mebatolism in ischaemic brain tissue. Some investigators in fact assumed that the circulatory improvement is secondary to the improved metabolism, rather than the reverse. The majority of the controlled studies have shown that hydergine (3-4.5 mg per day) is more effective than a placebo in aged patients with intellectual disorders (e.g. Rao and Norris 1972; Gaitz et al., 1977). It has not been clearly demonstrated, however, whether the improvement primarily concerned intellectual functions or primarily concerned the mood, with improved performance as secondary effect.

In the case of suspected (mild) arteriosclerotic dementia there are, therefore, arguments in favour of trying cyclandelate or hydergine. The side effects of these compounds are generally negligible although with some vasodilators the possibility of an untoward decrease in blood pressure is to be taken into account. If no effect is demonstrable after two months, medication should be discontinued.

Anticoagulants

These have proved to be of no value in intellectual disorders based on cerebral arteriosclerosis. The same applies to *central stimulants* (of which an indirect effect had been expected via an impoved degree of alertness and level of activity).

Procainamide

Developed in Romania, this has been recommended as a general rejuvenant, with an effect on cognitive functions. In the absence of controlled studies, its value cannot be estimated. The compound is a reversible inhibitor of the enzyme MAO, and this may explain the euphoretic action attributed to it.

Recent studies of the effects of certain *neuropeptides* on certain functions of memory in animals have yielded promising results. The value of these agents in the treatment of human individuals remains to be established. *Piracetam* (Nootropil) is a compound whose possible beneficial influence on intellectual functioning was discovered accidently. Its value in intellectual deterioration is disputed, but it certainly has been insufficiently investigated.

8. Conclusions

Drugs unequivocally able to delay or arrest the deterioration of neurons in the brain and the associated deterioration of intellectual functions are not available. We do, however, have drugs which are valuable in the treatment of: a) psychiatric symptoms secondary to intellectual deterioration, and b) psychiatric symptoms of senescence which do not seem to be directly related to the anatomical process of senescence.

In any case, it should always be borne in mind that psychological disorders in the aged are the result of the influence of a complex of factors: somatic (cerebral and extracerebral) as well as psychological and social. A good therapeutic program accounts for this and, in addition to the prescription of psychotropic drugs, if required, comprises:

1) Optimalization of the physical condition.
2) Activation aimed at abolition of social isolation, stimulation of productivity and, thus, promotion of feelings of self-respect.
3) Psychotherapy focused on the existential problems so commonly experienced in this phase of life, or on neurotic conflicts of recent or less recent date.
4) Advising relatives about the best way to deal with the patient in taking account of his abilities and inabilities.

BIBLIOGRAPHY

ALEXANDER, C. S. AND A. NINO (1969). Cardiovascular complications in young patients taking psychotropic drugs. *Am. Heart. J.* 78, 757.

ALTMAN, H., D. MEHTA, R. EVENSON AND I. W. SLETTEN (1973). Behavioral effects of drug therapy on psychogeriatric inpatients. I. Chlorpromazine and thioridazine. *J. Am. Geriatr. Soc.* 21, 241.

BALL, J. A. C. AND A. R. TAYLOR (1967). Effect of cyclandelate on mental function and cerebral blood flow in elderly patients. *Lancet* 3, 525.

BELVILLE, J. W., W. H. FOREST AND E. MILLER (1971). Influence of age on pain relief from analgesics. *J.A.M.A.* 217, 1835.

BENDER, A. D. (1974). Pharmacodynamic principles of drug therapy in the aged. *J. Am. Geriatr. Soc.* 22, 296.

BIRKETT, D. P. AND B. BOLTUCH (1972). Chlorpromazine in geriatric psychiatry. *J. Am. Geriatr. Soc.* 20, 403.

BUSSE, E. W. AND E. PFEIFFER (Eds.) (1969). *Behavior and Adaptation in Later Life.* Boston: Little, Brown.

DAVIS, J. M. (1974). Use of psychotropic drugs in geriatric patients. *J. Geriatr. Psychiat.* 7, 145.

DIMASCIO, A., D. L. BERNARDO, D. J. GREENBLATT AND J. E. MANDER (1976). A controled trial of amantadine in drug-induced extrapyramidal disorders. *Arch. Gen. Psychiat.* 33, 599.

Drugs for dementia (1975). *Drug and Therapeutics Bull.* 13, 85.

EISDORFER, C. (1975). Observations on the psychopharmacology of the aged. *J. Am. Geriatr. Soc.* 23, 53.

EISDORFER, C. AND W. E. FANN (1973). *Psychopharmacology and Aging.* New York: Plenum Press.

EL-YOUSEF, M. K., D. S. JANOWSKY, J. M. DAVIS AND H. J. SEKERKE (1973). Reversal of antiparkinsonian drug toxicity by physostigmine: a controlled study. *Am. J. Psychiat.* 130, 141.

FINE, E. W. (1971). The use of cyclandelate in chronic brain syndrome with arteriosclerosis. *Curr. Ther. Res.* 13, 568.

FLETCHER, G. F. AND N. K. WENGER (1969). Cardiotoxic effects of mellaril: conduction disturbances and supraventricular arrhythmias. *Am. Heart J.* 78, 135.

GAITZ, C. M., R. V. VARNER AND J. F. OVERALL (1977). Pharmacotherapy for organic brain syndrome in late life. *Arch. Gen. Psych.*, 34, 839.

GROF, P., B. SAXENA, R. CANTOR, L. DAIGLE, D. HETHERINGTON AND T. HAINES (1974). Doxepin versus amitriptyline in depression: a sequential double-blind study. *Curr. Ther. Res.* 16, 470.

HADER, M. (1965). The use of selected phenothiazines in elderly patients: a review. *Mt. Sinai J. Med.* N.Y. 32, 622.

HOLLISTER, L. O. (1975). Drugs for mental disorders of old age. *J.A.M.A.* 234, 195.

HURWITZ, N. (1969). Predisposing factors in adverse reactions to drugs. *Brit. Med. J.* 1, 536.

KEYES, J. W. (1965). Problems in drug management of cardiovascular disorders in geriatric patients. *J. Am. Geriatr. Soc.* 13, 118.

KIRVEN, L. E. AND E. F. MONTERO (1973). Comparison of thioridazine and diazepam on the control of nonpsychiatric symptoms associated with senility: double-blind study. *J. Am. Geriatr. Soc.* 21, 546.

LEAROYD, B. M. (1972). Psychotropic drugs and the elderly patient. *Med. J. Aust.* 1, 1131.

LIPPINCOTT, R. C. (1968). Depressive illness: identification and treatment in the elderly. *Geriatrics* 23, 149.

MacFarlane, D. M. and H. Besbris (1974). Procaine (gerovital H3) therapy: mechanism of inhibition of monoamine oxidase. *J. Am. Geriatr. Soc.* 22, 365.

Mindus, P., B. Cronholm, S. E. Lewander and D. Schalling (1976). Piracetam-induced improvement in mental performance. *Acta psychiat. Scand.* 54, 150.

Moir, D. C. (1973). Tricyclic antidepressants and cardiac disease. *Am. Heart J.* 84, 841.

Nelson, J. J. (1975). Relieving select symptoms of the elderly. *Geriatrics* 30, 133.

Pattison, J. H. and R. P. Allen (1972). Comparison of the hypnotic effectiveness of secobarbital, pentobarbital, methyprylon and ethchlorvynol. *J. Am. Geriatr. Soc.* 22, 398.

Post, F. (1972). The management and nature of depressive illnesses in late life: A follow-through study. *Brit. J. Psychiat.* 121, 393.

Praag, H. M. van and A. F. Kalverboer (Eds.) (1972). *Ageing of the Central Nervous System.* Haarlem: De Erven Bohn N.V.

Prien, R. F., P. A. Haber and E. M. Caffey (1975). The use of psychoactive drugs in elderly patients with psychiatric disorders: survey conducted in twelve veterans administration hospitals. *J. Am. Geriatr. Soc.* 23, 104.

Prien, R. F. (1973). Chemotherapy in chronic organic brain syndrome—a review of the literature. *Psychopharmacol. Bull.* 9, 5.

Rao, D. B. and J. R. Norris (1972). A double-blind investigation of hydergine in the treatment of cerebrovascular insufficiency in the elderly. *Johns Hopkins Med. J.* 130, 317.

Roubicek, J., C. H. Geiger and K. Abt (1972). An ergot alkaloid preparation (hydergine) in geriatric therapy. *J. Am. Geriatr. Soc.* 20, 222.

Salzman, C., R. I. Shader and M. Pearlman (1970). Psychopharmacology and the elderly. In: *Psychotropic Drug Side Effects*, edited by R. I. Shader and A. DiMascio. Baltimore: Williams & Wilkins.

Smith, W. L., J. B. Lowrey and J. A. Davis (1968). The effects of cyclandelate on psychological test performance in patients with cerebral vascular insufficiency. *Curr. Ther. Res.* 10, 613.

Stotsky, B. B. and J. Borozne (1972). Butisol sodium vs librium among geriatric and younger outpatients and nursing home patients. *Dis. Nerv. Syst.* 33, 254.

Terry, R. D. and H. M. Wisniewski (1970). The ultrastructure of the neurofibrillary tangle and senile plague. In: Wolstenhilme G. E. W., O'Connor M. (Eds.): *Alzheimer's Disease and Related Conditons.* London: J. & A. Churchill, p. 145.

Tobin, J. M., E. R. Brousseau and A. A. Lorenz (1970). Clinical evaluation of haloperidol in geriatric patients. *Geriatrics* 25, 119.

Tsuang, M. M., L. M. Lu, B. A. Stotsky and J. O. Cole (1971). Haloperidol vs thioridazine for hospitalized psychogeriatric patients: double-blind study. *J. Am. Geriatr. Soc.* 19, 593.

Vesell, E. S., G. T. Passananti and F. E. Greene (1970). Impairment of drug metabolism by allopurinol and nortriptyline. *N. Engl. J. Med.* 283, 1484.

De Wied, D. (1977). Neuropeptides and behavior. In: *Neurotransmission and Distrubed Behavior*, H. M. van Praag and J. Bruinvels (Eds.). Utrecht: Bohn Scheltema and Holkema.

Williams, R. B. and C. Sherter (1971). Cardiac complications of tricyclic antidepressant therapy. *Ann. Intern. Med.* 74, 395.

Zeman, F. (1969). Neuropsychiatric symptoms of somatic disorders in the aged. *Gerontologist* 9, 219.

XXVII

Emergency Cases: Some Practical Guidelines

1. Purpose of this chapter

In this chapter I discuss some emergencies in clinical psychiatry and possibilities of their pharmacotherapeutic control. I do this very briefly because all the drugs in question have already been discussed in earlier chapters. It seems useful, however, to survey them in the special context of psychiatric first aid.

The drugs mentioned by me of necessity indicate a good deal of personal preference. This is unavoidable, for each group of psychotropic drugs has many representatives and we are still far from a situation in which all individual drugs and their therapeutic merits have been properly compared in well-defined groups of patients.

I confine myself to pharmacotherapeutic first-aid measures. Since these situations often involve restive, anxious, suicidal patients, it is obvious that, apart from pharmacotherapy, great importance must be attached to calming, reassuring conversations and the creation of an environment in which the patient can sense at least a measure of safety and understanding.

I mention parenteral doses because we are dealing with emergency situations. Since this mode of administration entails greater risks, the switch to oral administration should be made as soon as possible.

2. States of motor agitation

These states are usually encountered in psychoses. The patient is not only agitated, anxious and/or aggressive, but in addition shows such symptoms as incoherence of thoughts, delusions and hallucinations. Consciousness is undisturbed or only slightly disturbed; otherwise the condition is more likely to be a delirium. There can be many causes: morphological brain lesions or psychosocial factors, and motor agitation also occurs in the group of the schizophrenic psychoses. An effort should be made to trace the causes via (hetero)anamnestic data and investigation.

In cases with predominance of motor agitation which is not evidently nourished by anxious and threatening delusions or hallucinations, the following compounds are suitable.

1) *Haloperidol* (Serenase; Haldol), 2.5-5 mg by intramuscular injection, which can be repeated after 60 minutes. The dose per 24 hours should not exceed 40 mg. Prophylactic administration of traditional anti-parkinson drugs is not recommendable. These are anticholinergics and, as such, can potentiate the tendency towards disintegration. In the case of severe extrapyramidal side effects, orphenadrine (Disipal, 40 mg intramuscularly) or biperiden (Akineton, 5 mg intramuscularly) can be given.

2) *Clozapine* (Leponex), 50 mg by intramuscular injection, which can be repeated after 60 minutes. The dose per 24 hours should not exceed 300 mg. Extrapyramidal symptoms rarely develop, and this is a major advantage of this compound over other neuroleptics. Unfortunately, the gravity of the risk of agranulocytosis with this compound is still uncertain. For the time being, the blood picture should be carefully monitored.

3) *Droperidol* (Inapsine; Innovar; Dehydrobenzperidol) has been used mostly as premedication before operations, but is also valuable in acute agitation. Experience within this range of indications has been limited, but results have been promis-

ing. The dose is 5-10 mg by intramuscular injection or, in very serious cases, by slow intravenous administration. If necessary, another 5-10 mg can be given after 15-20 minutes; the second injection should be intramuscular. The maximum parenteral dose per 24 hours is 45 mg. Extrapyramidal side effects are rare when the compound is used briefly. Hypotension does occur, particularly after intravenous administration.

In cases in which motor agitation is accompanied by distinct delusions and hallucinations, neuroleptics with an aliphatic side chain are to be preferred, such as the following.

1) *Chlorpromazine* (Largactil; Thorazine), 50-100 mg by intramuscular injection, which can be repeated after 60 minutes. The dose per 24 hours should not exceed 300 mg. The injections are painful and can cause muscle infiltrates. The sedative effect of chlorpromazine can be greatly enhanced by combination with a sedative antihistamine such as promethazine (Phenergan, 50-100 mg intramuscularly).

   A very strongly sedative combination can be obtained by combining chlorpromazine and promethazine with the barbiturate amobarbital (Amytal, 100-200 mg intramuscularly). In view of the risk of respiratory depression and hypotension, such a cocktail may be given only if there is no evidence of anatomical brain lesion or disturbed cardiac function. Pulse, respiration and level of consciousness are to be monitored. Not more than three cocktails should be given per 24 hours, and treatment should not be continued longer than three days. Amobarbital has to be injected separately: barbiturates in solution show an alkaline reaction and precipitate in the weakly acid milieu of the chlorpromazine/promethazine solution.

2) *Laevomepromazine* (Nozinan), 25-50 mg by intramuscular injection, which can be repeated after 60 minutes. The dose per 24 hours should not exceed 200 mg. Pain at the site of injection is the rule with this agent also, and muscle infiltrates are not unusual.

During parenteral administration of phenothiazines one should beware of hypotension, especially in elderly patients and those with a disturbed cardiac function.

3. Mania

In the maniacal syndrome, many psychological functions are disinhibited. The patient is talkative, agitated and uninhibited, starting all sorts of things and finishing nothing. His mood fluctuates between euphoria and dysphoria and he can be very irritable. Sleep requirements are reduced and appetite is increased. Self-criticism diminishes, and self-confidence increases. The purest syndromes are observed in the context of the bipolar depressions, but maniacal episodes can also occur in schizophrenics and in patients with anatomical brain lesions.

A specific therapeutic agent is lithium, which should be prescribed in doses sufficient to ensure a blood concentration of 1-1.5 mEq/l. The daily dose required to achieve this averages 1200-2000 mg. The therapeutic effect does not become manifest until after a latent period of about one week. To bridge this latent period, haloperidol can be given by mouth or by intramuscular injection, e.g. 3-8 × 3-5 mg per 24 hours. The possible risks of this combination have been pointed out on page 292.

4. Delirium

The cardinal symptoms of this syndrome are a lowered level of consciousness, motor unrest, disorientation and delusions and/or hallucinations which often generate anxiety but are not very systematized. The most common causes are the following:

1) cerebral arteriosclerosis or other anatomical brain lesions;
2) internal diseases, e.g. those associated with high fever;
3) chronic abuse of alcohol or "drugs" (sedatives, ataractics, opioids, stimulants) or acute withdrawal of these agents after chronic abuse.

re 1). The treatment of the (nocturnally) confused elderly patient is a serious problem, already discussed in chapter XXVI. Phenothiazines should be used with reluctance in view of the risk of hypotension, which can reduce the central circulation and so cause exacerbation of the delirium. Of the neuroleptics, haloperidol is to be preferred because it usually exerts little or no influence on blood pressure. In view of the risk of extrapyramidal side effects, dosage should initially be conservative, e.g. 1-2 mg by intramuscular injection, which if necessary can be repeated after 1-2 hours. Before prescribing neuroleptics, less drastic compounds should first be tried, e.g.

a) paraldehyde, 3-5 g intramuscularly (not more than 20 g per 24 hours), or

b) chloral hydrate, 1-3 g by suppository (not more than 6 g per 24 hours), or

c) diazepam (Valium), 10 mg intramuscularly (not more than 40 mg per 24 hours).

re 2). In these cases control of the internal disease is the first concern. A neuroleptic can be prescribed for a short time if necessary, dependent on the severity of motor unrest, e.g. haloperidol or chlorpromazine.

re 3). Delirium can be a symptom either of intoxication or of withdrawal. Withdrawal delirium is observed in particular upon acute withdrawal (as part of therapy) of such addictive agents as alcohol, opioids and stimulants; it is less likely to occur after gradual withdrawal of, for example, sedatives and ataractics.

There are two agents of choice in the treatment of alcoholic delirium; unfortunately, their merits have not been tested in comparative studies.

a. *Chlordiazepoxide* (Librium), 50 mg by intramuscular (or slow intravenous) injection, repeated after 30 minutes if necessary, to a maximum of 300 mg per 24 hours.

b. *Chlormethiazole* (Hemineurine; Distraneurine) in 0.8% solution by continuous drip; 100 ml of the solution contains 0.8 g chlormethiazole. The maximum dose is 8 g per 24 hours; 3 g as a rule suffices. The drip rate should be so adjusted that the patient falls asleep but remains readily arousable. Respiration, pulse, blood pressure and depth of sleep should be carefully monitored.

Both agents reportedly have a degree of specificity in the treatment of alcoholic delirium in the sense that their efficacy is superior to that of neuroleptics. Nevertheless, agents such as haloperidol and chlorpromazine are also effective.

Chlordiazepoxide and chlormethiazole are also recommended in drug-induced delirium. We do not know whether these compounds have advantages over such neuroleptics as haloperidol (2.5-5 mg by intramuscular injection, to a maximum of 40 mg per 24 hours) or chlorpromazine (50-100 mg by intramuscular injection, to a maximum of 300 mg per 24 hours).

5. Anxiety states

Acute panicky anxiety, which one would like to see arrested as quickly as possible, is frequently a result of abuse of "drugs" and particularly of a bad trip with LSD or amphetamines and, less frequently, marihuana.

Diazepam (Valium) is a good choice in these cases: 10 mg by intramuscular injection, repeated after 15-30 minutes if necessary, to a maximum of 50 mg per 24 hours. Slow intravenous injection is possible but rarely necessary. During parenteral administration of benzodiazepines, the blood pressure should be monitored.

In anxiety states following amphetamine abuse (often associated with paranoid ideas and sometimes with auditory hallucinations), haloperidol can be given (2.5-5 mg by intramuscular injection, repeated after 1 hour if necessary, to a maximum of 40 mg per 24 hours). Since haloperidol is a selective dopamine antagonist and since amphetamine-induced psychosis possibly involves dopaminergic hyperactivity in the brain, haloperidol is considered to be a specific antidote.

6. Suicidal tendencies

Acute suicidal tendencies usually imply acute, overwhelming problems of life, or an agitated vital depression. Acute suicidal risk on the basis of psychotic disorders is much less common.

There are no acutely effective antidepressants. Even if they are effective, there is a latent period of 10-20 days. This is why hospitalization is nearly always necessary. In the case of a personal depression, the patient can be calmed verbally as well as by medication, e.g. with diazepam (Valium), 10 mg by intramuscular injection which can be repeated once or twice if necessary. A neuroleptic is indicated only if the patient is really overwhelmed by his emotions and can no longer take any distance from them. In such cases, thioridazine (Mellaril) can be given by intramuscular injection (50 mg, to be repeated 3 or 4 times during the first 24 hours, if necessary). This agent produces few extrapyramidal side effects.

In agitated vital depressions, a subduing antidepressant is indicated, e.g. amitriptyline (Tryptizol; Elavil). There are no indications that parenteral administration of this agent reduces the latent period. In addition, one should give a strongly subduing neuroleptic, e.g. chlorpromazine, 50-100 mg by intramuscular injection, to be repeated 2 or 3 times during the first 24 hours, if necessary.

A suicidal psychotic patient is treated with a neuroleptic which, if necessary, can be given parenterally the first day(s).

BIBLIOGRAPHY

Andersen, W. H. and J. C. Kuehnle (1974). Strategies for the treatment of acute psychoses. *J. Am. Med. Ass.* 229, 1884.

Bellak, L. and L. Small (1965). *Emergency Psychotherapy and Brief Psychotherapy.* New York: Grune and Stratton.

Glick, R. A., A. T. Meyerson, E. Robbins and Y. A. Talbott (1976). *Psychiatric Emergencies*. New York, San Francisco, London: Grune and Stratton.

Harkoff, L. D. (1969). *Emergency Psychiatric Treatment. A Handbook of Secondary Prevention*. Springfield, Ill.: Charles C Thomas.

Resnik, H. L. P. and H. L. Ruben (1975). *The Management of Mental Health Crises.* Bowie, Md.: Charles Press.

Slaby, A. E., J. Lieb and L. R. Tancredi (1975). *Handbook of Psychiatric Emergencies*. Bern, Stuttgart, Vienna: Hans Huber Publishers.

Zonana, H., J. E. Henisz and M. Levine (1973). Psychiatric emergency services a decade later. *Psychiatry in Medicine* 4, 273.

Index